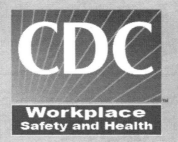

Workplace Safety and Health

Report on Respiratory Symptoms and Disease among Cemented Tungsten Carbide Workers

Nancy Sahakian, MD, MPH

Aleksandr Stefaniak, PhD, CIH

Gregory Day, PhD

Richard Kanwal, MD, MPH

Health Hazard Evaluation Report
HETA 2003-0257-3088
Metalworking Products
Huntsville, Gurley, and Grant, Alabama
August 2009

DEPARTMENT OF HEALTH AND HUMAN SERVICES
Centers for Disease Control and Prevention

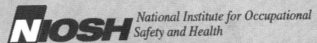

National Institute for Occupational Safety and Health

The employer shall post a copy of this report for a period of 30 calendar days at or near the workplace(s) of affected employees. The employer shall take steps to insure that the posted determinations are not altered, defaced, or covered by other material during such period. [37 FR 23640, November 7, 1972, as amended at 45 FR 2653, January 14, 1980].

CONTENTS

ABBREVIATIONS

ATS	American Thoracic Society
BMI	body mass index
Cr	chromium
Co	cobalt
Dae	aerodynamic diameter
DLCO	diffusing capacity of the lung for carbon monoxide
EBC	exhaled breath condensate
EDTA	ethylenediaminetetraacetic acid
EDX	energy dispersive x-ray
FEV1	forced expiratory volume in one second
FVC	forced vital capacity
g	gram
HEPA	high-efficiency particulate air
HLA	human leukocyte antigen
HSA	human serum albumin
ICP-AES	inductively coupled plasma-atomic emission spectrometry
ICP-MS	inductively coupled plasma-mass spectrometry
IgE	immunoglobulin E
IgG	immunoglobulin G
ILO	International Labor Organization
IL-8	interleukin-8
IARC	International Agency for Research on Cancer
kU	kilo units
LOD	limit of detection
LOQ	limit of quantitation
L	liter
LTβ4	leukotriene β-4
m^3	cubic meter
MDA	malondialdehyde
mg	milligram
ml	milliliter
mM	millimolar
mm	millimeter
MOUDI	micro-orifice uniform deposit impactor
NHANES	National Health and Nutrition Examination Survey
NIOSH	National Institute for Occupational Safety and Health
Ni	nickel
OSHA	Occupational Safety and Health Administration
PEFR	peak expiratory flow rate
PBZ	personal breathing zone
PC_{20}	provocative concentration causing a 20% fall in FEV1
PEL	permissible exposure limit
REL	recommended exposure limit
STEL	short-term exposure limit
SOD	superoxide dismutase
TLC	total lung capacity
TWA	time-weighted average
μg	microgram
μl	microliter
μm	micron
W	tungsten
WC	tungsten carbide

Highlights of the NIOSH Health Hazard Evaluation

In June 2003, the National Institute for Occupational Safety and Health (NIOSH) received a Health Hazard Evaluation (HHE) request from workers at three Metalworking Products plants in Alabama, after former workers had developed hard metal lung disease and occupational asthma.

What NIOSH Did

- Interviewed current workers

- Completed the following medical tests and analyses on workers:

  o Chest x-rays and lung function tests.
  o Urine analyses for cobalt and tungsten levels.
  o Blood analyses for cobalt, tungsten, nickel, and chromium levels.
  o Exhaled breath condensate analyses for cobalt, tungsten, and nickel levels, and for levels of biomarkers of inflammation and oxidative stress.
  o Blood analyses for total immunoglobulin E levels, for immunoglobulin G to specific metals (cobalt, nickel, and chromium), and for variants of a gene reported to be associated with hard metal disease.

- Measured levels of cobalt, nickel, endotoxin, bacteria, and fungi in metalworking fluids.

- Measured levels of metals (cobalt, nickel, and chromium), tungsten-containing fibers, dust, and metalworking fluid in the air of the plants.

- Measured amounts of cobalt, tungsten, nickel, and chromium on work surfaces and on workers' skin.

- Reviewed company measurements of cobalt air levels obtained from 1985 to 2003 and of cobalt blood levels obtained from 1998 to 2003.

What NIOSH Found

- One former worker had findings of hard metal disease on lung biopsy and two current workers had lung function test results indicating possible hard metal disease. One worker was working in pressing, another in sintering, and the third in grinding at the time they developed symptoms or were found to have abnormal lung function.

- The number of workers who reported having physician-diagnosed asthma (ever or currently) was about one-and-a-half to two times higher than expected compared to Alabama state population data and U.S. national population data, respectively.

- Based on information from workers who reported adult-onset (age 16 or older) physician-diagnosed asthma, workers developed asthma at a two-and-a-half times higher rate after being hired than before being hired.

- Based on criteria specified in this report, the four work areas with the highest rates of suspected occupational asthma were *product testing, pressing, milling/spray drying* (data from these two areas combined for analyses), and sintering.

- Workers with greater cobalt exposure over their work tenure (estimated cumulative total cobalt exposure) were more likely to have asthma-like symptoms than workers with lesser cobalt exposure.

- On average, workers in the following areas had urine and/or blood cobalt levels that indicated high exposures: *reclamation, powder mixing/reprocessing/blending* (data from these three areas combined for analyses), *milling, spray drying, pressing, and shaping/round cell* (data from these two areas combined for analyses).

- Cobalt levels in air were highest in *reprocessing* and *powder mixing*; those in *powder mixing, screening, reprocessing,* and *blending* exceeded the OSHA permissible exposure limit (PEL) of 100 micrograms per cubic meter of air ($\mu g/m^3$) for total cobalt; air concentrations in these areas and also in *spray drying* and *reclamation* exceeded the NIOSH recommended exposure limit (REL) of 50 $\mu g/m^3$ for total cobalt.

- Measured sizes of dust particles indicated they are small enough to deposit not only in the nose and throat, but also in the airways of the lung and the gas exchanging region (alveoli) of the lung.

- Surface wipe samples collected from all work surfaces in all three plants contained measurable amounts of cobalt.

- Skin wipe samples collected at mid-shift from all participating workers' hands and most of the same workers' necks contained measurable amounts of cobalt.

- In-use metalworking fluid contained low amounts of cobalt, and no detectable nickel, culturable fungi, or mycobacteria; some culturable bacteria and endotoxin were detected.

- Levels of airborne chromium and nickel were low.

- Results of genetic and antibody (immunoglobulin) analyses were not helpful in the assessment of asthma risk.

- Levels of biomarkers of inflammation and oxidative stress in exhaled breath condensate did not differ significantly between "healthy" workers and workers who met criteria for "current asthma."

What Metalworking Products Managers Can Do

- Reduce cobalt levels to below the OSHA PEL of 100 $\mu g/m^3$ and preferably below the NIOSH REL of 50 $\mu g/m^3$.

- Perform air sampling for cobalt annually and whenever there is a major change in work processes.

- Require all workers to use appropriate respirators when working in or entering work areas known to have cobalt air levels above the NIOSH REL.

- Provide protective clothing and nitrile gloves to prevent cobalt from getting on workers' skin.

- After implementation of exposure controls, obtain blood and/or urine cobalt levels in workers from work areas where past blood or urine results were above the upper limit of normal.

- Obtain spirometry tests and chest x-rays on all new and current employees who, in the course of their job duties, regularly work in or enter plant areas where cobalt exposures occur; repeat spirometry tests every year and chest x-rays every three years.

- Ensure that any newly hired worker with pre-existing lung disease, abnormal spirometry, or abnormal chest x-ray, or any worker who develops respiratory symptoms, chest x-ray abnormalities, or spirometry test abnormalities subsequent to hire, is medically evaluated; the evaluating physician should inform the worker and company of any individualized work restrictions or limitations recommended on the basis of findings from the medical evaluation.

What Metalworking Products Workers Can Do

- Wear the appropriate respirator provided by management when working in or entering work areas where respirator use is required due to high cobalt air levels.

- Wash hands frequently, keep work surfaces clean, and use nitrile gloves and protective clothing to reduce skin exposure to cobalt and metalworking fluids.

- Report any persistent or recurring cough, shortness of breath, wheeze, or chest tightness to your supervisor and your doctor. Provide your doctor with a copy of the highlights section of this report.

SUMMARY

Cobalt exposures in several areas exceeded the NIOSH REL and sometimes also the OSHA PEL. Urine and blood cobalt levels also revealed evidence of high cobalt exposures in many areas. A former worker had medical evaluation results consistent with hard metal lung disease due to cobalt exposure. Lung function test results in two current workers suggested possible hard metal disease. Results of analyses of medical and environmental survey data suggest that workers in some areas at each of the three plants were also at increased risk for occupational asthma. This report contains recommendations for minimizing occupational lung disease risk through exposure controls and other measures.

Background:

In June 2003, NIOSH received a Health Hazard Evaluation (HHE) request from employees at three cemented tungsten carbide manufacturing facilities in Alabama to investigate the risk of hard metal lung disease, asthma, and bronchitis among workers. The three facilities are owned by Metalworking Products and are located within 30 miles of each other in Huntsville, Gurley, and Grant, Alabama. Prior to the HHE request, two former workers had been diagnosed with hard metal disease and one former worker had been diagnosed with occupational asthma. Exposures of concern included cobalt, tungsten carbide, nickel, and metalworking fluids. From September 2003 through May 2005, NIOSH investigators conducted several medical and environmental surveys to identify if particular exposures, production processes, and work practices were associated with increased occupational lung disease risk in these facilities. NIOSH investigators were particularly interested in analyzing relationships between cobalt exposures and respiratory health outcomes because of cobalt's known ability to cause hard metal lung disease and asthma.

Assessment:

NIOSH investigators conducted a walkthrough of all three facilities in July 2003, and conducted three medical surveys in September 2003, January/February 2005, and April/May 2005. These surveys included: standardized questionnaires; chest x-rays; lung function tests; measurement of metals levels in blood (cobalt, tungsten, nickel and chromium), urine (cobalt and tungsten), and exhaled breath condensate (cobalt, tungsten, and nickel); measurement of levels of biomarkers of inflammation and oxidative stress in exhaled breath condensate; and blood analyses for antibodies to metals and for variants of the gene HLA-DPβ1, which has been associated with hard metal lung disease. NIOSH investigators conducted three environmental surveys in May 2004, October/November 2004, and November 2004. Environmental samples collected included: bulk metalworking fluid samples for cobalt, nickel, endotoxin, and microbial analyses; air and wipe samples (work area surfaces and workers' skin) for cobalt, tungsten, nickel and chromium levels; and air samples for analyses of particle shape, chemistry, and size. The different particle sizes included particles small enough to enter the nose, mouth, and throat (inhalable-size); particles small enough to enter the large air passageways or deep regions of the lungs (thoracic-size); and particles small enough to enter the deepest regions of the lung (respirable-size). NIOSH investigators also reviewed company air sampling results for total cobalt obtained from 1985 to 2003 and worker blood cobalt levels obtained from 1998 to 2003.

Main Findings:

1. Exposures:

   a. Based on NIOSH air samples, the *powder mixing area* had the highest average (mean) personal breathing zone (PBZ) total cobalt concentration (574 micrograms per cubic meter of air [$\mu g/m^3$]), the highest mean PBZ thoracic cobalt concentration (304 $\mu g/m^3$), and the highest mean PBZ respirable cobalt concentration (78 $\mu g/m^3$). Based on combined NIOSH and company air sampling results, mean total cobalt levels were highest in reprocessing (427 $\mu g/m^3$) and *powder mixing* (414 $\mu g/m^3$); air concentrations in *powder mixing, screening, reprocessing, and blending* exceeded the OSHA PEL of 100 $\mu g/m^3$ for total cobalt; air concentrations in these areas and also in *spray drying* and *reclamation* exceeded the NIOSH REL of 50 $\mu g/m^3$ for total cobalt.

   b. Wipe samples detected measurable levels of cobalt on all work surfaces across the three facilities. Results of skin wipe samples identified measurable levels of cobalt on all of the hands and most of the necks of participating workers. The two work areas where workers had accumulated the most cobalt on their necks over approximately four hours of work were *metal separation and powder mixing.*

   c. In-use metalworking fluid (MWF) contained low levels of cobalt, and no detectable nickel, culturable fungi, or mycobacteria; culturable bacteria and endotoxin were detected. (Recommended or regulatory limits for levels of endotoxin and microbial contaminants in metalworking fluids have not been established.) Levels of metalworking fluid in air in the *grinding* work area were below the NIOSH REL. (NIOSH recommends a MWF aerosol exposure limit of 0.4 mg/m³ (thoracic particulate mass) as a 10-hour time-weighted average

Keywords: NAICS 335991 (Carbon and Graphite Product Manufacturing), cemented tungsten carbide, hard metal disease, asthma, cobalt, tungsten, metalworking fluids.

(TWA). This corresponds to approximately 0.5 mg/m^3 for total particulate mass).

d. Blood cobalt measurements obtained by the company from 1998 through 2003 on workers in areas with potential high risk for cobalt exposure indicate that most workers had exposures above the NIOSH REL. NIOSH measurements of cobalt in blood and urine in 2005 showed that the average blood and/or urine cobalt levels in several work areas indicated exposures above the NIOSH REL. These areas included *reclamation, powder mixing/reprocessing/blending* (data from these three areas combined for analyses), *milling, spray drying, pressing, and shaping/round cell* (data from these two areas combined for analyses).

2. Medical findings:

a. Survey participation: For the 2003 medical survey, 249 current workers with possible exposure to cobalt at the three facilities were invited to participate. Of these 249 workers, 171 (69%) participated in the 2003 medical survey; an additional 26 of the 249 workers participated for the first time in the 2005 survey, for a total participation rate of 79% in the original invited group.

b. Respiratory symptoms and asthma: Data analyses after the 2003 survey showed that the numbers of workers reporting respiratory symptoms and physician-diagnosed asthma were approximately twice as high as expected when compared to national data. In workers who reported adult-onset (age 16 or older) physician-diagnosed asthma, the estimated post-hire asthma incidence rate was approximately two-and-a-half times higher than the pre-hire rate. Information from the questionnaire and medical test results from both the 2003 and 2005 surveys was used to identify workers with possible ("suspected") occupational asthma. The work areas with the highest estimated rates of suspected occupational asthma were *milling/spray drying* (data from these two areas combined for analyses), *pressing, sintering,* and *product testing.*

c. Hard metal lung disease: One former worker had lung biopsy findings consistent with hard metal disease and two current workers had findings on lung function tests indicating possible hard metal disease. One worker was working in *pressing*, another in *sintering*, and the third in *grinding* at the time they developed symptoms or were found to have abnormal lung function. No current workers had chest x-ray findings indicating possible hard metal disease.

3. Relationships between exposures and health outcome data:

a. Statistical models showed relationships between some exposure measures and some health outcomes. There was a statistically significant association between estimated cumulative total cobalt air concentration and reporting three or more asthma-like symptoms. The amounts of cobalt in the urine, on the wrist, and in exhaled breath condensate were also associated with reporting three or more asthma symptoms. In statistical models that included cobalt and tungsten levels, lung function on spirometry tests was negatively correlated with current and estimated cumulative respirable cobalt air concentration (i.e., lung function declined as exposures increased).

b. Three of the areas with the highest rates of suspected occupational asthma had mean total cobalt exposures that were below the NIOSH REL. The former worker with hard metal lung disease and both current workers with possible hard metal lung disease had worked in areas where air sampling results showed exposures below the NIOSH REL, though urine and blood cobalt levels in one of these areas (*pressing*) indicated exposures above the REL.

4. Findings from other analyses:

a. Genetic analyses: There was no association found between the genetic allele HLA-DPβ1^{E69} and post-hire physician-diagnosed asthma. The low number of cases of suspected hard metal lung disease did not permit analyses of an association between this outcome and HLA-DPβ1^{E69}.

b. Antibody analyses: There were no statistically significant differences in the levels of total immunoglobulin E among workers with pre-hire physician-diagnosed asthma, workers with suspected occupational asthma, and other workers. Of 140 workers tested, none had immunoglobulin G specific to cobalt, nickel, or chromium.

c. Exhaled breath condensate (EBC) analyses: Statistical models showed a weak correlation between levels of cobalt in EBC and total cobalt air concentrations. EBC cobalt levels were moderately correlated with urine and blood cobalt levels. EBC levels of malondialdehyde (MDA), a biomarker of lung oxidative stress, were weakly correlated with total cobalt air concentrations but were not correlated with EBC cobalt or tungsten. Levels of LTB-4 and IL-8 (biomarkers of inflammation) and MDA did not differ significantly between "current asthma" cases (workers who reported currently-active physician-diagnosed asthma or who had airways hyperresponsiveness on methacholine challenge testing with a PC_{20} of less than or equal to 4 mg/m) and "healthy" workers (workers who did not have an asthma history, respiratory symptoms, or findings suggestive of asthma on NIOSH lung function tests).

Conclusions:

Among workers at three cemented tungsten carbide facilities owned by Metalworking Products in Alabama, a former worker had evidence of hard metal disease on lung biopsy and two current workers had findings on lung function tests that suggested possible hard metal disease. Cobalt exposures in two of the three areas where these workers worked were below the NIOSH REL. Because some workers may still be at risk for hard metal disease even when exposures are below recommended and regulatory limits, it is important to regularly monitor the health of all exposed workers to identify those who may be potentially affected. Several work areas in these facilities had cobalt exposures that exceeded the NIOSH REL and sometimes also the OSHA PEL, indicating a need for additional exposure controls in these areas.

Our finding of an elevated rate of post-hire asthma compared to pre-hire asthma strongly suggests that exposures in these facilities at the time of the medical survey were putting workers at risk for asthma. Some of our analyses showed associations and correlations between different measures of cobalt exposure and respiratory symptoms and lung function. Studies conducted in other cemented tungsten carbide plants in other countries have utilized controlled cobalt inhalation in a laboratory setting to identify workers who had developed asthma due to cobalt exposure; antibody analyses indicated that some of those workers had developed cobalt asthma due to an allergic mechanism. We did not utilize the controlled cobalt inhalation approach to determine if any workers had asthma due to cobalt exposure, and our antibody analyses did not identify evidence of an allergic response to cobalt in any Metalworking Products workers. Therefore, while it is possible that some workers we identified with suspected occupational asthma may have asthma due to cobalt exposures, it is also possible that, in some Metalworking Products workers, respiratory symptoms or asthma may be due to other workplace exposures.

INTRODUCTION

In June 2003, NIOSH received a confidential worker request to investigate the risk of hard metal lung disease, asthma, and bronchitis among workers at three cemented tungsten carbide facilities owned by Metalworking Products in Alabama. Exposures of concern included cobalt, tungsten carbide, nickel, and metalworking fluids. Prior to this request, two former workers had been diagnosed with hard metal lung disease, and one former worker had been diagnosed with occupational asthma. NIOSH investigators performed an initial walkthrough survey of the three facilities in July 2003. From September 2003 through May 2005, NIOSH investigators conducted several medical and environmental surveys at the three facilities to determine if specific exposures, production processes, and work practices were associated with increased occupational lung disease risk. After each survey, we provided requestors and company management with preliminary results and recommendations in detailed interim letter reports (see Appendix A). This final report summarizes major findings previously reported in the interim letters and provides information from additional analyses.

Respiratory Disease Associated with Cemented Tungsten Carbide Production

Exposures to cobalt related to the production of cemented tungsten carbide can cause alveolitis, hard metal lung disease, and occupational asthma [Cugell 1992; Lison 1998]. Alveolitis is an inflammation of the air sacs (alveoli) in the lungs. Symptoms, including fever, cough, and shortness of breath with exertion, improve with removal from exposure; chest x-rays may show abnormal opacities (spots). Alveolitis can progress to hard metal lung disease, a condition in which scarring makes the lungs stiff and less able to perform gas exchange. Hard metal lung disease is a type of interstitial lung disease. Typical symptoms include progressive shortness of breath on exertion and cough. Chest x-rays may show small opacities; lung function tests may show a restrictive pattern, wherein the individual has difficulty taking a deep breath, and low diffusing capacity for carbon monoxide (DL_{CO}), evidence of poor gas exchange in the lungs. A lung biopsy showing multi-nucleated giant cells within the alveoli is a finding frequently seen in hard metal lung disease. The mechanisms involved in the development of hard metal lung disease are incompletely understood. Hard metal lung disease displays some of the characteristics of hypersensitivity pneumonitis [Cugell 1992], a lung disease in which an individual's immune system responds to a particular exposure. There is also evidence that cobalt can be directly toxic to lung tissue through the production of highly reactive oxygen molecules, a process that is markedly enhanced in the presence of tungsten carbide [Lison 1998].

Occupational asthma is defined as variable airways obstruction or airways hyperreponsiveness (sensitive airways) due to occupational exposures. Symptoms include wheezing, shortness of breath, coughing, and chest tightness. Occupational asthma may occur with exposure to sensitizing agents (allergic asthma) and non-specific irritants (non-allergic asthma). Allergic asthma requires a period of time (from weeks to several years) between the first exposure and the onset of symptoms. Once occupational asthma develops, symptoms generally follow one of two patterns: symptom onset within an hour of the start of exposure (immediate onset), with improvement away from work; or symptom onset several hours after the start of exposure, even after leaving work for the day (delayed onset). Airways obstruction may not totally resolve before the affected individual's next work shift. Both patterns have been observed in workers with asthma due to cobalt exposure [Bernstein et al. 2006]. In some workers with occupational asthma due to cobalt, there is evidence that the disease is allergic; in others, the disease mechanism is unknown [Lison 1998]. In addition to asthma caused by cobalt, workers in the cemented tungsten carbide industry may be at risk for asthma caused by occupational exposure to other agents known to cause asthma, such as nickel, chromium, and metalworking fluids.

Process Description

Cemented tungsten carbide is composed of approximately 80% tungsten carbide, 5–20% cobalt, and smaller amounts of other metals (e.g., chromium, nickel, titanium, tantalum, niobium, and molybdenum). Because of its strength, heat-resistance, and extreme hardness, cemented tungsten carbide is used for high-speed cutting tools and drills, saw tips, and armor-piercing shells.

The three Metalworking Products facilities investigated as part of this Health Hazard Evaluation request are located within 30 miles of each other in Huntsville, Gurley, and Grant, Alabama. The production processes at these facilities include the manufacture of base powders at the Huntsville facility, formulation of powder mixtures at the Gurley facility, and manufacture of cemented tungsten carbide products at the Grant facility (see Table 1).

Table 1. Cemented tungsten carbide production work areas and production support activities at the three Metalworking Products facilities

Huntsville Facility	Gurley Facility	Grant Facility
Tungsten Oxide Reduction	Powder Mixing	Pressing
Tungsten Carbide Production	Reprocessing	Extrusion
Reclamation	Blending	Shaping
Metal Separation	Milling	Round Cell
Powder Laboratory	Spray Drying	Sintering
Shipping	Screening	Grinding
Maintenance	Shipping	Sandblasting
	Maintenance	Product Testing
		Shipping
		Maintenance

Production Processes at the Huntsville Facility

In the *tungsten oxide reduction* area, tungsten oxide is manually placed or automatically augered into containers called "boats" that are placed in a hydrogen atmosphere furnace to reduce tungsten oxide to tungsten metal powder. In the *tungsten carbide production* area, tungsten metal powder is combined with carbon black powder and the mixture is ball-milled and then carburized by heating in a hydrogen atmosphere furnace to form aggregated tungsten carbide "bricks." The bricks of tungsten carbide are then milled into powder which is screened to achieve a desired particle size.

In the *reclamation* area, sintered cemented tungsten carbide pieces that do not meet customer specifications are reacted in furnaces that produce a cake that is crushed and milled, yielding metal powder which is screened and then shipped to the Gurley facility for reuse. In the *metal separation* area, floor sweepings, grinding sludge, and dust collections are processed in a calcining furnace to convert tungsten carbide into tungsten oxide which is further processed chemically to produce a pure tungsten oxide for reuse in the reduction process. Because the *reclamation work area* is very dusty and workers in *metal separation* are exposed to strong alkaline and acid vapors, some workers in these two work areas choose to wear respirators; however, at the time of our initial walkthrough survey in July 2003, respirator use in these work areas was not required by management. (Management implemented mandatory respirator use in reclamation shortly after our walkthrough visit.)

Workers in the *powder laboratory* test all powders produced in the Huntsville facility's *tungsten oxide reduction, tungsten carbide production, reclamation,* and *metal separation* departments, as well as the Gurley facility's *screening* and *reprocessing* departments.

Production Processes at the Gurley Facility

In the *powder mixing* area, large amounts of cobalt powder and smaller quantities of other metals (such as chromium, nickel, titanium carbide, tantalum carbide, and vanadium) are manually scooped and added to large hoppers containing tungsten carbide (Figure 1). In the adjacent *reprocessing* area, metals are manually added to scrap powder mixtures. The materials are mixed and screened in the *blending* area to make reprocessed powder mixtures. Workers are required to use respirators and protective disposable coveralls in the *powder mixing* and *reprocessing/blending* work areas.

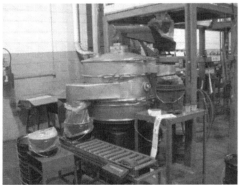
Figure 1. Powder mixing (Gurley facility)

Powder mixtures are sent to *milling*, where they are ball-milled with heptane and other liquids to form a slurry. The slurry is pumped into the spray dryer, where liquids are evaporated off and hard metal powder is produced. The hard metal powder is discharged onto a conveyor belt and dropped into a storage container. Workers in the *spray drying* area stand in close proximity to the location where the metal powder is discharged onto the conveyor belt. The hard metal powder is then sent to *screening*, where machines with different sized screens are used to collect metal powder with the desired particle size (Figure 2).

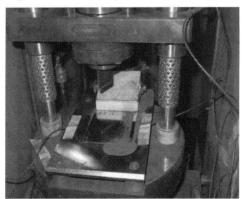
Figure 2. Screening (Gurley facility)

Production Processes at the Grant Facility

In the *pressing area*, workers use large scoops to manually load hard metal powder into hoppers that gravity-feed the dies of pressing machines (Figure 3). Other workers use large scoops to manually fill large forms with hard metal powder and operate a hydraulic press. In the *extrusion area*, plasticizers are added to the hard metal powder to form cylindrical rods of material with a clay-like consistency. Pieces produced in the *pressing area* and the *extrusion area* are friable. Workers in the *pressing area* use brushes to collect hard metal powder from work surfaces and to dry-sweep their work stations at the end of the day. Collected hard metal powder is sent to the Huntsville facility, where tungsten oxide is recovered and reused.

In the *shaping area*, the friable forms are hand polished, machined

Figure 3. Pressing (Grant facility)

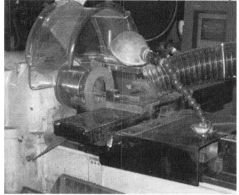

Figure 4. Shaping (Grant facility)

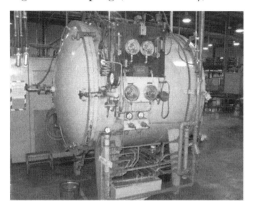

Figure 5. Sintering (Grant facility)

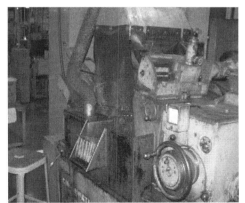

Figure 6. Centerless grinding (Grant facility)

(Figure 4), or cut using water under high pressure. In the *round cell* area, workers operate machinery for slicing and shaping and also operate a dry bag press.

In the *sintering area*, pressed and extruded forms (held on graphite trays within a graphite box) are placed in furnaces (Figure 5) where they are heated at reduced pressure (i.e., vacuum) to fully densify them. In some cases, an over-pressure of argon is used at the end of the furnace cycle to complete densification. Following sintering, the fully dense cemented tungsten carbide pieces have very high hardness.

Final finishing of the cemented tungsten carbide pieces occurs in the *grinding* and *sandblasting* areas. Workers use surface and centerless grinders (Figure 6) to finish the cemented tungsten carbide pieces. With surface grinders, the cemented tungsten carbide pieces are loaded into the machines where they are ground in the presence of metalworking fluids that cover the surface of the carbide pieces. Centerless grinders require the worker to hand-feed small cylindrical cemented tungsten carbide pieces into the machine. Workers manually wash off any remaining metalworking fluid from finished pieces. Workers who operate surface grinders wear nitrile gloves; some also wear Tyvek™arm cuffs. Workers who operate centerless grinders wear nitrile gloves and sometimes wear oil-resistant aprons. Large industrial fans, positioned with the grinding machine between the fan and the worker, are used to cool off workers who operate the centerless grinders. (Metalworking Products removed these fans after NIOSH recommended this in an interim letter.) A Torit air-filtering system routes air through high-efficiency particulate filters and back into the grinding work area. The metalworking fluid used in grinding is water-based (RichGrind 662™) and contains a biocide and cobalt inhibitor (agglomerator). Workers add an anti-foaming agent to the metalworking fluid in the sump as needed. Used metalworking fluid is pumped to a sump pump and passed through a cellulose filter on a wedge wire grid. Filtered metalworking fluid is recirculated to the grinding machines. Workers perform abrasive blasting of cemented tungsten carbide pieces in a sealed glove box with silicon carbide as the abrasive. At the time of our walk-through visit, the gloves of the box had been repaired with duct tape.

Workers in *product testing* test the finished pieces for tensile strength, density, etc. Workers who maintain the Torit air-filtering system and others who prepare sintering trays use half-facepiece air-purifying respirators.

ASSESSMENT

Walkthrough Survey

NIOSH investigators performed walkthrough surveys at the three Metalworking Products facilities in Alabama on July 7 and 8, 2003, at which time they interviewed workers and (at the Grant facility) obtained bulk samples of metalworking fluid. Bulk samples obtained included unused metalworking fluid, in-use metalworking fluid from the centerless grinder, and liquid and solid sludge from the sump system. The metalworking fluid in the sump had last been changed one to three years prior to our visit, though additional metalworking fluid had been added to the sump several days before and on the day of our visit. These samples were analyzed for cobalt, nickel, endotoxin (a component of the cell wall of Gram-negative bacteria), fungi, and bacteria (including *Mycobacteria*).

Medical Surveys

The medical surveys were designed and conducted to determine the percentage of the workforce in different work areas that had findings consistent with asthma or hard metal lung disease. Medical analyses that would provide information on workers' exposures and on possible biologic mechanisms involved in illness development were also included. This information was analyzed in relation to exposure measurements (see below) to determine if certain exposure levels or other aspects of exposures were associated or correlated with findings suggestive of asthma or hard metal lung disease in the workforce.

Two medical surveys, one in 2003 and the other in 2005, were conducted of workers currently employed at the three facilities. Methods for the different components of these medical surveys are described in detail in the subsections below and in Appendix A (Interim Letters) and Appendix C (Methods). NIOSH investigators obtained Human Subjects Review Board review and approval for the various medical survey components (see Appendix C, Methods, for more details). Signed informed consent was obtained from all survey participants. Survey participants were provided with their individual test results in letters mailed to their home addresses. NIOSH provided Metalworking Products management and workers with interim findings and recommendations in 13 interim letters from February 2004 through January 2007. Figure 7 shows a timeline of the medical and environmental surveys from July 2003 through June 2005.

Figure 7. Timeline for medical and environmental survey

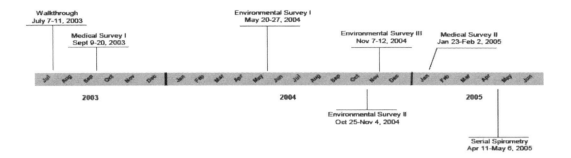

The following workers were invited to participate in the first NIOSH medical survey conducted in 2003: current workers at the Gurley and Grant facilities who had current or past cobalt exposure; and current workers at the Huntsville facility with current cobalt exposure. (Information on past exposures was not available prior to the survey for workers at the Huntsville facility.) The medical survey included a health questionnaire, chest x-ray, and spirometry (breathing) test. If a worker's spirometry test was abnormal, NIOSH technicians administered a bronchodilator medication, repeated the spirometry test to determine if the results improved, and then performed a diffusing capacity test (DLCO), a measurement of the lung's capacity to transfer gases (additional details on these medical survey components are provided below).

All current workers at all three facilities were invited to participate in the second NIOSH medical survey conducted in 2005. The same questionnaire that was used in the 2003 survey was administered to workers hired after that. It was also administered to workers who were working at one of the three facilities in 2003 but did not participate in the 2003 survey. An abbreviated questionnaire was administered to those workers who had previously participated in the 2003 survey (see Appendix B, Questionnaires I and II). Spirometry tests were administered by NIOSH technicians, who also obtained medical specimens for analyses as follows: urine and blood samples for metals levels; blood samples to measure total immunoglobulin E and specific antibodies to metals; blood samples for genetic analyses; exhaled breath condensate samples to measure levels of metals and biomarkers of inflammation and oxidative stress; and wrist wipe samples to measure amounts of metals on the skin. To identify potential asthma cases and controls for serial spirometry testing, selected workers were offered a methacholine challenge test to detect airways hyperresponsiveness. From April 11–May 6, 2005, 11 employees completed serial spirometry over a three-week period. Additional details on these medical survey components are provided below.

Health Questionnaires

The questionnaires included questions on symptoms, medical diagnoses, smoking history, work history, and occupational exposures. Some questions were derived from the American Thoracic Society (ATS) standardized respiratory symptom questionnaire [Ferris 1978] and the 3rd National Health and Nutrition and Examination Survey (NHANES III) [CDC 1996]; additional asthma symptom questions previously demonstrated to be predictive of airways hyperresponsiveness were also included [Venables et al. 1993]. For most workers, NIOSH interviewers administered the questionnaires using a laptop computer. Some workers who participated during short off-work periods during the 2003 survey completed a shorter self-administered paper questionnaire.

Chest X-rays

Chest x-rays consisted of a single posteroanterior view. Two NIOSH-approved B Readers independently scored each chest x-ray for opacities according to the International Labor Organization (ILO) classification system for pneumoconioses [ILO 2002]. If the B Readers' scores differed, the film was sent to a third B Reader for an additional classification. The median category was taken as the final determination of opacity category. In the ILO system, the profusion of small opacities is graded on a 12-point scale ranging from 0/- (abnormal small opacities absent), which is normal, to 3/+ (indicative of very severe disease). We considered a final determination of category 1/0 or higher as suggestive of hard metal disease. Category 1/0 indicates that sufficient opacities were present to classify the chest x-ray as Category 1, though serious consideration was given to classifying the x-ray as Category 0. Any higher category indicates that no serious consideration was given to classifying the chest x-ray as Category 0.

Lung Function Tests

In lung function testing with spirometry, a device (spirometer) is used to measure exhaled volume and airflows when an individual performs a series of forceful exhalations. In both the 2003 and 2005 medical surveys, a NIOSH technician administered spirometry tests using a dry rolling-seal spirometer interfaced to a personal computer following ATS guidelines [ATS 1995]. Spirometry results were compared to reference values generated from NHANES III data [Hankinson et al. 1999]. Each participating worker's largest forced vital capacity (FVC) and forced expiratory volume in one second (FEV_1) were selected for analysis. We defined obstruction as an FEV_1/FVC ratio and FEV1 below their respective lower limits of normal. We defined borderline airways obstruction as an FEV_1/FVC ratio below the lower limit of normal with a normal FEV_1. We defined restriction as an FVC below the lower limit of normal with a normal FEV_1/FVC ratio. Workers with evidence of airways obstruction (or borderline airways obstruction) were administered albuterol, a bronchodilator medication used to treat obstructive lung diseases such as asthma, and were then retested to see if the obstruction was reversible. We defined reversible obstruction (and reversible borderline obstruction) as an improvement in the FEV_1 of 12% and at least 200 milliliters (mL). For workers who had abnormal spirometry results in the 2003 survey, NIOSH technicians administered a DL_{CO} test to measure the efficiency of gas exchange in the lungs. We estimated total lung capacity (TLC), the maximum amount of air that the lungs can hold, from DL_{CO} results. We considered a DL_{CO} result as abnormally low if it was below the lower limit of normal and an estimated TLC result as abnormally low if it was less than 80% of the predicted value [Miller et al. 1983].

Methacholine Challenge Test

Methacholine challenge, a test commonly used in the evaluation of asthma symptoms, causes temporary limitation of airflow in some individuals. People with sensitive airways, such as asthmatics, react to low concentrations of inhaled methacholine, whereas most people react only at higher concentrations. This test is performed by having workers breathe increasingly higher concentrations of methacholine, with spirometry testing after each administered dose. We defined airways hyperresponsiveness as a 20% or greater drop in FEV_1 at a methacholine concentration less than or equal to 16.0 mg/mL. (The methacholine concentration causing a 20% or greater drop in FEV_1 is referred to as the PC_{20}.) We used methacholine challenge testing to identify suspect asthma cases and non-cases (i.e., controls) for further testing with serial spirometry.

Serial Spirometry Testing

Workers performed serial spirometry using a portable spirometer (EasyOne™, ndd Medical Technologies, Chelmsford, MA). NIOSH technicians instructed workers to blow forcefully into the portable spirometer a minimum of three times per test session, with five test sessions per day over a 3-week period. Workers were asked to perform spirometry upon awakening, on arrival at work, right before lunch, at the end of the work shift, and at bedtime. Workers were asked to perform tests at comparable times on non-work days during the 3-week period. Two NIOSH physicians and another NIOSH researcher independently reviewed the serial spirometry records to determine if the peak expiratory flow rate (PEFR) or FEV_1 decreased, or the daily variation in PEFR or FEV_1 increased, in a pattern temporally related to the work schedule. A worker was considered to have a work-related pattern of serial spirometry if at least two of the three reviewers found evidence of work-relatedness.

Urine, Blood, Exhaled Breath Condensate, and Wrist Wipe Metal Levels

NIOSH investigators collected urine, blood, exhaled breath condensate, and wrist wipe samples during the last two hours of an employee's shift on one of the last two days of their work week. Urine samples were analyzed for cobalt, tungsten, creatinine, and specific gravity. Whole blood samples were analyzed for cobalt, tungsten, nickel, and chromium. Exhaled breath condensate samples were analyzed for cobalt, tungsten, and nickel. Wrist wipe samples were analyzed for cobalt, tungsten, nickel, and chromium.

Urine and whole blood analyses for cobalt and tungsten used inductively coupled plasma-mass spectrometry (ICP-MS). In the analysis of chromium in blood, samples were initially tested using ICP-MS. However, due to technical problems with this technique, remaining samples were analyzed using inductively coupled plasma-atomic emission spectrometry (ICP-AES). In this report, only blood chromium results for samples analyzed with ICP-AES are included.

For urine collection, workers were instructed to wash their hands, remove the sterile collection container from a plastic bag, put on a pair of nitrile gloves (also in a plastic bag), and then collect their urine sample in the sterile container provided. Whole blood samples for metals were drawn using disodium EDTA-containing blood tubes. Urine and whole blood samples were refrigerated on-site, packed in insulated containers with cold-packs, and shipped to a NIOSH-contracted laboratory for analysis. In our statistical analysis of metal concentrations in urine and blood, we excluded results for 13 workers who reported working in more than one work area; two workers who provided samples at the beginning of their work shift; one worker who worked in a different work area two days prior to the collection of the sample; and one worker who had recently returned to work after an extended absence. We report results for work areas for which we received at least three samples. Additional details including limits of detection (LOD) and quantitation (LOQ) are provided in Appendix A, Interim Letter IX.

NIOSH investigators collected exhaled breath condensate samples over a 20-minute period using a TURBO DECCS™ unit (Ital Chill, Parma, Italy) with a chilling temperature of -5° Centigrade. Workers rinsed their mouth with water prior to collection and wore a pair of nitrile gloves during collection of the sample. Individual samples were transferred on-site to Eppendorf tubes, packed with dry ice, and shipped to a collaborating research laboratory for analysis.

To obtain a wrist wipe sample, a NIOSH technician put on a clean pair of nitrile gloves and wiped the underside of the employee's wrist for 30 seconds with a Wash 'n Dri™ moist disposable towellette (First Brands Corporation, Danbury, CT). Wipes were subsequently placed in individual zip-lock plastic bags and shipped to a NIOSH-contracted laboratory for analysis.

Biomarkers of Inflammation and Oxidative Stress in Exhaled Breath Condensate

A collaborating research laboratory analyzed exhaled breath condensate samples for biomarkers of inflammation (leukotriene β-4 [LTB-4] and interleukin-8 [IL-8]) and a biomarker of oxidative stress (malondialdehyde [MDA]). We used Pearson correlations and multiple linear regression models to analyze associations between exhaled breath condensate results, cobalt air concentrations, and cobalt levels in blood and urine. In our statistical analyses we used all MDA values, as all values were greater than the LOQ. For LTB-4 and IL-8, we used: 1) values greater than the LOQ; or 2) all values, with the use of one-half the LOD for values less than the LOD (see Appendix A, Interim Letter IX).

We used Student's t-test and the Wilcoxon Rank Sum test to compare biomarker levels from "healthy" workers and current asthma cases. We defined "healthy" workers as those: 1) whose most recent spirometry test (from either the 2003 or 2005 survey) was normal; 2) who did not have airways hyperreponsiveness on methacholine challenge testing (i.e., PC_{20} of less than or equal to 16 mg/ml); and 3) who reported that they had never been diagnosed with asthma, did not have asthma-like symptoms, were not troubled by shortness of breath, did not have shortness of breath when hurrying on level ground, did not have a usual cough, had never been diagnosed with chronic bronchitis, and were not currently using breathing medication. We defined "current asthma" cases as workers who reported current physician-diagnosed asthma or who had a PC_{20} of less than or equal to 4 mg/ml on methacholine challenge testing.

Blood Antibody Levels

Blood samples were centrifuged on-site to separate the serum from the blood cells. The serum was transferred to cryogenic vials, packed in insulated containers with dry ice, and shipped to NIOSH for analysis.

Blood samples were analyzed for total immunoglobulin E (IgE). We considered 100 kilo units (kU) or more of total IgE per liter of serum to be elevated and to be suggestive of atopy (allergic asthma, hayfever, or eczema). We calculated geometric mean total IgE levels for the following groups: 1) suspected occupational asthma cases (see case definition in Statistical Analyses section below); 2) pre-hire asthma cases; and 3) the remainder of the workforce. We then tested whether there were any statistically significant differences among these three geometric mean values.

Blood samples were also screened for immunoglobulin G (IgG) against cobalt, nickel, and chromium bound to two proteins found in human blood: human serum albumin (HSA) and superoxide dismutase (SOD). HSA is the main binding protein in the blood; SOD is an important antioxidant enzyme. IgE against cobalt bound to HSA has been identified in workers with cobalt asthma

[Shirakawa et al. 1988, 1989]. We chose to screen for specific IgG because individuals often produce IgG in addition to IgE against a substance to which they are allergic; IgG is usually produced in larger amounts and is therefore potentially more sensitive as a marker of exposure and immune system response.

Genetic Analyses

The HLA-DPβ1^{E69} allele has been reported to be associated with hard metal lung disease [Potolicchio et al. 1997]. We sought to determine whether or not this allele was associated with post-hire asthma among Metalworking Products workers. Whole blood samples for genetic analysis were drawn in CPT™ tubes containing sodium citrate (100 mM, 450 μl) and a Ficoll Hypaque® gel, refrigerated on-site, packed in insulated containers with cold-packs, and shipped to the NIOSH laboratory for analysis. Blood samples were analyzed for the well known lysine (K)/glutamic acid (E) polymorphism at position 69 of the HLA-DPβ1 gene. This was done by fractionating the blood and isolating the white blood cells, extracting DNA, amplifying the target gene (HLA- DPβ1), and identifying the coding sequence at position 69 [McCanlies et al. 2004].

We calculated the percentage of individuals with one or two HLA-DPβ1^{E69} alleles and the HLA-DPβ1^{E69} allelic frequencies for two worker groups – workers with post-hire physician-diagnosed asthma and workers who did not have asthma (non-asthmatics). We defined post-hire physician-diagnosed asthma as physician-diagnosed asthma with a reported onset date that was later than the hire date. We defined non-asthmatic workers as those who did not report asthma. We defined HLA-DPβ1^{E69} allelic frequency as the number of HLA-DPβ1^{E69} alleles in a worker group divided by the total number of HLA-DPβ1 alleles. We also tested the Hardy-Weinberg equilibrium of HLA-DPβ1 alleles in these worker groups. Hardy-Weinburg equilibrium in a population is defined as the presence of proportional numbers of individuals with a single allele (heterozygous for a specific allele) and with two of the same allele (homozygous) that would be expected in the absence of non-random influences.

Environmental Surveys

From May 20–27, 2004, we performed a preliminary environmental survey to understand levels of metals in general workplace air as a basis for planning subsequent detailed surveys to monitor personal μexposures. General work area air samples were collected with micro-orifice uniform deposit impactor (MOUDI) samplers (Model 110, MSP Corporation, Shoreview, MN) (17 samples), Marple Series 290 8-stage cascade impactor samplers (11 samples), and cassette samplers (26 samples). The MOUDI and 8-stage cascade impactor samplers collect and separate particles by size (see below). The cassette sampler is used to collect all ("total") airborne particles without regard to particle size. All samples were analyzed for cobalt, nickel, and chromium. In specific work areas, optical particle counters (Model 1.108, GRIMM Technologies Inc., Douglasville, GA) were used to estimate the sizes of airborne particles in the physical size range 0.30μm to >20 μm in 15 channels: >0.30 μm, >0.40 μm, >0.50 μm, >0.65 μm, >0.80 μm, >1.0 μm, >1.6 μm, >2.0 μm, >3.0 μm, >4.0 μm, >5.0 μm, >7.5 μm, >10 μm, >15 μm, and >20 μm.

In our second environmental survey from October 25–November 4, 2004, we obtained air samples as follows: 108 PBZ samples for metal analyses were collected with Marple 8-stage cascade impactor samplers; 252 PBZ samples for metal and dust analyses were collected with 37-mm cassette samplers; 8 PBZ (*grinding* workers) and 8 area samples (*grinding* work area) for metalworking fluid analysis were collected with 37-mm cassette samplers; and 7 PBZ samples and 62 area samples for tungsten fiber analysis were collected with 25-mm cassette samplers. One sample, a 37-mm cassette sample for metal analyses, was discarded because of equipment failure.

The 50% aerodynamic diameter cut points (D_{50}) for the 10-stage MOUDI and 8-stage Marple impactor samplers are summarized in Table 2. For a given impactor stage, the D_{50} differed between the samplers because of differing sampler design and operating flow rate.

Table 2. 50% aerodynamic diameter cut points (D_{50}) for the 10-stage MOUDI and 8-stage Marple impactor samplers

Size-fraction	D_{50} (μm) 10-stage MOUDI	D_{50} (μm) 8-stage Marple
pre-filter	> 18	--
stage 1	10	> 21.3
stage 2	5.6	14.8
stage 3	3.2	9.8
stage 4	1.8	6.0
stage 5	1.0	3.5
stage 6	0.56	1.55
stage 7	0.32	0.93
stage 8	0.18	0.52
stage 9	0.10	--
stage 10	0.056	--
final filter	< 0.056	< 0.52

In our third environmental survey from November 7–12, 2004, we collected wipe samples from work surfaces (156 samples) and from the skin of 41 workers. For each wipe sample of a work surface routinely touched by workers, we outlined the area to be sampled using a 10-centimeter by 10-centimeter disposable template (in accordance with NIOSH Method 9100) and wiped the area with a Wash 'n Dri™ moist disposable towellette (ASTM Method E1792). Skin wipe samples were collected prior to the work shift (baseline samples) and before lunchtime (follow-up samples). Workers were instructed to wipe both hands (palm and back) from the top of the wrist to the fingertips with a Wash 'n Dri™ towellete and then place the towellette in a zip-lock plastic bag. Then the workers were asked to put on a clean pair of nitrile gloves and use another Wash 'n Dri™ towellete to wipe their necks from the chin down to the top of the Adam's apple and from ear to ear and place the sample in a separate zip-lock plastic bag. All surface and skin wipe samples were analyzed for cobalt, nickel, chromium, and tungsten. MOUDI samplers were used to collect 16 samples of airborne particles from 13 different work areas for subsequent analysis using transmission electron microscopy to determine particle shape, and energy dispersive x-ray spectrometry to determine particle chemistry.

For tungsten fiber analysis, we used a direct transfer method (NIOSH Method 7402) and a transmission electron microscope (Philips, Model CM 12, Eindhoven, Netherlands). We defined a fiber as a particle with an aspect ratio (length to diameter) of at least 5:1and length greater than 0.50 μm. Elemental composition of fibers was determined using an energy dispersive x-ray (EDX) spectrometer (Gresham Light Element Detector, Model 510 with IXRF software, Houston, TX) connected to a transmission electron microscope. This EDX spectrometer is able to identify elements having atomic numbers greater than 4.

Air and wipe samples for metals were analyzed for cobalt, nickel, and chromium using NIOSH Method 7300, and for tungsten using NIOSH Method 7074. Air samples for metals collected during the first environmental survey and 37-mm cassette air samples for metals collected during the second environmental survey from the Huntsville facility were analyzed only for cobalt, nickel, and chromium. Air samples collected for metalworking fluids were analyzed using NIOSH Method 5524. Air samples collected for dusts were analyzed using NIOSH Method 0500.

For the purposes of statistical analyses, we defined "total" particulate mass as encompassing particles of all sizes captured by the 37-mm cassette sampler or the sum of masses of particles collected on all stages of the impactor samplers. By convention, airborne particulate mass includes several health-relevant sub-fractions that can be selectively sampled on the basis of particle aerodynamic diameters. From largest to smallest diameters, these fractions are: inhalable particulate, representing particles that enter as far as the nose, mouth, and throat when inhaled; thoracic particulate, representing particles that enter as far as the airways of the lung when inhaled; and respirable particulate, representing particles that enter as far as the deepest (alveolar) regions of the lung when inhaled.

We calculated work-area mean, median, and highest recorded concentrations for: (1) total cobalt and tungsten from cassette samples (251 samples); and (2) inhalable, thoracic, and respirable cobalt and tungsten air concentrations from the Marple impactor samples (105 samples). These cassette and Marple impactor samples were collected during our second environmental survey. We used previously published prediction equations to estimate the inhalable, thoracic, and respirable particle concentrations [Hinds 1986]. For total airborne cobalt, we also calculated mean, median, and highest recorded concentrations using our samples (251 cassette samples collected during our second environmental survey) and historical company samples (72 cassette samples collected from 1985 to 2003). An arithmetic mean (mean), commonly referred to as the "average" of a group of measurements, is the sum of all the measurements in a list divided by the total number of measurements. The median value is the middle value in a list of ordered measurements for which half of the measurements are higher and half the measurements are lower. The geometric mean is an average value that uses multiplication rather than addition to summarize data values. Both the geometric mean and the median are less influenced by extremely high or low measurements compared to the arithmetic mean. Additional information regarding sampling media, work areas that were sampled, and LODs and LOQs are provided in Appendix A (Interim Letters II, III, IV, V, VI, VII, VIII, X, XI, and XII).

Additional Statistical Analyses

We used prevalence ratios to compare the proportions of survey participants who reported respiratory symptoms, physician-diagnosed chronic bronchitis and asthma, and who had abnormal spirometry test results, to expected numbers based on general population data from the NHANES III survey [CDC 1996]. We also compared the proportion of survey participants who reported physician-diagnosed asthma to general population data for Alabama from the Behavior Risk Factor Surveillance System (BRFSS) [CDC 2003]. We calculated prevalence ratios by dividing the number of persons with an observed health outcome by the expected number derived from the NHANES III survey. A prevalence ratio greater than "1" indicates the number of workers with that particular health outcome is greater than expected compared to the general public. A ratio greater than "1" with a 95% confidence interval (CI) that excludes "1" indicates a less than 5% chance that the elevated prevalence ratio was a random occurrence. We grouped workers by smoking history (ever-smokers and never-smokers), age (17–39 years-old and 40–69 years-old), gender, and race to take these factors into account in our comparisons.

We calculated estimates of asthma incidence (the occurrence of new cases) in two separate analyses. In each analysis, the incidence of asthma was calculated by dividing the number of new cases by the total time at risk (expressed as person-years) for all individuals who could potentially develop the disease. In one analysis, we estimated the incidences of pre-hire and post-hire adult-onset asthma based on worker reports of physician-diagnosed asthma on the questionnaire; workers had to have been at least 16 years-old at the time of diagnosis to be considered as an asthma case in this analysis. We excluded asthma cases with no known diagnosis date, and person-time subsequent to diagnosis for asthma cases with a known diagnosis date.

In a second analysis, we estimated the incidence of suspected occupational asthma in different work areas. We identified workers as having suspected occupational asthma if they met at least one of the following: 1) post-hire onset, currently active, physician-diagnosed asthma; 2) three or more asthma-like symptoms with post-hire onset of wheeze or shortness of breath (see Appendix B, Questionnaires I and II); 3) current use of asthma medication with post-hire onset of wheeze or shortness of breath; or 4) reversible obstruction or reversible borderline obstruction on spirometry with post-hire onset of wheeze or shortness of breath. We only considered workers who were working at the time of the 2003 medical survey and who participated in either the 2003 or 2005 medical survey. We excluded the following from our analysis: 1) workers with pre-hire asthma; 2) workers who otherwise met the suspected occupational asthma case definition but who had unknown symptom or asthma onset dates; 3) work tenure of suspected occupational asthma cases subsequent to the development of symptoms or disease; 4) work tenure of workers who developed asthma post-hire but did not currently have asthma; and 5) work tenure of workers in the 2003 survey who had airways obstruction (one worker) or borderline obstruction (one worker) but who did not perform a bronchodilator trial and did not meet the other criteria for suspected occupational asthma. We considered estimated incidence rates for work areas with total person-time at risk of less than 50 person-years to be less reliable than incidence rates for areas with more than 50 person-years at risk.

To identify potential high-risk work areas for hard metal disease, we identified workers as having suspected hard metal disease if they met at least one of the following criteria: 1) DL_{CO} and TLC both less than 80% of predicted; 2) restriction on spirometry with a body mass index (BMI) greater than or equal to 18.5 and less than 30 and a TLC less than 80% of predicted; or 3) a chest x-ray with a small opacity profusion category of 1/0 or greater. Because the DL_{CO} test was only performed on participants who had an abnormal or borderline abnormal spirometry test, it is possible that workers who had normal spirometry test results might have had DL_{CO} and TLC abnormalities that we did not identify. BMI was calculated as: weight in kilograms ÷ (height in meters)^2. We excluded workers who only participated in the 2005 medical survey because neither DLCO measurements nor chest x-rays were obtained during that survey. We reviewed the medical records of two former workers who reported having been diagnosed with hard metal lung disease to determine if they met our case definition for suspected hard metal disease. We identified as high-risk work areas for hard metal disease the areas where suspected hard metal disease cases worked when they first developed symptoms or when they underwent testing that identified them as having suspected hard metal disease, whichever occurred first.

We used statistical regression models to determine whether any exposure measures for metals or dust were correlated with health effects (exposure-response relationships). Greater detail is available in Appendix C (Methods). For continuous outcomes we used SAS PROC GLM. For categorical outcomes we used SAS PROC LOGISTIC. Because exposure measurements did not follow a normal statistical distribution, we used natural logarithm transformations of the exposure variable measurements in our regression models. Total cobalt air concentration data were derived from air samples collected by NIOSH during the second environmental survey and from historical company data. Total tungsten, nickel, and chromium, and size-selected metal and total dust air concentration data were derived from air samples collected by NIOSH during the second environmental survey. NIOSH Marple impactor data (for size-selected particles), NIOSH cassette data (for total metal and dust particles), and company cassette data (for total cobalt particles) were all from full-shift samples.

All statistical analyses were performed using SAS®, version 9.1 (SAS Institute Inc., Cary, NC). We defined statistical significance as a p value of ≤0.05 and marginal statistical significance as a p value >0.05 and ≤0.10.

Results

Walkthrough Survey

Metalworking Products had previously obtained blood cobalt levels for workers in specific work areas in the Gurley facility that had known high cobalt air levels. From 1998 to 2003, individual blood cobalt levels for these workers ranged from 7.8 to 18.6 µg/L blood.

Table 3 summarizes the results of analyses for bulk metalworking fluid samples obtained by NIOSH from the Grant facility. In-use metalworking fluid contained approximately 1µg cobalt/g metalworking fluid, whereas solid sludge in the sump system contained 6600 µg cobalt/g sludge. Levels of nickel were below the limit of detection in liquid metal working fluid samples and over 80 µg/g in the solid sludge. Although levels of cobalt and nickel were highest in sludge, workers are generally not exposed to this material. Endotoxin and culturable fungi, bacteria, or mycobacteria were not detected in the sample of unused metalworking fluid. The in-use metalworking fluid sample had detectable endotoxin and bacteria as noted in Table 3. (Recommended or regulatory limits for levels of endotoxin and microbial contaminants in metalworking fluids have not been established.)

Table 3. Metalworking fluid analysis of four bulk samples, Grant facility, July 2003

Sample Type	Cobalt (µg/g)	Nickel (µg/g)	Endotoxin (EU/mL)	Fungi (culture)	Bacteria (culture)	*Mycobacteria* (culture)
Unused Rich Grind 662™ MWF	(1)	ND	< 0.5	No growth	No growth	No growth
In-use liquid MWF from centerless grinder	(1)	ND	200	No growth	Staphylo-coccus 1700 CFU/mL	No growth
Liquid sludge in sump system	74	(2)	NA	NA	NA	NA
Solid sludge in sump system	6600	82	NA	NA	NA	NA

EU/ml – endotoxin units per milliliter; CFU/ml – colony forming units per milliliter; MWF – metalworking fluid; ND – not detectable; NA – not analyzed.
Limits of detection (LOD) and quantification (LOQ) for cobalt were 0.8 and 3 µg/g, respectively; LOD and LOQ for nickel were 1 and 4 µg/g, respectively; LOD for endotoxin was 0.005 EU/ml (LOQ is not available); LOD for fungal and bacterial growth was 100 CFU/ml; parentheses indicate semi-quantitative values between the LOD and LOQ.

Medical Surveys

Participation and Demographics

Table 4 shows the numbers of workers who participated in the different components of the 2003 and 2005 NIOSH medical surveys. Workers in cobalt-exposed areas at the three facilities were invited to participate in the 2003 survey. All workers at the three facilities were invited to participate in the 2005 survey. Some of the numbers of participants for some of the tests shown in Table 4 are slightly higher than the corresponding provisional numbers previously reported in the interim letters.

Table 4. Participation in the 2003 and 2005 NIOSH medical surveys

Participation	2003 Survey (249 Workers Invited)*	2005 Survey (267 Workers Invited)
Questionnaire	171[a]	150[b]
Spirometry	171[c]	79
DLco	28	ND
CXR	172	ND
Methacholine Challenge	ND	44
Serial Spirometry	ND	11
Urine	ND	142
Blood	ND	140
EBC	ND	121
Wrist Wipe	ND	135
Total Participants	174[d]	150[e]

*Twenty-five additional workers from areas of the Huntsville facility without cobalt exposures requested to participate in the survey; all 25 participated in the questionnaire and spirometry components of the survey; 24 had a chest x-ray performed; and three underwent DL_{co} measurement. These 25 uninvited participants are not included in this table or in any data analyses presented in this report or in the interim letters.
ND – Test or analysis not performed during survey.
[a]133 participants completed the interviewer-administered computerized questionnaire; 38 participants completed the short self-administered questionnaire; 3 workers completed a questionnaire but did not complete spirometry.
[b]46 participants completed the interviewer-administered computerized questionnaire used in 2003; 104 participants completed the short follow-up questionnaire.
[c]3 workers completed spirometry but did not complete a questionnaire.
[d]Total number of participants who completed the questionnaire or spirometry
[e]Total number of participants who completed questionnaire.

Of 249 workers with a history of cobalt exposure who were invited to participate in the 2003 NIOSH survey, 197 (79%) completed a questionnaire in either the 2003 survey or the follow-up survey

RESULTS (CONTINUED)

in 2005 (171 in the 2003 survey and 26 additional workers in the 2005 survey). Table 5 shows demographic data for these survey participants. Most were male and about one-half had never smoked. The median age was 44 years. The median work tenure was 9 years.

Table 5. Demographics of workers who worked in one of the three facilities during the 2003 medical survey and who participated in either the 2003 or 2005 medical survey (N=197)

Characteristic	Value
Age (years)	
- Median	44.0
- Range	25.0–70.5
Male (percent)	70.6
Smoking status (percent)	
- Current smokers	32.0
- Former smokers	22.8
- Never smokers	45.2
Pack-years (for smokers)	
- Median	20.1
- Range	0.4–120.0
Tenure (years)	
- Median	8.9
- Range	0.2–37.2
Race (percent)	
- White	74.1
- Black	14.7
- Native American	2.0
- Asian or Native Hawaiian	1.0
- White and Native American*	8.1
Ethnicity (percent)	
- Hispanic	3.0
- Non-Hispanic	97.0

*Some workers indicated that they were both White and Native American.

Lung Function Test and Questionnaire Results

Of 172 workers who had chest x-rays in our September 2003 survey, none had findings suggestive of hard metal disease. Of 171 workers tested with spirometry, 5 (3%) had a restrictive pattern and 12 (7%) had airways obstruction. When compared to data from NHANES III, the prevalences of restriction and airways obstruction among all workers was not higher than expected. However, of 53 white never-smokers, 4 (8%) had airways obstruction, which was 3 times higher than expected (statistically significant). Compared to national data from NHANES III, the questionnaire data from the NIOSH medical survey showed that the overall Metalworking Products workforce prevalences were significantly higher than expected for

Page 22

the following health outcomes: shortness of breath when hurrying on level ground or walking up a slight hill; usual cough on most days for three consecutive months or more during the year; wheeze or whistling in the chest in the last 12 months; ever having been diagnosed with chronic bronchitis; and having been diagnosed by a physician with asthma (Table 6). In this workforce, these health outcomes were approximately twice as common as would be expected based on the general population survey results. Of 171 workers who completed a questionnaire, 28 (16%) reported having been diagnosed by a physician with asthma and 11 (6%) reported that their asthma began post-hire. The number of workers who reported having been diagnosed by a physician with asthma was 2.1 times higher than expected, based on national data (Table 6); and 1.5 times higher than expected when compared to Alabama state data. Eighteen (11%) workers reported that they had currently-active physician-diagnosed asthma. Compared to national data, the prevalence of currently-active physician-diagnosed asthma was 2.1 times higher than expected; compared to Alabama state data, the prevalence was 1.6 times higher than expected.

Table 6. Adjusted prevalence ratios* with 95% confidence intervals compared to NHANES III, 2003 medical survey participants (N=167)

Category	N	Shortness of breath[a]	Usual cough[b]	Wheeze[c]	Physician-diagnosed chronic bronchitis	Physician-diagnosed asthma
Huntsville Facility	31	1.4 (0.7–2.8)	2.7* (1.3–5.6)	1.8 (1.0–3.4)	2.0 (0.6–7.4)	1.3 (0.4–3.8)
Gurley Facility	36	2.3* (1.4–3.7)	0.8 (0.3–2.5)	1.8* (1.1–3.2)	2.4 (0.9–6.2)	2.2 (1.0–4.7)
Grant Facility	100	1.7* (1.2–2.3)	1.7* (1.1–2.8)	2.0* (1.4–2.8)	2.1* (1.2–3.6)	2.2* (1.4–3.5)
Entire Workforce	167[d]	1.8* (1.4–2.3)	1.7* (1.2–2.5)	1.9* (1.5–2.5)	2.1* (1.3–3.3)	2.1* (1.4–3.0)

*Adjusted for age, race, gender, and smoking (ever vs. never).
[a] Are you troubled by shortness of breath when hurrying on level ground or walking up a slight hill?
[b] Do you usually cough on most days for 3 consecutive months or more during the year?
[c] Have you had wheezing or whistling in your chest at any time in the last 12 months?
[d] One Asian survey participant was excluded from these analyses due to lack of information on expected prevalences for adjustment of prevalence ratios.
N – number.
* Asterisked/bolded prevalence ratios indicate statistical significance.

RESULTS (continued)

The estimated pre-hire adult-onset asthma incidence rate was 2.1 cases per 1000 person-years, identical to that estimated from NHANES I data [McWorter et al. 1989]. In contrast, the estimated post-hire adult-onset asthma incidence rate was 5.5 cases per 1000 person-years, or 2.6 times higher. This post-hire/pre-hire incidence rate ratio had a 95% confidence interval of 1.2 to 6.2, indicating a statistically higher incidence rate in the post-hire compared to the pre-hire period.

Using data from the 2003 medical survey as well as information from the medical records of two former workers, we identified one former worker and two current workers with suspected hard metal disease based on lung function test abnormalities. The former worker had a lung biopsy that (according to the reviewing pathologist) showed the presence of multi-nucleated giant cells. One worker was working in *pressing*, another in *sintering*, and the third in *grinding* at the time they developed symptoms or were found to have abnormal lung function.

In the request for this HHE, it had been reported that a former worker had occupational asthma. A NIOSH investigator spoke with this individual, who reported onset of episodic wheezing and shortness of breath while working in the pressing area at the Grant facility soon after being hired. The affected individual reported that, within one month of being hired at the plant, a personal physician had diagnosed the asthma. Symptomatic relief was obtained from treatment with inhaler medications.

Table 7 shows the estimates of incidence of suspected occupational asthma in different work areas. Among work areas with more than 50 person-years at risk, the four highest estimates of incidence of suspected occupational asthma were in *product testing, pressing, milling/spray drying* (data from these two areas combined for analyses), and *sintering*. (Note: Due to correction of some person-year calculations from the work history data, the person-years and estimates of incidence are slightly different from those provisionally reported in Interim Letter IX (Appendix A).)

Table 7. Incidence rates of suspected occupational asthma, 2003 and 2005 surveys (N=164)

Work area(s)	Number of cases	Person-years	Incidence rate (cases per 1000 person-years)
Screening	1	11	90.9
Gurley Facility Maintenance	2	36	55.6
Product Testing	2	79	25.3
Pressing	7	313	22.4
Milling and Spray Drying	3	129	22.3
Sintering	2	91	22.0
Reclamation	3	177	16.9
Shaping and Round Cell	2	119	16.8
Powder Mixing, Reprocessing, and Blending	1	60	16.7
Other*	4	298	13.4
Grant Facility Shipping	1	82	12.2
Grinding	1	226	4.4
Gurley Facility Powder Laboratory	0	42	0
Gurley Facility Shipping	0	37	0
Sandblasting	0	12	0
Grant Facility Maintenance	0	96	0
Metal Separation	0	86	0
All Work Areas	29	1894	15.3

*Participants at the Huntsville facility were included in this analysis only if they currently worked in Reclamation or Metal Separation; the "Other" category includes minimal person-time from other work areas at the Huntsville facility (such as tungsten oxide reduction and tungsten carbide production).

Of 15 employees with suspected occupational asthma and who completed a methacholine challenge test, 5 (33%) had airways hyperreponsiveness. Two of 29 (7%) employees without suspected occupational asthma who completed a methacholine challenge test had airways hyperreponsiveness. Of eight workers with suspected occupational asthma who completed serial spirometry of sufficient quality to allow interpretation, 2 (25%) had a work-related pattern. Both of these employees worked in pressing at the onset of their suspected occupational asthma. Of the six suspected occupational asthma cases who did not have a work-related pattern on serial spirometry, three used an asthma inhaler multiple times (range: 13–26) during the three weeks of serial spirometry testing. (The use of an asthma inhaler can obscure work-related changes in FEV_1 and PEFR.)

Exhaled Breath Condensate Biomarker Results

There was a low but statistically significant correlation between natural log exhaled breath condensate (EBC) cobalt levels and

RESULTS (CONTINUED)

natural log total cobalt air concentrations (Pearson correlation coefficient = 0.33, p=0.0023); natural log EBC cobalt levels were not correlated with natural log respirable cobalt air concentrations. There were statistically significant correlations between natural log EBC cobalt levels and natural log urine and blood cobalt levels; the correlation with blood cobalt was moderate (0.47; p=0.0002) and the correlation with urine cobalt was low (0.35; p=0.0005). Stepwise regression analysis did not identify any possible confounders (current or former smoking, race, gender, or age) of these correlations.

EBC MDA levels were not correlated with either EBC cobalt levels or EBC tungsten levels. There were statistically significant but low correlations between EBC MDA levels and the natural logs of total cobalt air concentrations (0.33, p=0.0018) and respirable cobalt air concentrations (0.22, p=0.04). Stepwise regression analysis of possible confounders (current or former smoking, race, gender, and age) showed that smoking status was a possible confounder (p<0.25). In multiple linear regression models for MDA levels where smoking status was included, total cobalt air concentration remained significant (p=0.005), while respirable cobalt air concentration was marginally significant (p=0.08). MDA levels were not significantly correlated with blood or urine cobalt levels.

Geometric mean values of LTB-4, IL-8, and MDA in EBC did not differ significantly between "healthy" workers and "current asthma" cases. (See above Methods subsection, *Biomarkers of Inflammation and Oxidative Stress in Exhaled Breath Condensate*, for criteria for "healthy" workers and "current asthma" cases. Additional details of results are shown in Table 12 in Interim Letter IX in Appendix A.)

Total Immunoglobulin E and Metal Antibody Results

Of 140 workers tested, 32 (23%) had IgE levels of at least 100 kU/L. Geometric means were 81.4 kU/L for workers with pre-hire physician-diagnosed asthma, 28.0 kU/L for workers with suspected occupational asthma, and 40.3 kU/L for other workers. There were no statistically significant differences among these geometric mean values. Of 140 workers tested, none had antibodies specific to cobalt, nickel, or chromium bound to HSA or SOD.

Genetic Analyses

We did not find an association between the genetic allele HLA-DPβ1^{E69} and post-hire physician-diagnosed asthma. Only two of 9 (22%) workers with post-hire physician-diagnosed asthma had one or more HLA-DPβ1^{E69} alleles compared to 39 of 101 (39%) non-asthmatic workers (Table 8). Additionally, the allelic frequency for HLA-DPβ1^{E69} was lower among workers with post-hire physician-diagnosed asthma compared to non-asthmatic workers. Hardy-Weinberg equilibrium was present among workers with post-hire physician-diagnosed asthma, but not among non-asthmatic workers. The lack of Hardy-Weinberg equilibrium in the non-asthmatic worker group may be due to the small number of workers and possibly multiple members of the same families working in the three facilities.

Table 8. Frequency of workers with different allelic combinations of the HLA-DPβ1 gene by asthmatic status, 2005 medical survey

Worker Group	# of Workers (KK)	# of Workers (KE)	# Workers (EE)	# Workers (Total)	% of Workers with $\geq$1 HLA-DPβ1^{E69} Allele	HLA-DPβ1^{E69} Allelic Frequency[a]	Hardy-Weinberg Equilibrium[b]
Post-hire asthma[c]	7	2	0	9	22%	0.11	Yes (p=0.708)
Non-asthmatic[d]	62	27	12	101	39%	0.25	No (p=0.003)

KK – Two alleles that are either HLA-DPβ1^{K69} (or HLA-DPβ1^{R69}).
KE – One HLA-DPβ1^{K69} (or HLA-DPβ1^{R69}) allele and one HLA-DPβ1^{E69} allele.
EE – Two HLA-DPβ1^{E69} alleles.
[a]The number of HLA-DPβ1^{E69} alleles in the specified worker group divided by the total number of HLA-DPβ1 alleles in the worker group multiplied by 100.
[b]Hardy-Weinberg p-values are based on chi-square test.
[c]Participants who reported physician-diagnosed asthma with post-hire onset on the NIOSH survey questionnaire in 2005.
[d]Participants who did not report asthma on the NIOSH survey questionnaire in 2005.

Exposure Measurements

Using the MOUDI and 8-stage cascade impactor samplers in May 2004, we found that airborne particles capable of reaching the large airways (thoracic size) were generated in the *scrap reclamation, powder mixing,* and *spray drying* areas. Smaller particles capable of reaching the deepest part of the lung (respirable size) were found in the *grinding* area at the Grant facility. Of all airborne particles collected, the weight (expressed as a percent) that was respirable in size ranged from 9% (*scrap reclamation*-ball mill) to approximately

50% (*pressing* and *grinding*). The respirable mass of cobalt-containing particles ranged from 7% (*scrap reclamation*-ball mill) to 37% (*grinding*).

When results from NIOSH air samples collected using 37-mm cassette samplers in 2004 (251 cassette samples) were aggregated with company data (72 cassette samples) from 1985 to 2003, the two highest area-specific mean total cobalt concentrations were in *reprocessing* (427.2 µg/m^3) and *powder mixing* (414.3 µg/m^3)(see Table 9 on page 49). Considering only results from the 2004 NIOSH air samples (251 samples from 37-mm cassette samplers and 105 samples from 8-stage Marple impactors), the highest mean air concentrations of total cobalt (574.5 µg/m^3), thoracic cobalt (304.5 µg/m^3), and respirable cobalt (77.6 µg/m^3) were all from the *powder mixing area*, as were the highest individual concentrations of total cobalt (1,622.1 µg/m^3), thoracic cobalt (849.0 µg/m^3), and respirable cobalt (213.2 µg/m3)(see Table 10 on page 50). In all work areas, air samples contained particles with a range of sizes that could potentially deposit anywhere along the respiratory tract if inhaled, from the upper airway (nose and throat) to the deepest regions of the lung. Levels of airborne chromium and nickel were generally low among all facilities (see Appendix A, Interim Letter II); the highest individual measurement of airborne nickel (445 µg/m^3, also from the *powder mixing area*) was above the NIOSH REL but only half the legally enforceable PEL set by OSHA.

During our second survey in October 2004, we found that within each work area, the shape and chemistry of airborne particles was similar among all sizes of particles we studied. However, there was no consistent shape or chemistry for airborne particles among work areas. In work areas that prepare and handle feedstock powders (*powder mixing*), the particles were generally round and usually consisted of only one metal or compound (e.g., cobalt or tungsten). In work areas that compressed powders into different forms (*pressing, extrusion*), the particles were a mixture of round particles and compacted particles (data not shown) containing one or more metals or compounds. In work areas that handle sintered product (*sintering, grinding, sandblasting*), the particles had irregular edges and appeared to be more compact than particles from previous production steps, and nearly all were composed of multiple metals and compounds (tungsten carbide, cobalt, tantalum, nickel, chromium, etc.)[Stefaniak et al. 2007].

The NIOSH REL for metalworking fluids is 0.4 mg/m^3

thoracic particulate matter, which corresponds to an exposure concentration of 0.5 mg/m³ when using a 37-mm cassette sampler. All PBZ and area sample measurements for airborne metalworking fluids collected using 37-mm cassette samplers in the October 2004 survey were below 0.5 mg/m³.

Tungsten oxide fibers were detected in 9 of 12 work areas sampled with PBZ and area air samplers (see Appendix A, Interim Letter XII). (It is unknown if there any potential adverse health effects related to human exposure to airborne tungsten oxide fibers.)

Wipe samples collected from routinely-handled work surfaces contained measurable amounts of cobalt in all areas across the three facilities. Mid-shift wipe samples from workers' skin (neck and hand) contained measurable amounts of cobalt on all hand samples and most neck samples. The highest median mid-shift neck wipe measurements occurred among workers in *metal separation* and *powder mixing* [Day et al. 2009](see Appendix A, Interim Letter VIII).

Geometric mean urine cobalt levels (µg/L) or blood cobalt levels in excess of biological levels comparable to the NIOSH REL of 50 µg cobalt /m³ air were present in *reclamation, powder mixing/ reprocessing/blending* (data from these three areas combined for analyses), *milling, spray drying, pressing,* and *shaping/round cell* (data from these two areas combined for analyses) (Table 11). Among work areas with suspected hard metal lung disease cases or with relatively high estimates of incidence of suspected occupational asthma, *sintering, grinding,* and *product testing* had comparatively low urine and blood cobalt levels, whereas *milling, spray drying,* and *pressing* had levels in excess of biological levels comparable to the NIOSH REL.

Table 11. Geometric mean urine and blood cobalt concentrations* by work area, January 2005

Facility	Work Area(s)	Urine Cobalt (µg/g creatinine) (N)	Urine Cobalt (µg/g creatinine) (GM)	Urine Cobalt (µg/g creatinine) (95% CI)	Urine Cobalt (µg/L urine) (N)	Urine Cobalt (µg/L urine) (GM)	Urine Cobalt (µg/L urine) (95% CI)	Blood Cobalt (µg/L blood) (N)	Blood Cobalt (µg/L blood) (GM)	Blood Cobalt (µg/L blood) (95% CI)
Huntsville	Reclamation**	7	25 2	8 7–73 2	6**	30 5**	9 6–101 8**	7**	4 0**	1 2–13 2**
	Metal Separation	8	4 2	2 3–7 8	5	8 3	3 1–22 7	7	1 4	0 9–2 27
Gurley	Powder Mixing, Reprocessing, & Blending**	5	14 5	2 5–84 9	4	26 6	3 4–207 5	5**	3 7**	0 6–23 6**
	Milling**	5	134 7	95 8–189 4	4**	185 1**	112 8–303 8**	5**	15 6**	11 2–21 7**
	Spray Drying**	2	20 0	0 9–438 4	2**	44 9**	2 7–743 6**	2**	3 2**	1 8–5 8**
Grant	Pressing **	10	30 3	14 9-61 8	7**	46 8**	20 9–104 8**	11**	3 7**	2 6–5 2**
	Shaping and Round Cell**	4	25 7	5 0–133 5	4	26 0	3 8–176 4	4**	3 3**	2 2–5 1**
	Sintering	3	4 7	1 7–13 0	2	5 4	4 8–6 0	3	0 9	0 2–4 7
	Grinding	12	3 2	2 2–4 7	11	4 8	2 9–7 7	12	0 9	0 6–1 5
	Product Testing	4	3 1	1 1–9 3	1	2 1	-	4	0 7	0 2–2 9
	Shipping	2	3 5	0 3–38 1	2	3 1	0 1–167 5	2	1 2	<0 1–9629 6
	Maintenance	2	4 9	0 1–257 3	2	11 8	1 4–100 3	2	1 7	<0 1–1475 2
All	Other	20	6 1	3 5–10 0	11	9 7	4 3–21 9	21	1 3	0 8–2 3
	Total	84	9 6	7 1–12 8	61	15 2	10 7–21 7	85	2 0	1 5–2 5

*Reported urine and blood cobalt concentrations are from employees who denied the use of multivitamins (or vitamin B_{12}) and artificial joint implants. Reported urine cobalt concentrations were for urine samples that had specific gravity levels between 1.010 and 1.030 and creatinine concentrations between 0.3 and 3.0 g/L. Blood and urine cobalt concentrations (µg/L) which correspond to the NIOSH recommended exposure limit for cobalt in workplace air of 50 µg/m³ are 2.5 and 30 µg/L, respectively [Lauwerys and Hoet 2001]; **/boxes shaded in grey indicate work areas with geometric mean blood or urine cobalt levels in excess of these values.
N – number of samples; GM – geometric mean; CI – confidence interval.

We compared geometric mean EBC metal concentrations for workers in work areas with the four highest estimates of incidence of suspected occupational asthma and in work areas with suspected hard metal lung disease cases to EBC metal concentrations for workers in other work areas. Among work areas with more than 50 person-years at risk, the four highest estimates of incidence of suspected occupational asthma were in *product testing, pressing, milling/spray drying* (data from these two areas combined for analyses), and *sintering*. *Pressing, sintering,* and *grinding* had suspected hard metal lung disease cases. Table 12 shows the geometric mean EBC metal concentrations for workers in these areas compared to workers in other areas.

Table 12. Geometric mean exhaled breath condensate metal concentrations among participating workers in *product testing, pressing, milling/spray drying, sintering,* **and** *grinding* **compared to workers in other work areas**

Metal in EBC	Product Testing, Pressing, Milling/Spray Drying*, Sintering, and Grinding	All Other Work Areas
Cobalt (µg/L)	6.2	5.5
Tungsten (µg/L)	2.3**	10.2

*Data from the *milling* and *spray drying* areas combined for analyses.
**Statistically significant difference from corresponding value for "All Other Work Areas."

Exposures among Workers with Suspected Occupational Lung Disease and Workers without Evidence of Lung Disease

Table 13 shows current total cobalt exposures and estimated cumulative exposures (total cobalt, respirable cobalt, and total tungsten) for the three suspected hard metal lung disease cases, for the group of suspected occupational asthma cases, and for a group of workers who did not have evidence of lung disease (i.e., those survey participants who did not report respiratory symptoms or physician-diagnosed asthma or chronic bronchitis and who did not have pulmonary function test abnormalities). Workers suspected of having hard metal disease did not have higher indices of cobalt or tungsten exposure, compared to the group of workers who did not have evidence of lung disease. Similarly, workers suspected of having occupational asthma did not have higher indices of exposure.

Table 13. Current total cobalt exposures and estimated cumulative exposures (total cobalt, respirable cobalt, and respirable tungsten) among workers with suspected occupational lung disease and workers without evidence of lung disease

Worker / Group	Current Total Cobalt µg/m³	Estimated Cumulative Exposures* Total Cobalt µg/m³-yrs	Estimated Cumulative Exposures* Respirable Cobalt µg/m³-yrs	Estimated Cumulative Exposures* Respirable Tungsten µg/m³-yrs
Suspected Hard Metal Lung Disease, Case 1	9.4	95.6	--	--
Suspected Hard Metal Lung Disease, Case 2	11.1	66.6	24.5	217.4
Suspected Hard Metal Lung Disease, Case 3	42.7	71.7	2.7	16.2
Suspected Occupational Asthma cases, n=29	48.3 (2.7–414.3)**	319.4 (0–1605)**	35.2 (0–180)**	253.1 (0–1722)**
"Healthy" Workers†, n=36	43.6 (3.7–414.3)**	395.1 (1.4–1969)**	45.7 (0.1–369)**	312.8 (0.7–1167)**

*Exposure at time of symptom development or when case was identified at time of NIOSH medical survey (for suspected hard metal lung disease cases), at time of symptom development (for suspected occupational asthma cases), or at time of NIOSH questionnaire (for healthy workers).

**Mean (range).

~ Could not be calculated due to missing data.

†Survey participants whose (1) most recent spirometry test (from either the 2003 or 2005 survey) was normal; 2) who did not have airways hyperreponsiveness on methacholine challenge testing (i.e., PC_{20} of less than or equal to 16 mg/ml); and 3) who reported that they had never been diagnosed with asthma, did not have asthma-like symptoms, were not troubled by shortness of breath, did not have shortness of breath when hurrying on level ground, did not have a usual cough, had never been diagnosed with chronic bronchitis, and were not currently using breathing medication.

Exposure-Response Models

Among workers who participated in the 2005 survey, we found marginally significant associations between the presence of three or more asthma-like symptoms and individual test results for the amount (µg) of cobalt on the wrist, the concentration (µg/g creatinine) of cobalt in the urine, and the concentration (µg/L) of cobalt in exhaled breath condensate (Table 14). The odds for these symptoms increased 1.3- to 1.4-fold for every one-unit increase in the natural log of these exposure metrics (a unit increase in the natural log of an exposure metric corresponds to a 2.7-fold increase in the unlogged exposure metric). For an analysis based on dichotomized exposure metrics, we selected cutpoints using a binary decision tree called Classification and Regression Tree (CART) (JMP®, version 5.1, SAS Institute Inc., Cary, NC). We found that the odds of having three or more asthma-like symptoms were 9-fold greater if the amount of cobalt on the wrist was greater than 250 µg compared to lower levels. Likewise, the odds of having three or more asthma-like symptoms were 5-fold greater if the amount of urine cobalt was greater than 24.45 µg/g creatinine compared to lower levels; and the odds of having three or more asthma-like symptoms were 6-fold greater if the amount of cobalt in exhaled breath condensate was greater than 0.9 µg/L compared to lower levels. All of these results were statistically significant (Table 14).

Table 14. Associations between three or more asthma-like symptoms and current personal exposure measurements (2005 participants)

Current personal exposure measurements	Number	Continuous Exposure Data[a] Odds Ratio[b] (95% CI)	Dichotomized Exposure Data Cutpoint	Dichotomized Exposure Data Odds Ratio[b] (95% CI)
Wrist cobalt (µg)	129	<u>1.35</u> (0.96–1.92)	<250 vs. ≥250	**9.26*** (1.98–48.20)
Urine cobalt (µg/g creatinine)	91	<u>1.43</u> (0.96–2.20)	<24.45 vs. ≥24.45	**5.09*** (1.43–19.67)
Cobalt in exhaled breath condensate (µg /L exhaled breath)	110	<u>1.34</u> (0.99–1.85)	<0.9 vs ≥0.9	**6.48*** (1.02–131.76)

*/Bold font – statistically significant association (p value ≤0.05).
Underlined odds ratio indicates marginally significant association (p value ≤0.10 and >0.05).
[a] Continuous exposure variables were transformed using the natural log.
[b] Odds ratios were adjusted for gender, age, tenure, smoking (pack-years), and currently active physician-diagnosed asthma. Profile likelihood confidence intervals were used.

Among the 2003 and 2005 survey participants, when current work area respirable cobalt and respirable tungsten levels were both included in models (as either the highest recorded exposures or the mean exposures) both were, in general, significantly or marginally significantly associated with FEV_1 and FVC modeled either as percent predicted values or as absolute volumes (see Table 15 on page 51). The statistically significant association for FEV_1 showed that for every one-unit increase in the natural log of mean respirable cobalt exposure there was a 0.14 L decline in FEV_1 and an absolute decline of 4% in percent predicted FEV_1. However, when mean respirable cobalt was the only exposure variable included in the models, the associations were not statistically significant (p values: 0.23 and 0.70 for FEV_1 and percent predicted FEV_1 declines, respectively)(data not shown). Five workers who were unlike other workers (due to much higher cobalt than tungsten exposure) were responsible for the statistically significant relationships in models that included both current respirable cobalt and current tungsten exposures. When we explored associations between the mean respirable cobalt/mean respirable tungsten ratio for current exposures and lung function, we found that a one-unit increase in the ratio was significantly associated with a 0.44 L decline in FEV_1 and an absolute decline of nearly 13% in percent predicted FEV_1 (see Table 15 on page 51).

Among the 2003 and 2005 survey participants, a similar pattern was found in models based on estimated cumulative exposures, where every one-unit increase in the natural log of mean respirable cobalt (modeled together with mean respirable tungsten) was significantly associated with an absolute decline of 5% in percent predicted FEV_1 (see Table 16 on page 52). When estimated cumulative mean respirable cobalt was the only exposure variable in the model, the result was not statistically significant (p=0.39) (data not shown). Additionally, estimated cumulative mean total cobalt was significantly associated with three or more asthma-like symptoms. For every one-unit increase in the natural log of estimated cumulative mean total cobalt exposure, the odds of having three of more asthma-like symptoms increased 1.4-fold (OR=1.44; 95% CI: 1.06–2.03; p=0.03)(data not shown). When we compared workers in the highest quartile of estimated cumulative mean total cobalt exposure to workers in the lowest quartile, we found an odds ratio of 4.43 (95% CI: 1.24–19.24; p=0.03) for having three or more asthma-like symptoms (data not shown).

DISCUSSION

With the report that former workers of the three Metalworking Products facilities in Alabama had been diagnosed with occupational asthma and hard metal lung disease, we conducted several medical and environmental surveys at these facilities from September 2003 through May 2005. These surveys were intended to measure exposures, to identify possible relationships between exposures and worker health to assess the extent of risk among the workforce, and to provide company management and workers with specific prevention recommendations to minimize the risk.

High exposures measured in the Metalworking Products facilities indicated a need for additional exposure controls. Based on combined NIOSH and company air sampling results, geometric mean total cobalt levels were highest in *reprocessing* (427 μg/m³), *powder mixing* (414 μg/m³), *blending* (119.8 μg/m³), and *screening* (142.8 μg/m³). These mean levels provide strong evidence that exposures in these four areas typically exceeded the OSHA PEL of 100 μg/m³ for total cobalt. Individual total dust samples exceeding 100 μg/m³ cobalt were obtained in a total of 12 work areas. Along with the four areas with mean exposures exceeding 100 μg/m³, two additional areas, *spray drying* (86.2 μg/m³) and *reclamation* (67.6 μg/m³), had geometric mean exposures that exceeded the NIOSH REL of 50 μg/m³ for total cobalt. Individual total dust samples exceeding 50 μg/m³ cobalt were obtained in a total of 14 work areas. In many of the work areas where air concentrations exceeded the REL, elevated geometric mean cobalt levels in urine and/or blood samples were consistent with exposures above the NIOSH REL.

As a basis for our analyses to identify exposure characteristics that might be associated with lung disease risk, we used symptom and medical test data to identify Metalworking Products workers likely to have occupational asthma or hard metal lung disease (i.e., suspected cases). Although no current workers had chest x-rays showing evidence of hard metal lung disease, one former worker (already clinically diagnosed with the disease) and two current workers met our criteria for suspected hard metal lung disease. Especially because the affected former worker had evidence of hard metal lung disease on lung biopsy, and in light of the documented excessive cobalt exposures at the Metalworking Products facilities, it can reasonably be concluded that workers at Metalworking Products facilities are at risk for hard metal lung disease. Our medical survey data showed that, compared to the general population, the current Metalworking Products workforce

DISCUSSION (CONTINUED)

in Alabama had elevated rates of respiratory symptoms and self-reported physician-diagnosed asthma; the data also showed that, among current workers at Metalworking Products, the incidence rate of adult-onset physician-diagnosed asthma was 2.6 times higher after hire than before hire. These findings suggested likely ongoing risk of work-related lung disease for current workers.

Based on our medical survey data, 29 of 164 workers (18%) met our criteria for suspected occupational asthma. It is possible that our criteria for suspected occupational asthma overestimated the actual prevalence of occupational asthma. These criteria, designed to identify all possible cases, were purposely more sensitive than specific; some individuals who met our case definition may have had work-related chest symptoms but not asthma. Also, exposures to production materials besides cobalt may have contributed to symptoms among those with suspected occupational asthma. The results of studies at two other cemented tungsten carbide facilities, though not directly comparable to our study results due to the different assessment methods used, suggested a lower occupational asthma prevalence than we found in our study. At one of these facilities, investigators found an 11% prevalence of work-related wheeze [Sprince et al. 1988]. In another study, of 319 workers exposed to dusts generated during production of hard metal, 18 (5.6%) were found to have occupational asthma [Kusaka et al. 1986].

In our analyses we observed that both higher current and higher estimated cumulative respirable cobalt exposure were associated with decreased lung function; higher estimated cumulative total cobalt was also associated with three or more asthma symptoms. Of greater significance is the observation that suspected hard metal lung disease cases and some suspected occupational asthma cases had exposures that were below the NIOSH REL for cobalt (50 μg/m^3). Similar findings have been reported by other researchers. One study noted very low exposures (<8 μg/m^3) for three workers with evidence of lung disease [Sprince et al. 1988]. In workers with confirmed cobalt asthma and available exposure data at another facility, four of eight had exposures below the NIOSH REL [Kusaka et al. 1986]. Thus, even the REL is probably not completely health-protective for some workers. The occurrence of lung disease in workers with relatively low cobalt exposures emphasizes the importance of not only monitoring and maintaining exposures below recommended and regulatory limits, but also of monitoring the health of potentially exposed workers to identify evidence of early disease. With hard metal disease, workers may show evidence of lung disease on medical tests before they become symptomatic. In another study by Sprince et al., four of nine hard metal-exposed workers who had evidence of interstitial lung disease on their chest x-rays did not have respiratory symptoms [Sprince et al. 1984]. Identifying affected workers before they become symptomatic provides an opportunity to prevent further progression of disease by minimizing further exposures.

In addition to controlling inhalation exposures to decrease the likelihood that workers will develop cobalt-related lung disease, minimizing skin exposures may be an important prevention consideration. Animal studies of lung disease development with exposures to beryllium and isocyanates have shown that skin exposure can lead to an immunologic response (sensitization) that can later result in respiratory disease [Bello et al. 2007; Redlich et al. 2008]. Recent evaluation of a chronic beryllium lung disease prevention program showed a decrease in the rate of worker sensitization to beryllium after skin protection was added [Cummings et al. 2007]. Most cobalt-related asthma likely involves immunologic sensitization to cobalt that might be prevented by skin protection.

Our January 2005 medical survey at Metalworking Products included collection of blood samples to determine possible immunological mechanisms involved in the development of cobalt-related lung disease. We looked for IgG (a type of antibody) against cobalt, nickel, and chromium. Other investigators who had previously evaluated workers with occupational asthma at another cemented tungsten carbide facility found that some affected workers had IgE against cobalt bound to HSA [Shirakawa et al. 1988, 1989]. IgE is the antibody type involved in the allergic process known as immediate hypersensitivity, which occurs in many individuals who have asthma. Along with IgE, individuals often produce IgG against any substances to which they are allergic; IgG is usually produced in larger amounts, potentially making this antibody easier to detect in blood analyses.

Our blood analyses did not identify IgG against cobalt, nickel, or chromium in any survey participant. Compared to our survey, Shirakawa et al. specifically looked for antibodies in workers who had cobalt asthma confirmed in a controlled inhalation challenge exposure to cobalt chloride in a laboratory setting. Of the 12 workers identified by Shirakawa et al. as having cobalt asthma among the approximately 400 workers at a hard metal plant, seven had IgE against cobalt. There are several possible explanations for our negative antibody findings. One possible reason that our blood analyses did not identify antibodies to cobalt might relate to the infrequent occurrence of true cobalt asthma, even among hard metal workers, and the smaller size of the workforce we assessed compared to that assessed by Shirakawa et al. Also, the fact that Shirakawa et al. did not find IgE in all cobalt asthma cases indicates that other disease mechanisms not dependent upon antibodies to cobalt may be involved in some cobalt asthma cases. Finally, while our serial spirometry data established a high likelihood of occupational asthma in two Metalworking Products workers, we did not conduct inhalation challenge studies to confirm that cobalt was the cause. Thus, the suspect occupational asthma cases we identified might have been caused by workplace exposures other than cobalt, nickel, or chromium; blood analyses would not be expected to show antibodies to these metals in this situation.

We included blood analyses for the HLA-DPβ1^{E69} gene allele in our 2005 survey because a previous study by other researchers had shown an association between this allele and hard metal lung disease [Potolicchio et al. 1997]. However, the very low number of suspected hard metal lung disease cases in our survey did not allow us to determine if this association was evident in our data. We also conducted an analysis to see if suspected occupational asthma was associated with the HLA- DPβ1^{E69} allele, but did not identify an association.

We collected exhaled breath condensate from participants in the 2005 survey to assess the potential of this technique to provide useful information on exposures and possible health effects. In a study of diamond tool and hard metal parts workers in Italy, EBC levels of MDA, a biomarker of oxidative stress, increased with EBC cobalt levels and were enhanced by co-exposure to tungsten [Goldoni et al. 2004]. This finding is consistent with results of animal studies showing greater toxicity of cobalt when mixed with tungsten carbide and with the potential for mixtures of cobalt and tungsten carbide particles to generate reactive oxygen species [Lison 1998]. In our EBC results, EBC MDA was not correlated with EBC cobalt or tungsten, nor were EBC levels of MDA or two biomarkers of inflammation (LTB-4 and IL-8) statistically different between workers with current asthma and a comparison group of "healthy" workers.

CONCLUSIONS

At three cemented tungsten carbide production facilities owned by Metalworking Products in Alabama, cobalt exposures in several areas exceeded the NIOSH REL and/or the OSHA PEL. Urine and blood cobalt levels also revealed evidence of high cobalt exposures in many areas. A former worker had evidence of hard metal disease on lung biopsy and two current workers had findings on lung function tests that suggested possible hard metal disease. Our medical surveys identified an elevated rate of post-hire asthma compared to pre-hire. This suggests that exposures in these facilities at the time of the medical survey were putting workers at risk for asthma as well. Because these diseases can become severe and disabling, the risk that Metalworking Products workers might develop them should be minimized through exposure control measures such as process isolation and ventilation improvements, administrative and work practice changes, and respiratory and skin protection. Worker education and regular medical monitoring are also important components of a comprehensive prevention strategy, because some workers may be at risk even when exposures are below the NIOSH REL.

RECOMMENDATIONS

The following is a summary of the recommendations we have provided in letters to company management from February 2004 through January 2007.

General Measures:

- Reduce cobalt exposure levels to below the OSHA PEL of 100 µg/m³ and preferably below the NIOSH REL of 50 µg/m³.

- Make efforts to further reduce potential air and skin exposures in work areas with the highest estimates of incidence of suspected occupational asthma and where workers with suspected hard metal lung disease worked (*milling/spray drying, pressing, sintering, grinding,* and *product testing*).

- To reduce worker exposures to cobalt, follow the principles of the industrial hygiene hierarchy of controls, prioritizing control methods from most preferred to least preferred: engineering > work practices > personal protective equipment.

- Limit migration of cobalt from areas of higher contamination to areas of lower contamination. Possible routes of cross-contamination include the transfer of cobalt from shoes, clothing, hands, equipment, and paperwork to less contaminated work areas.

- Improve general cleanliness of both production and non-production areas through good housekeeping measures. Designate lunch rooms as "Clean Areas" and prevent the migration of cobalt into these areas through the use of tacky mats and by requiring workers to wash their hands prior to entry.

Engineering Controls:

- Minimize cobalt exposures through the implementation of engineering controls. Examples of engineering controls include enclosing machines, improving local exhaust ventilation, and automating powder handling processes.

- Minimize the generation of metalworking fluid mists through appropriate operation and control of the metalworking fluid delivery system (see for example, *Mist Control Considerations for the Design, Installation, and Use of Machine Tools Using Metalworking Fluids,* American National Standards Institute Technical Report B11 TR 2-1997).

RECOMMENDATIONS
(CONTINUED)

Work Practices:

- Ensure that the company's current written metalworking fluid management plan specifies procedures for maintenance of fluid chemistry (e.g., pH, temperature, viscosity; storage, mixing and diluting metalworking fluid concentrate; preparing additives such as biocides and cobalt inhibitor; and monitoring tramp oil contamination) and maintenance of the fluid filtration and delivery systems (e.g., fluid level in sump tank).

- Instruct workers in the *grinding* work area to stand a reasonable distance away from grinding machines during operation that still allows workers to oversee machine processes. Along with appropriate usage of respiratory protection, maximizing the distance between the operator and the machine will reduce exposure to aerosolized metalworking fluids.

- Reposition cooling fans in work areas so that they blow potentially contaminated air away from the worker's breathing zone.

- Dedicate equipment (e.g., hand tools) to specific work areas to prevent cobalt migration from an area of higher cobalt contamination to an area of lower cobalt contamination.

- Replace contaminated shop packets (plastic folders containing paperwork that accompany orders throughout production) with clean packets before bringing paperwork into administrative areas for processing.

- Provide a vacuum equipped with high-efficiency particulate air (HEPA) filtration in the pressing area for employees to clean off their machines and work area and thereby eliminate the need for dry sweeping/brushing.

- Instruct workers to: 1) periodically wash skin contaminated with metalworking fluid and metals with mild soap and water and use clean towels to dry off; 2) wash their hands before eating, smoking, or using the rest room; and 3) shower soon after work.

Personal Protective Equipment:

Skin Protection
- Implement a skin protection program to minimize contamination of skin with metal powders and metalworking fluids.

RECOMMENDATIONS
(CONTINUED)

- Instruct workers to wear long-sleeved shirts when passing through or working in production areas.

- Instruct workers to wear nitrile gloves when working in production areas. When performing activities that require durable protection, workers should additionally use over-gloves made of a resilient material.

- Instruct workers to not place their bare hands into metalworking fluid.

- Instruct workers to not reuse disposable protective gloves. Workers should replace nitrile gloves with new gloves when they become damaged or torn.

- Instruct workers to put on clean gloves before they handle contaminated equipment. For example, workers should put on gloves prior to handling work shoes or respirators.

Respiratory Protection

- Ensure that the company's current respiratory protection program is in compliance with the OSHA respiratory protection standard. The program should be documented in writing and should include medical evaluation, fit testing, filter and cartridge change-out protocol, training, and record keeping.

- Ensure that all necessary respirator sizes, filters, and cartridges are always available.

- Require the mandatory use of respirators: 1) in work areas with known high cobalt air concentrations until engineering and work practice controls decrease these levels below the NIOSH REL; and 2) for all cleaning and maintenance activities that involve surfaces or equipment potentially contaminated with cobalt.

- The NIOSH *Pocket Guide to Chemical Hazards* recommends the following minimum levels of respiratory protection for exposure to cemented tungsten carbides:

  o Up to 0.25 mg Co/m³: Any quarter-mask respirator.
  o From 0.25 to 0.5 mg Co/m³: Any particulate respirator equipped with any N, R, or P filter (includes filtering facepieces but not quarter-mask respirators) or any supplied-air respirator.
  o From 0.5 to 1.25 mg Co/m³: Any supplied-air respirator operated in continuous-flow mode; or any powered,

air-purifying respirator with a high-efficiency particulate air (HEPA) filter.

  o   From 1.25 to 2.5 mg Co/m^3: Any air-purifying, full-facepiece respirator with an N100, R100, or P100 filter; any self-contained breathing apparatus with a full facepiece; or any supplied-air respirator with a full facepiece.

  o   From 2.5 to 20 mg Co/m^3: Any supplied-air respirator that has a full facepiece and is operated in a pressure-demand or other positive-pressure mode.

- NIOSH recommends the following levels of respiratory protection for exposure to metalworking fluids:

  o   From 0.5 to 5.0 mg/m^3: Any air-purifying, half-mask respirator equipped with any P-or R-series particulate filter.

  o   From 5.0 to 12.5 mg/m^3: Any powered air-purifying respirator equipped with a hood or helmet and a HEPA filter.

- Respiratory protection may not perform as intended if not donned, used, and maintained properly. Therefore, respiratory protection should be used as an interim measure until engineering controls that successfully reduce exposure levels have been implemented.

Exposure Monitoring:

- Assess exposures to metalworking fluid and to cobalt annually and whenever any major process change occurs.

- Assess workers' inhalational exposures on results of air samples collected in workers' personal breathing zones.

Employee Training:

- Provide yearly training on the potential adverse health effects associated with cobalt exposure and how exposure can be minimized through appropriate work practices and effective use of engineering controls and respiratory and skin protection.

- Provide yearly training on the potential adverse health effects associated with exposure to metalworking fluids, how to detect potentially hazardous situations (e.g., bacterial overgrowth and degradation of metalworking fluid), and appropriate work practices (e.g., minimizing skin contact with metalworking fluid).

Medical Surveillance:

Spirometry tests, Chest x-rays, and Respiratory Symptoms

- Obtain spirometry tests and chest x-rays on all new and current employees who, in the course of their job duties, regularly work in or enter plant areas where cobalt exposures occur; repeat spirometry tests every year and chest x-rays every three years. Spirometry tests should be of high quality to enable valid comparison of results over time. Have all chest x-rays interpreted by a NIOSH-approved B Reader according to the *International Classification of Radiographs of Pneumoconioses* [ILO 2000]).

- Ensure that any newly hired worker with pre-existing lung disease, abnormal spirometry, or abnormal chest x-ray, or any worker who develops respiratory symptoms, chest x-ray abnormalities, or spirometry test abnormalities subsequent to hire, is medically evaluated; the evaluating physician should inform the worker and company of any individualized work restrictions or limitations recommended on the basis of findings from the medical evaluation.

- Designate a safety person in each plant and encourage workers to report respiratory symptoms to this person. The company's director of safety and environment should establish a mechanism to monitor respiratory symptoms and disease reported by workers.

Cobalt urine and blood tests

- After improvements in engineering controls, work practices, general housekeeping, and personal protective clothing and equipment have been instituted, repeat urine or whole blood cobalt tests for workers the following areas: reclamation, powder mixing, reprocessing, blending, milling, spray drying, pressing, shaping, and round cell. Obtain urine and whole blood samples at the end of the work shift on the last day of the work week.

- Workers found to have urine or whole blood cobalt levels greater than or equal to 30 μg/L and 2.5 μg/L, respectively (i.e., levels comparable to the NIOSH REL) should wear a respirator at work . If a worker was already wearing a

RECOMMENDATIONS
(CONTINUED)

respirator at work when the urine or blood sample with high cobalt level was obtained: 1) evaluate the affected worker's respirator fit and ensure compliance with respirator use; and 2) remind the affected worker of the importance of frequently washing hands and wearing nitrile gloves while at work.

REFERENCES

American Thoracic Society (ATS) [1995]. Standardization of spirometry: 1994 update. Am J Resp Crit Care Med 152:1107–1136.

Bello D, Herrick CA, Smith TJ, Woskie SR, Streicher RP, Cullen MR, Liu Y, Redlich CA [2007]. Skin exposure to isocyanates: Reasons for concern. Environ Health Perspect 115:328–335.

Bernstein I, Merget R [2006]. Metals. In: Bernstein I, Chan-Yeung M, Malo J, and Bernstein D, eds. Asthma in the Workplace, 3rd ed. New York, NY: Taylor and Francis Group. pp. 525–554.

CDC [1996]. Third National Health and Nutrition Examination Survey, 1988–1994, NHANES III Examination Date File [CD-ROM]. Hyattsville, MD: U.S. Department of Health and Human Services, Public Health Service, Centers for Disease Control and Prevention. (Public use data file documentations No. 76300).

CDC [2003]. Behavioral Risk Factor Surveillance System Survey Data. Atlanta, GA: U.S. Department of Health and Human Services, Centers for Disease Control and Prevention.

Cugell D [1992]. The hard metal diseases. In: Occupational Lung Diseases. Clinics in Chest Medicine 13:269–279.

Cummings KJ, Deubner DC, Day GA, Henneberger PK, Kitt MM, Kent MS, Kreiss K, Schuler CR [2007]. Enhanced preventive programme at a beryllium oxide ceramics facility reduces beryllium sensitization among new workers. Occup Environ Med 64:134–140.

Day GA, Virji MA, Stefaniak AB [2009]. Characterization of exposures among cemented tungsten carbide workers. Part II: Assessment of surface contamination and skin exposures to cobalt, nickel and chromium. J Expos Sci Environ Epidemiol, 19:423-434.

Ferris BG [1978]. Epidemiology standardization project. Am Rev Respir Dis 118:Suppl:1–53.

Goldoni M, Catalani S, De Palma G, Manini P, Acampa O, Corradi M, Bergonzi R, Apostoli P, Mutti A [2004]. Exhaled breath condensate as a suitable matrix to assess lung dose and effects in workers exposed to cobalt and tungsten. Environ Health Perspect 112:1293–1298.

Hankinson JL, Odencrantz JR, Fedan KB [1999]. Spirometric reference values from a sample of the general U.S. population. Am J Respir Crit Care Med 159:179–187.

Hinds WC [1986]. Data analysis. In: Cascade impactor sampling and data analysis. Lodge JP and Chan TL, eds. Akron, OH: American Industrial Hygiene Association, pp. 45–77.

International Labour Office (ILO) [2002]. Guidelines for the Use of the ILO International Classification of Radiographs of Pneumoconioses, Revised Edition 2000 (Occupational Safety and Health Series, No. 22). International Labour Office: Geneva.

Kusaka Y, Yokoyama K, Sera Y, Yamamoto S, Sone S, Kyoto H, Shirakawa T, Goto S [1986]. Respiratory diseases in hard metal workers: an occupational hygiene study in a factory. Br J Ind Med 43:474–485.

Lauwerys RR, Hoet P [2001]. Industrial chemical exposure: guidelines for biological monitoring. 3rd ed., Boca Raton, FL: Lewis Publishers. p. 93.

Lison D [1998]. Hard metal disease. In: Rom N, ed. Environmental and Occupational Medicine, 3rd ed. Philadelphia, PA: Lippincott-Raven Publishers. pp. 1037–1043.

McCanlies E, Ensey J, Schuler C, Kreiss K, Weston A [2004]. The association between HLA-DPβ1^{Glu69} and chronic beryllium disease and beryllium sensitization. Am J Ind Med 46:95–103.

McWorter W, Polis M, Kaslow R [1989]. Occurrence, predictors, and consequences of adult asthma in NHANES I and follow-up survey. Am Rev Respir Dis 139:721–724.

Meyer-Bisch C, Pham QT, Mur J-M, Massin N, Moulin J-J, Teculescu D, Carton B, Pierre F, Baruthio F [1989]. Respiratory hazards in hard metal workers: a cross sectional study. Br J Ind Med 46:302–309.

Miller A, Thornton J, Warshaw R, Anderson H, Teirstein AS, Selikoff IJ [1983]. Single breath diffusing capacity in a representative sample of the population of Michigan, a large industrial state. Am Rev Respir Dis 127:270–277.

NIOSH [1994]. NIOSH manual of analytical methods (NMAM®). 4th ed. Schlecht PC, O'Connor PF, eds. Cincinnati, OH: U.S. Department of Health and Human Services, Centers for Disease Control and Prevention, National Institute for Occupational Safety and Health, DHHS (NIOSH) Publication 94-113 (August, 1994); 1st Supplement Publication 96-135, 2nd Supplement Publication 98-119; 3rd Supplement 2003-154. [http://www.cdc.gov/niosh/nmam/]

Potolicchio I, Mosconi G, Forni A, Nemergy B, Seghizzi P, Sorrentino R [1997]. Susceptibility to hard metal lung disease is strongly associated with the presence of glutamate 69 in HLA-DPβ chain. Eur J Immunol 27:2741–2743.

Redlich CA, Herrick CA [2008]. Lung/skin connections in occupational lung disease. Curr Opin Allergy Clin Immunol 8:115–119.

Shirakawa T, Kusaka Y, Fujimura N, Goto S, Morimoto K [1988]. The existence of specific antibodies to cobalt in hard metal asthma. Clin Allergy 18:451–460.

Shirakawa T, Kusaka Y, Fujimura N, Goto S, Kato M, Heki S, Morimoto K [1989]. Occupational asthma from cobalt sensitivity in workers exposed to hard metal dust. Chest 95:29–36.

Sprince NL, Chamberlin RI, Hales CA, Weber AL, Kazemi H [1984]. Respiratory disease in tungsten carbide workers. Chest 86:549–557.

REFERENCES (CONTINUED)

Sprince NL, Oliver LC, Eisen EA, Greene RE, Chamberlin RI [1988]. Cobalt exposure and lung disease in tungsten carbide production. Am Rev Respir Dis 138:1220–1226.

Stefaniak AB, Day GA, Harvey CJ, Leonard SS, Schwegler-Berry DE, Chipera SJ, Sahakian NM, Chisholm WP [2007]. Characteristics of dusts encountered during the production of cemented tungsten carbides. Ind Health 45:793–803.

Venables KM, Farrer N, Sharp L, Graneek BJ, Newman Taylor AL [1993]. Respiratory symptoms questionnaire for asthma epidemiology: validity and reproducibility. Thorax 48:214–219.

ADDITIONAL TABLES

Table 9. Total cobalt air concentrations in micrograms per cubic meter air ($\mu g/m^3$) based on NIOSH (251 samples) and historical company (72 samples) full-shift personal breathing zone cassette air sample results, 1985–2004

Work Area	MeanT Co	Mean Th Co	Mean R Co	MedianT Co	MedianTh Co	MedianR Co	Highest Recorded Level T Co	Highest Recorded Level Th Co	Highest Recorded Level R Co	# of samples T Co	# of samples R or Th Co
Huntsville Facility											
WC Production (Carbide plant)	-	-	-	-	-	-	-	-	-	0	0
WC Reduction (Auto)	-	-	-	-	-	-	-	-	-	0	0
WC Reduction (Manual)	-	-	-	-	-	-	-	-	-	0	0
Reclamation	60.3	32.5	5.0	43.8	37.8	5.4	155.5	55.6	9.1	23	15
Metal Separation	40.1	10.7	2.1	13.2	4.6	1.2	278.9	35.1	6.1	30	8
Gurley Facility											
Powder Mixing	574.5	304.5	77.6	429.3	199.0	35.2	1622.1	849.0	213.2	8	7
Powder Mixing LP	17.3	11.0	3.7	17.1	11.0	3.7	18.9	13.5	4.8	4	2
Milling	51.3	19.3	3.3	38.8	19.3	3.3	134.1	24.8	3.9	10	2
Spray Drying	62.3	15.6	3.1	55.5	16.3	2.8	160.7	21.2	4.9	16	4
Spray Drying LP	21.0	-	-	21.0	-	-	21.9	-	-	2	0
Screening	98.3	55.8	7.3	97.8	72.9	7.5	161.4	75.3	9.6	8	5
Reprocessing	427 2	254.2	44.9	427.2	254 2	44.9	500.5	448.5	78.8	2	2
Blending	-	-	-	-	-	-	-	-	-	0	0
Production Control (Clerk)	8.0	2.4	0.6	4 3	2.4	0.6	22.9	2.6	0.6	5	2
Custodian	43.9	30.1	8.6	43.9	30 1	8.6	61.2	48.3	14.3	2	2
Maintenance	15.9	9.1	1.9	17.6	9.1	1.9	20.2	9.1	1.9	3	1
Maintenance LP	2.6	-	-	2.6	-	-	2.6	-	-	1	0
Grant Facility											
Pressing	26.4	11.3	1.9	23.6	9.3	1.7	58.5	21.0	3.2	13	7
Shaping	33.2	25.5	10.5	12.4	9.9	2.7	197.0	172.3	79.8	20	10
Round Cell	12.9	6.3	2.0	13.6	6.5	1.7	18.5	7.4	3.4	7	3
Extrusion	29.6	3.8	1.2	11.6	3.8	1.2	107.2	6.1	2.1	5	2
Sintering	-	-	-	-	-	-	-	-	-	0	0
Utility Breakdown	29.0	4.1	0.8	29.0	4.1	0.8	29.0	4.1	0.8	1	1
Grinding	7.4	15.3	4.1	4 1	9.0	2.1	28.0	56.0	11.9	15	7
Honing	-	-	-	-	-	-	-	-	-	0	0
Sandblasting	2.0	1.9	0.5	2 2	1.4	0.4	3.3	3.8	1.0	8	4
Product Testing	3.2	3.1	0.9	2 9	3.2	1.0	8.6	5.5	1.5	15	5
Shipping	2.8	3.9	0.6	0.7	1.5	0.6	31.7	11.9	1.0	16	3
Maintenance	7.1	2.0	0.5	1 8	1.4	0.5	46.1	4.2	1.1	10	5
Huntsville and Gurley Facilities											
Powder Laboratory	3.7	8.8	2.1	0 9	9.0	1.3	15.6	16.2	5.5	18	4
Shipping	13.8	6.7	1.8	13.9	7.5	1.9	20.2	8.4	2.3	9	4
Total										251	105

Table 10. Cobalt air concentrations in micrograms per cubic meter air (µg/m³) based on results from full-shift personal breathing zone air samples collected by NIOSH in October/November, 2004

Work Area	Mean	Median	Highest recorded level	Number of samples
Huntsville Facility				
WC Production (Carbide plant)	3.6	3.3	6.1	6
WC Reduction (Auto)	1.3	1.3	1.4	3
WC Reduction (Manual)	3.7	1.3	8.9	3
Reclamation	67.6	44.3	264.0	29
Metal Separation	39.9	15.2	278.9	33
Gurley Facility				
Powder Mixing	414.3	350.4	1,622.1	20
Powder Mixing Lead Person	17.3	17.1	19.0	4
Milling	48.4	34.0	134.1	14
Spray Drying	86.2	53.8	620.0	21
Spray Drying Lead Person	21.0	21.0	21.9	2
Screening	142.8	128.3	438.0	12
Reprocessing	427.2	427.2	500.5	2
Blending	119.8	31.4	280.0	5
Production Control (Clerk)	8.0	4.3	22.9	5
Custodian	43.9	43.9	61.2	2
Maintenance	15.9	17.6	20.2	3
Maintenance Lead Person	2.6	2.6	2.6	1
Grant Facility				
Pressing	42.7	28.7	180.2	17
Shaping	42.1	17.4	197.0	26
Round Cell	39.8	13.6	260.0	9
Extrusion	29.6	11.6	107.2	5
Sintering	9.4	9.4	9.4	1
Utility Breakdown	29.0	29.0	29.0	1
Grinding	11.1	7.3	41.4	19
Honing	7.4	7.4	7.4	1
Sandblasting	11.3	2.2	96.5	10
Product Testing	3.2	2.9	8.6	15
Shipping	2.7	0.7	31.7	17
Maintenance	7.1	1.8	46.1	10
Huntsville and Gurley Facilities				
Powder Laboratory	3.7	0.9	15.6	18
Shipping	13.8	13.9	20.2	9
Total				323

T – total; Th – thoracic; R – respirable; LP – lead person. Thoracic and respirable cobalt air concentrations were calculated based on results of 105 Marple 8-stage impactor samples; total cobalt air concentrations were calculated based on results of 251 cassette samples.

Table 15. Associations* between lung function and work area metal air sampling results for current work area (2003 and 2005 participants)

Current Work Area Exposure Variable[a]	N	FEV$_1$ % Predicted Estimate	FEV$_1$ % Predicted p value	FEV$_1$ Liters Estimate	FEV$_1$ Liters p value	FVC % Predicted Estimate	FVC % Predicted p value	FVC Liters Estimate	FVC Liters p value	FEV$_1$/FVC[b] Estimate	FEV$_1$/FVC[b] p value
Highest recorded respirable cobalt	178	-3.19*	0.05	-0.11**	0.05	-2.60**	0.09	-0.12**	0.05	-0.005	0.52
Highest recorded respirable tungsten	178	+2.88*	0.04	+0.09**	0.10	+2.61**	0.05	+0.12*	0.04	+0.0001	0.98
Mean respirable cobalt	178	-4.22*	0.03	-0.14*	0.04	-3.18**	0.09	-0.14**	0.08	-0.01	0.30
Mean respirable tungsten	178	+3.83*	0.03	+0.11	0.103	+3.20**	0.06	+0.12	0.11	+0.01	0.46
Median respirable cobalt	178	-3.48**	0.10	-0.13**	0.08	-2.24	0.26	-0.08	0.34	-0.02**	0.09
Median respirable tungsten	178	+3.59**	0.06	+0.11	0.12	+2.93	0.11	+0.08	0.34	+0.02	0.10
Mean respirable cobalt/mean respirable tungsten ratio[c]	157	-12.61*	0.03	-0.44*	0.03	-	-	-	-	-	-

*Models for percent predicted FEV$_1$ and FVC were controlled for smoking (pack-years) and tenure; models for FEV$_1$, FVC, and FEV$_1$/FVC were controlled for age, gender, race, height, smoking (pack-years), and tenure.
* /Bold font – statistically significant association (p value ≤0.05).
** /Underlined – marginally significant association (p value≤0.10 and >0.05).
Cells with dash mark (–) indicate that FVC and FEV$_1$/FVC were not included in model.
[a]Metal air concentrations were measured in µg/m^3 and were modeled as the natural log.
[b]FEV$_1$/FVC expressed as a proportion.
[c]Excludes workers who currently worked in more than one work area.

Table 16. Associations* between lung function and estimated cumulative exposures (2003 and 2005 participants)

Basis for Estimation of Cumulative Exposure Variable[a]	N	FEV$_1$ % Predicted Estimate	FEV$_1$ % Predicted p value	FEV$_1$ Liters Estimate	FEV$_1$ Liters p value	FVC % Predicted Estimate	FVC % Predicted p value	FVC Liters Estimate	FVC Liters p value	FEV$_1$/ FVC[b] Estimate	FEV$_1$/ FVC[b] p value
Highest recorded respirable cobalt	137	-2.50	0.11	-0.09	0.14	-1.97	0.18	-0.11	0.06	<-0.01	0.93
Highest recorded respirable tungsten	137	+2.95	0.07	+0.10	0.09	+2.37	0.12	**+0.15***	0.02	<+0.01	0.91
Mean respirable cobalt	137	**-5.02***	0.03	_-0.15**_	0.08	_-3.82_	0.07	-0.14	0.12	-0.01	0.30
Mean respirable tungsten	137	**+4.74***	0.04	_+0.15**_	0.08	+3.40	0.11	_+0.16**_	0.09	+0.01	0.38

*Models for percent predicted FEV$_1$ and FVC were controlled for smoking (packyears); models for FEV$_1$, FVC, and FEV$_1$/FVC were controlled for age, gender, race, height, and smoking (packyears).
* / Bold font – statistically significant association (p value ≤0.05).
** / Underlined – marginally significant association (p value ≤0.10 and >0.05).
[a] Estimated cumulative exposures, measured in μg cobalt/m^3-years, were modeled as the natural log; workers with 10% or more of their work history missing an exposure estimate were excluded.
[b] FEV1/FVC expressed as a proportion.

APPENDIX A: INTERIM LETTER I (FEBRUARY 20, 2004)

DEPARTMENT OF HEALTH & HUMAN SERVICES

Phone: (304) 285-5751
Fax: (304) 285-5820

Public Health Service

Centers for Disease Control
and Prevention (CDC)
National Institute for Occupational
Safety and Health (NIOSH)
1095 Willowdale Road
Morgantown, WV 26505-2888

February 20, 2004
HETA 2003-0257
Interim Letter 1

Mr. Steve Robuck
Director of Safety and Environment
Metalworking Products
1 Teledyne Place
La Vergne, Tennessee 37086

Dear Mr. Robuck:

This letter contains the results from the National Institute for Occupational Safety and Health (NIOSH) visits to the Alldyne Powder Technologies plants located in Huntsville and Gurley, Alabama and the Firth Sterling plant located in Grant, Alabama. NIOSH visited these plants in response to a confidential employee request concerning respiratory health effects and exposure to cobalt, nickel, chromium, tungsten carbide, and metalworking fluids. Three workers (index cases) were known to have developed lung disease within the preceding year. Two of these workers had developed scarring lung disease (hard metal pneumoconiosis) and one worker had developed cobalt asthma. We performed a walk-through visit of the three plants on July 7 through July 8, 2003. From July 9 through July 11, 2003 we visited Dr. Robert Johnson (the company physician) and his staff and reviewed medical records on plant employees in general, as well as on the three index cases. We conducted a medical survey from September 9 through September 20, 2003. Findings from the walk-through visit, medical record review, and medical survey are included in this letter and the attached appendices.

BACKGROUND

The three plants are hard metal manufacturing plants. Work areas in the Gurley plant include: a charging area, where workers measure and combine component metal powders; a mill area, where the metal powder mixtures are mixed with heptane to form a slurry; a spray-dry area, where the heptane slurry is aerosolized to form small metal powder beads; screening, where the metal powder is size-sorted; reprocessing, where metal powder waste (such as floor sweep) is reprocessed; and blending, where the reprocessed waste powder is mixed with other metal powders for reuse. Work areas in the Grant plant include: pressing, where metal powder from the Gurley plant is pressed into soft metal forms; shaping, where the pressed forms are shaped by abrasive wheels; sintering, where the shaped forms are heated in furnaces; grinding, where sintered forms are ground using a diamond wheel and metalworking fluid; sandblasting, where sintered forms are sandblasted in a glove box; and product testing, where the finished forms are tested for quality. Work areas of interest in the Huntsville plant include: zinc, where hard metal scrap is combined with zinc, crushed, and reprocessed; and Ammonium Paratungstate (APT) where scrap metal is reprocessed using a filtration system.

METHODS

Industrial Hygiene

We obtained bulk samples of metalworking fluid (MWF) and liquid and solid samples from the MWF filter system on July 7, 2003 during our walk-through visit. MWF bulk samples consisted of samples of unused MWF from a supply drum and MWF from the centerless grinder. Duplicate samples were simultaneously collected from the same sites by the company for independent analysis. An American Industrial Hygiene Association (AIHA)-accredited laboratory analyzed the bulk samples for cobalt, nickel, endotoxin (a component of gram-negative bacteria), and microbial content.

We reviewed company industrial hygiene air sampling records from 1985 to 2003 and employee blood cobalt level records from 1998 to 2003. We calculated average blood cobalt levels for workers tested during each testing period. The limit of detection for this test was 1 microgram cobalt per liter blood (μg/L). In our calculations we used the value of half the limit of detection for individual blood cobalt levels that were recorded as non-detectable.

Medical Survey

Plant lists of worker names, addresses, and work histories were used to identify workers from the three plants with potential cobalt exposure. For the Grant and Gurley plants, workers who currently or previously worked in either production or engineering jobs were considered potentially exposed to cobalt. For the Huntsville plant, workers who currently worked in either the Zinc or APT departments were considered potentially exposed to cobalt. We mailed invitations to 235 workers with potential cobalt exposure, requesting that they participate in a medical survey.

At the request of the company, all testing was performed during non-work time. We tested workers during regularly scheduled 15-minute work breaks, lunch breaks, before or after work, and on non-work days. The testing schedule was designed to include workers from all shifts. Testing before or after work and on non-work days included: administration of a medical questionnaire; chest x-ray; a baseline breathing test (spirometry); and, if the spirometry test was abnormal, administration of a medication (bronchodilator) to help open the airways, repeat spirometry test, and a test designed to measure how well the lungs exchange gases (lung diffusing capacity for carbon monoxide (DLCO)). Abbreviated testing was used on workers scheduled during 15-minute work breaks and lunch breaks. This testing included a short written questionnaire (completed at home), chest x-ray, and a baseline spirometry test.

A signed informed consent was obtained from all participants. We used a standardized questionnaire to collect information on worker symptoms, medical diagnoses, smoking history, and work history at any of the three Metalworking Products plants. Chest x-rays, which consisted of a single posteroanterior view, were sent to two or more B-readers for interstitial lung disease scoring. If the first two B-readers disagreed on the reading of a film, the film was sent to a third B-reader for resolution. Interstitial lung disease scores (profusion scores) range from 0/0, which is normal, to 3/+, which indicates very severe disease. A score of 0/1 indicates that the film was likely normal, but early interstitial lung disease is possible. A score of 1/0 indicates that there probably is early interstitial lung disease. We used a score of 1/0 or greater to define interstitial lung disease.

Spirometry tests were rated A to F for quality, using the 1995 recommendations of the American Thoracic Society.[1] Criteria included reproducibility of curves, absence of cough and hesitation, and expiration of at least 6 seconds. We chose the largest forced vital capacity (FVC) and forced expiratory volume in one second (FEV1) from a minimum of three trials. We calculated worker predicted and lower limits of normal values using reference values derived from asymptomatic never-smokers in the 3rd National Health and Nutrition Examination Survey (NHANES III).[2,3] Test results were compared to the lower limit of normal values to identify workers with abnormal spirometry patterns.[4] Obstruction is defined as a FEV1 and FEV1/FVC ratio below the lower limits of normal. Borderline obstruction is defined as a FEV1 lower than predicted but above the lower limit of normal with a FEV1/FVC ratio below the lower limit of normal. Restriction is defined as a FVC less than 98% of the lower limit of normal with a normal FEV1/FVC ratio and borderline restriction as an FVC within 2% of the lower limits of normal (either greater or lower than) with a normal FEV1/FVC ratio. Abnormal spirometry is defined as obstruction and/or restriction. Lung diffusing capacity for carbon monoxide and total lung capacity (TLC) measurements were considered abnormally low if their percent predicted values were lower than the lower limit of normal.[5] The TLC was calculated from the lung diffusing capacity test results.

We compared workers in the three plants with regard to age, gender, smoking status, amount of cigarettes smoked over their lifetime, and years tenure. For each plant, we calculated prevalence rates for reported respiratory and non-respiratory symptoms, physician diagnoses, and spirometry test abnormalities.

We compared observed numbers of individuals with respiratory symptoms, physician-diagnosed chronic bronchitis and asthma, and abnormal spirometry test results to expected numbers derived from the 3rd National Health and Nutrition Examination Survey.[3] A prevalence rate ratio (# observed ÷ # expected) greater than "1" indicates that a greater proportion of Metalworking Products workers, compared to the general public, have that particular health outcome. A prevalence rate ratio greater than "1" with a 95% confidence interval (CI) that excludes "1", indicates a 95% chance that the prevalence rate is greater than 1. Prevalence rate ratios were all adjusted for smoking status (categorized as ever-smokers or never-smokers), age (categorized as 17-39 and 40-69 years of age), gender, and race, to increase comparability. Using an indirect adjustment method, we calculated the expected number of events by applying the smoking status, age, gender, and race rates from NHANES III to the number of people in the study in specific matching groups. Analyses were performed for individual plants and for the entire workforce.

Hard metal pneumoconiosis is an interstitial lung disease. Suspected interstitial lung disease is defined as restriction, borderline restriction, or low DLCO with the following qualifiers: 1) cases were included only if the Body Mass Index (BMI) was greater than or equal to 18.5 and less than 30 and the total lung capacity (if known) was below the lower limit of normal; 2) cases of borderline restriction were included only if FVC was below the lower limit of normal. BMI is calculated as: weight in kilograms ÷ (height in meters)^2. The underweight, normal, overweight, and obese ranges for BMI are less than 18.5, 18.5 to 24.9, 25.0 to 29.9, and 30 and greater, respectively. Both underweight and obese BMIs are associated with low FVC lung function measurements. We did not include, as a suspected interstitial lung disease case, one worker with borderline restriction whose BMI was less than 18.5. Although this worker may have restriction due to interstitial lung disease, the worker was excluded so that we could be more certain that workers without disease were not included.

Suspected post-hire asthma is defined as one or more of the following: a current post-hire diagnosis of asthma; 3 or more asthma symptoms from the questionnaire developed by Venables et al;6 use of asthma medication; or obstruction or borderline obstruction on spirometry; AND no known pre-hire asthma diagnosis.

We assumed that work areas where symptoms began represented work areas that caused the lung disease. We reviewed work histories on workers with suspected asthma and suspected interstitial lung disease in a case-by-case analysis. Using date of symptom(s) onset, we determined the work area where the symptoms began. We included workers who had worked in only one work area even if they lacked symptoms or had symptoms but lacked symptom onset dates. We included one asymptomatic worker with suspected interstitial lung disease who had worked in two work areas, but who had worked for a much longer time in one of these areas. We then compared the number of affected workers whose symptoms were associated with a certain work area to the number of workers who had ever worked in that work area. We included index cases in both the numerator and denominator. For this and all subsequent work area analyses, we combined the work areas of charging, blending, and reprocessing into a category we call "charging"; and we combined round cell and shaping work areas and refer to this as "shaping".

We compared crude health outcome rates for workers who ever worked in certain work areas compared to workers who never worked in those work areas and for workers who currently work in certain work areas compared to workers who currently work in other areas. Ten work areas were considered.

The healthy worker effect occurs when symptomatic workers transfer to different jobs in a workplace or leave the workplace, resulting in a healthier workforce in jobs which are responsible for worker symptoms and disease. We evaluated the healthy worker effect by comparing prevalence rates of symptoms, airways obstruction, and disease in past workers and current workers in work areas identified as being responsible for disease in the case-by-case analysis. Past workers were defined as ever-workers who were not current workers in that work area. This comparison was not performed for zinc workers because there were very few prior zinc workers.

We calculated odds ratios which took into account age, gender, and pack years of smoking, in order to determine whether workers with certain health outcomes or suspected post-hire asthma were more likely to have ever worked or to currently work in any particular work areas.
We compared workers who had ever worked in specific work areas compared to workers who had never worked in those work areas for difference in lung function values. We controlled for age, gender, height, weight, and pack-years smoked for FEV1/FVC and controlled for weight and pack-years smoked for percent predicted FEV1 and FVC.

Statistical analyses were performed using Chi-Square and Fisher's exact tests, and linear and logistic regression. A Poisson distribution was used to determine confidence intervals of prevalence rates. We chose the probability values of 0.05 and 0.10 as criteria for statistical significance and marginal statistical significance, respectively.

Small Cell Numbers and Incomplete Medical Evaluation

Data is not reported for work areas with fewer than 6 workers. Individuals who did not complete the entire medical evaluation were not included in ratios where the missing test was required. For example, airways obstruction on spirometry was part of the suspected post-hire asthma definition, so workers without a spirometry test were excluded from both the numerator and denominator for the corresponding prevalence rate ratios.

RESULTS

Industrial Hygiene

Metalworking Fluid Samples

The metalworking fluid was replaced 1 ½ years prior to our visit. In-use metalworking fluid cobalt and nickel levels were 1 µg/gram and non-detectable, respectively (Table 1). No significant amounts of endotoxin or culturable fungi or bacteria (including mycobacteria) were found in any of the metalworking fluid samples.

Company Environmental Measurements

Company environmental sampling from 1985 to 2003 indicated that historically there have been elevated cobalt air levels in pressing, shaping/round cell, grinding, charging/blending, reprocessing, spray dry, screening, Zinc A, Zinc B, and APT (Table 2). The most current sampling indicates that cobalt air levels are elevated in charging/blending, reprocessing, spray dry, screening, and Zinc B.

Historical Worker Blood Cobalt Levels

From 1998 to 2003, Gurley workers (in approximately 20 jobs identified to be at high risk for cobalt exposure) have had their blood cobalt level monitored. Average blood cobalt levels for these workers ranged from 7.8 to 18.6 micrograms cobalt per liter (µg cobalt/L) (Table 3). The American Conference of Governmental Industrial Hygienists (ACGIH) has set the biological exposure index (BEI) cobalt blood level at 1µg cobalt/L for an end of shift, end of work week blood sample. Worker cobalt blood levels greater than the BEI reflect exposures above currently recommended exposure limits. Almost all tested workers (21 of 22) had blood cobalt levels in excess of the BEI during the most recent testing period. The median and upper values for this testing period also were higher than corresponding values for other testing periods.

Medical Survey

Demographic Data

One hundred sixty-five of 243 (68%) "invited" plant employees participated in the survey. "Invited" refers to workers who had received a mailed invitation as well as 8 current Zinc and APT workers who inadvertently had not received one. Participation rates by plant were: 97 of 135 (72%) workers from the Grant plant; 37 of 63 (59%) workers from the Gurley plant; and 31 of 45 (69%) workers from the Huntsville plant.

Most employees (70%) were male (Table 4). The percent of workers that were male ranged from 53% to 100% for the Grant and Huntsville workforces, respectively. Median age was 44 years and median tenure was 10 years. Workers were almost equally divided among those who had never smoked cigarettes and those who had ever (currently or previously) smoked. Ever-smokers had smoked a median of 20 pack-years. Individual plant workforces were comparable with regard to all demographic parameters, other than gender.

Workforce Prevalence Rates of Health Outcomes

Of the entire workforce participants, 34% answered "yes" to the question "Do you ever have trouble with your breathing?" and 38% reported shortness of breath when hurrying on level ground or walking up a slight hill (Table 5). Usual cough with onset since hire was present in 16% of workers. Fever, chills, or night sweats (symptoms commonly reported by workers with hypersensitivity pneumonitis) was present in 37% of workers. Prevalence rates for skin, eye, and nasal irritation were 36%, 47%, and 62%, respectively.

Hard Metal Pneumoconiosis Prevalence:
None of the workers had a chest x-ray with a profusion score of 1/0 or greater. Eight workers had low DLCO's and/or restriction or borderline restriction on spirometry. After excluding both workers with low DLCO's who had normal TLC's and one worker with borderline restriction who had a low BMI, 5 workers with suspected interstitial lung disease remained (Table 6). Restriction was present in 3 of 162 (2%) workers and suspected interstitial lung disease was present in 5 of 162 (3%) workers.

Among former workers, one ill worker with restriction on spirometry underwent a lung biopsy which showed giant cells within the air sacs (alveoli) of the lung, a finding frequently seen in hard metal pneumoconiosis and rarely due to other lung conditions.

Asthma Prevalence:
Airways obstruction was present in 12 of 162 (7%) workers. Ever-diagnosed and current asthma were present in 16% (27 of 165) and 11% (18 of 165) workers, respectively. Post-hire conditions of chronic bronchitis, asthma, and suspected asthma were present in 8% (13 of 165), 6% (10 of 165), and 29% (47 of 162) of the workforce, respectively. Of the 47 workers identified with suspected post-hire asthma, 10 (21%) had physician-diagnosed asthma, 31 (66%) had 3 or more Venables' asthma symptoms, 20 (43%) had airways obstruction, and 5 (11%) reported current use of asthma medication.

Health Outcome Prevalence Rate Ratios (NHANES III Comparisons)

Shortness of breath (with hurrying on level ground or walking up a slight hill), cough on most days, chronic bronchitis, wheeze or whistling in the chest in the last 12 months, and ever having been diagnosed with asthma were all reported about 2 times more often by this workforce than expected, based on a national survey (Table 7). These comparisons, which took into account smoking status, age, gender, and race, were all statistically significant. At the plant level, Grant workers showed a statistically significant excess for all the above health outcomes.

White workers who had never smoked had a three fold higher statistically significant prevalence rate of airways obstruction, compared to the national survey (Table 8). When analyzed at the plant level, white never-smokers in the Grant plant (but not in the Gurley and Huntsville plants) also had a statistically significant three-fold higher rate of airways obstruction (Table 9) compared to national rates. Restrictive lung disease rates were not elevated in the workforce as a whole or in any individual plants, when compared to national rates.

Work Areas Responsible for Cases of Suspected Interstitial Lung Disease and Suspected Post-Hire Asthma

When we reviewed work histories for workers with suspected lung disease, grinding, pressing, and possibly zinc and sintering were associated with suspected interstitial lung disease (Table 10). Shaping, pressing, zinc, and possibly maintenance were associated with suspected post-hire asthma (Table 11). We were able to identify associated work areas for all 3 index cases, all 5 workers with suspected interstitial lung disease, and 38 of 47 (81%) workers with suspected post-hire asthma. The small numbers of workers with suspected interstitial lung disease associated with zinc and sintering and with suspected post-hire asthma associated with maintenance make these last associations less reliable.

Comparison of Past-Worker and Current-Worker High Risk Work Area Health Outcome Rates

Current grinders had lower prevalence rates than past grinders for having had bronchitis since hire (17% versus 55%), shortness of breath when walking with others the same age (25% versus 36%), ever having wheezed (17% versus 86%), and of having a current asthma diagnosis (8% versus 18%) (Figure 1). Current pressers had lower prevalence rates than past pressers for having had bronchitis since hire (42% versus 54%), shortness of breath when walking with others the same age (21% versus 29%), ever having wheezed (32% versus 66%), and airways obstruction (0% versus 18%) (Figure 2). A lower percentage of current shapers than past shapers had bronchitis since hire (18% versus 47%) (Figure 3).

Health Outcomes Associated with Ever Working in a Work Area

Tables 12 and 13 compare selected respiratory symptoms, diagnoses, spirometry abnormalities, and suspected post-hire asthma prevalence rates in workers who had ever worked in certain areas to workers who had never worked in those areas. A significantly greater percentage of ever-grinders than never-grinders (32% versus 14%) reported shortness of breath when walking with others the same age. Suspected post-hire asthma was present in 43% of ever-shapers versus 25% of never-shapers (marginally significant).

Odds ratios that take into account age, gender, and pack-years of smoking indicate that shortness of breath when walking with others the same age was 3 times more likely to occur in ever-grinders compared to others (Table 14). Post-hire physician-diagnosed bronchitis was about 3 times more likely to occur in ever-pressers than in workers who had never worked in that work area. Suspected post-hire asthma was about 2 times more likely in workers who had ever worked in shaping than in other workers (Table 15).

In a linear regression model which took into account age, gender, height, weight, and pack-years of smoking, workers who had ever worked in shaping had significantly decreased FEV1/FVC, compared to never-shapers (Table 16). Although the amount of decline in FEV1/FVC was small and not clinically significant, ever-shapers had a 5 times higher rate of airways obstruction than never-shapers (Table 12).

Health Outcomes Associated with Ever Having Worked in Sandblasting

Among 14 ever-sandblasters 11 (79%) reported having ever wheezed compared to 70 of 151 (46%) never-sandblasters (Table 12). Known post-hire asthma was present in 2 of 14 (14%) ever-sandblasters compared to 7 of 151 (5%) never-sandblasters. However of the 2 ever-sandblasters with a post-hire asthma diagnosis, one started wheezing prior to hire and the other began wheezing while assigned to several jobs, of which sandblasting was only a minor component. Post-hire bronchitis was seen in 9 of 14 (64%) ever-sandblasters compared with 42 of 151 (28%) never-sandblasters.

Odds ratios that take into account age, gender, and pack-years of smoking indicate that ever having wheezed, current asthma diagnosis, and post-hire physician-diagnosed bronchitis were about 5, 4, and 4 times, respectively, more likely in ever-sandblasters than in never-sandblasters (Table 14). In a linear regression model which took into account age, gender, height, weight, and pack-years of smoking, ever-sandblasters had a significantly decreased FEV1/FVC and a significantly decreased percent predicted FEV1 than never-sandblasters (Table 16). However, not one of the 14 ever-sandblasters had airways obstruction on spirometry.

Health Outcomes Associated with Currently Working in a Work Area or Plant

Current shapers are more likely to have airways obstruction and current zinc workers were more likely to have a usual cough than workers in other work areas (Tables 17 and 18). However, these relationships were marginally significant and were not duplicated in odds ratio analyses that took into account age, gender, and pack-years of smoking. The odds ratio analysis did indicate that usual cough was about 4 times more likely in current zinc workers (data not shown).

Suspected post-hire asthma was present in 50% of current shapers compared to 27% of workers currently working in other work areas (Table 17). When age, gender, and pack-years of smoking are taken into account, suspected post-hire asthma was about 3 times more likely to be found in current shapers than other workers (marginal statistical significance) (Table 19).

DISCUSSION AND CONCLUSIONS

Cobalt Exposure

Representative cobalt air measurements are achieved with a sampling strategy using full-shift personal air breathing samples on workers from all shifts and over several days.
In contrast, only a small number of cobalt air samples have routinely been obtained in each work area during company industrial hygiene surveys. Given the small number of samples, it is not advisable to ignore single elevated cobalt levels, assuming them to be unrepresentative. Work areas where the most recently measured cobalt air levels exceeded the NIOSH Recommended Exposure Limit (REL) were charging, reprocessing, spray drying, screening, and Zinc B operation where respective cobalt air levels are as much as 16, 6, 12, 6, and 3 times higher than the NIOSH REL of 0.05 milligrams cobalt per cubic meter air (mg/m^3).

Cobalt absorption occurs as a result of inhaling cobalt in the air, ingesting cobalt on lips and/or from hands when eating food, and contamination of the skin. Cobalt is also present in small quantities in food and vitamin supplements. Worker cobalt blood tests are used to identify high work exposures. Gurley worker cobalt blood levels have been consistently elevated since 1998. Blood samples for these tests were drawn mostly before shift and on all different days of the work week. Had the blood samples been drawn at the appropriate time (end of work week, end of shift), worker cobalt blood levels would probably have been higher.

The health impact of a persistently elevated cobalt level is not known. Since cardiomyopathy and thyroid gland enlargement have been associated with cobalt exposure, it would be prudent to retest worker blood cobalt levels after exposure control measures have been implemented, both to assure the company that over-exposure is not continuing and to assure the individual workers that their blood cobalt levels are no longer elevated.

Cobalt is excreted from the body over a period of up to two years; most is excreted within several weeks and the remainder is mostly excreted over several months. If a worker is removed from exposure (such as during a long vacation) and the cobalt blood test is repeated immediately prior to return to work, then the degree to which that worker's level exceeds 1 µg/L mostly indicates excessive prior exposure. If the blood test is then repeated one to two weeks later at the end of the shift at the end of the work week, the difference from the after-vacation level would reflect current exposure. Should this be elevated, engineering controls need to be implemented; the respiratory protection program needs to be critically examined; and non-respiratory exposures (such as related to personal hygiene and skin contamination) need to be addressed.

Hard Metal Pneumoconiosis/Hypersensitivity Pneumonitis

Interstitial lung disease in the hard metal industry may be due to hard metal pneumoconiosis or hypersensitivity pneumonitis (HP). Both lung diseases may result in lung fibrosis with restriction on spirometry and a low DLCO. However, unlike with hard metal pneumoconiosis, individuals with HP frequently experience non-respiratory symptoms (such as fever, chills, fatigue, decreased appetite, and weight loss).

In hard metal workers HP may be caused by metalworking fluid contaminants (endotoxin, fungi, and mycobacteria) or possibly cobalt. The metalworking fluid samples obtained during our walk-through survey did not contain substantial amounts of any of the known causes of HP. However, our sampling was limited and does not exclude the possibility that higher levels may have existed previously. Fever, chills, or night sweats as well as unusual fatigue were present in over one-third of the workforce. Frequent (weekly or more frequently) unusual fatigue was reported by 33 of 165 (20%) workers and frequent fever, chills, or night sweats was reported by 9 of 165 (5%) workers. We do not believe that HP exists in this workforce as a result of exposure to metalworking fluid contaminants. Because of the nonspecific symptoms currently experienced by this workforce, we cannot rule out cobalt-related HP.

Only 3 out of 162 current workers (2%) had restriction on spirometry. The prevalence rate of restriction in this workforce is not elevated when compared to the general population prevalence rate of 7%. We suspect that the low prevalence of restriction and the absence of chest x-rays with evidence of pneumoconiosis in the current workforce is due to workers ill with hard metal pneumoconiosis leaving the workforce. This is known to be true for at least 2 former workers within the last year. One of these former workers had giant cells on lung biopsy. When giant cells are detected in a lung biopsy or in lung fluid of a hard metal worker, we are virtually certain that the lung disease in the affected individual is caused from exposure to cobalt.

Grinding and pressing were most highly associated with suspected interstitial lung disease, based on a review of work histories and symptom-onset dates. The two index cases included in this analysis, developed their disease while working in grinding. The small numbers of cases with restriction and/or suspected interstitial lung disease prevented meaningful statistical analysis by work area.

Cobalt Asthma
Compared to national rates there was a statistically significant 3-fold excess of airways obstruction in white never-smokers and a 2-fold excess of ever-diagnosed asthma in the entire workforce. When analyzed at the plant level, there was a statistically significant 3-fold excess of airways obstruction in white never-smokers at the Grant plant and greater than 2-fold excess of ever-diagnosed asthma, also statistically significant, in workers at the Grant and Gurley plants.

Post-hire asthma was present in 6.1% of the workforce which is consistent with an industry-wide rate of 5.6% for cobalt-induced occupational asthma (defined as asthma with post-hire onset and which improved away from work), published in 1988.[7]

Suspected post-hire asthma was present in 29% of the workforce. Shaping, pressing, and zinc work were most highly associated with suspected post-hire asthma, based on a review of work histories and symptom-onset dates. In a controlled analysis of the entire workforce, current shapers were about 3 times more likely to have suspected-post hire asthma than workers in other areas (marginal statistical significance); and ever-shapers were about 2 times more likely to have this diagnosis than workers who had never worked in this area (marginal statistical significance).

Sandblasting appeared to be a risk area in the statistical analyses. Despite a 3-fold increase in known post-hire asthma in ever-sandblasters, compared to never-sandblasters, the increased prevalence rate is based on two cases in only 14 ever-sandblasters; these small numbers make the risk estimate uncertain. The work history analysis in relation to symptom onset casts doubt on the association of wheezing and sandblasting (details in results).

We conclude that work-related asthma is very prevalent in this workforce; that **shaping, pressing, and zinc** are high risk areas (giving the greatest weight of evidence to the work history review); and that **shaping** is a current high risk area.

Asthma is known to occur in workers exposed to cobalt and metalworking fluids. Because suspected post-hire asthma is associated with work areas with presumably low levels of MWF exposure and is not associated with the grinding work area, we suspect that most of the work-related asthma cases are due to exposure to cobalt and not MWFs. However, some of these cases may have been due to MWF exposure.

Cobalt Exposures in High Risk Areas

Of the 9 current workers and one index case with suspected post-hire asthma associated with pressing, 9 of these 10 workers were exposed during or after 1988 when cobalt air levels were at or below 0.04 mg/m^3 (Table 2). Of the 7 workers who had suspected post-hire asthma with onset of their disease in the shaping area, 2 (29%) were exposed during or after 2001 when cobalt levels were about 0.01 mg/m^3.

Of the 1 current worker and 2 index cases with suspected interstitial lung disease associated with grinding, 1 was exposed during or after 1999 when cobalt air levels were at or below 0.04 mg/m^3. Two workers with suspected interstitial lung disease associated with pressing were exposed after 1988, when levels were at or below 0.04 mg/m^3.

The number of environmental samples obtained during these time periods is very limited and the degree to which these samples reflect actual average daily cobalt exposure is not known. However, if we assume that they accurately represent historical cobalt air levels, then at least 14 cases of suspected lung disease possibly occurred at air cobalt levels below the NIOSH REL. This may indicate that the current exposure limits are not protective and/or that some other unmeasured exposure indicator is important (for example ultra-fine size particles or skin exposure) in predicting risk.

Grinding, pressing, shaping, and zinc areas are associated with interstitial lung disease and asthma. Workers who currently work in grinding, pressing, and shaping have lower prevalence rates for a number of symptoms, post-hire diagnosed bronchitis, current asthma diagnosis, and airways obstruction than workers who previously worked in those areas. This can be explained by either an improvement in the work environments or a healthy worker effect where symptomatic workers leave these work areas and transfer to other work areas. Historical company cobalt air level measurements from 1988 onward do not demonstrate a reduction in cobalt air levels in grinding or pressing. We believe that the better health of the current workers compared to past workers is due to the healthy worker effect.

Strengths

An overall participation rate of 68% indicates that study participants adequately represent the workforce. Accuracy of medical tests is ensured by the superior quality of the spirometry tests and a study design that required agreement among physicians' chest x-ray profusion scores. No single respiratory symptom is able to distinguish between asthma, pneumoconiosis, asthmatic bronchitis, and non-allergic airways irritation. However, our definition for suspected post-hire asthma used a set of symptoms previously shown to be highly predictive of asthma.6

Limitations

Our sampling of MWF for contaminants was limited to one grinding machine and may not be representative of all grinding operations or past conditions.

Studies in which the current workforce is studied at a single point in time (cross-sectional studies) can be strongly affected by the healthy worker effect, where symptomatic workers leave the workforce or transfer to other work areas. This may result in relatively low prevalence rates of disease. Studies where workers are followed over time (longitudinal studies) can estimate incidence rates of disease (the number of workers who develop disease over a period of time) and may more accurately reflect the true disease burden if a sizeable proportion of symptomatic workers is leaving the workforce.

In our calculation of disease risk by work areas ever worked, ill workers who worked in a number of different work areas will contribute their "risk" to all the jobs ever worked. This underestimates risk for truly risky work areas and overestimates risk for others. Calculations of disease risk by current work area are limited due to the smaller number of workers in these categories which makes it difficult to demonstrate statistically significant relationships. Current work area analysis is also flawed by the healthy worker effect where ill workers transfer out of a given job.
When work histories were reviewed on a case-by-case basis, it was not possible in all cases to identify when the worker first developed symptoms or, in the case where a number of different symptoms were reported, which symptom most accurately reflected the identified suspected lung disease. Workers may have inaccurately recalled dates that they worked specific jobs and/or dates when their symptoms began. If either of these dates was inaccurate it may have resulted in an inappropriately assigned high risk work area for that particular worker.

Statistical significance was difficult to demonstrate with the small numbers in comparison groups (as was true of ever-workers and current workers). Low statistical power also existed for associations involving low prevalence outcomes (such as suspected interstitial lung disease). Power was less of a problem when a prevalence rate for a more common outcome (such as airways obstruction) in the entire workforce was compared to a national rate.

RECOMMENDATIONS

1.   **Engineering Controls:**

- Mechanize the charging process.
- Reduce cobalt exposures in the grinding, pressing, shaping, and zinc work areas (where an elevated risk of cobalt-associated lung disease has been identified). We will be returning to further characterize cobalt exposures in these work areas in order to help direct how these cobalt exposures should be reduced.
- Reduce cobalt exposures in the charging, reprocessing, spray dry, screening, and zinc B work areas (where cobalt air levels currently exceed the NIOSH REL).
- Dedicate the charging/reprocessing floor sweeper for sole use in those work areas, so as to prevent

contamination of other areas of the plant.

- Ensure and routinely check the integrity of the sandblasting glove box air hoses and gloves.

- Store extrusion department liquid solvents in chemical safety cabinets.

2.   Respiratory Protection:

- Implement a respiratory protection program, which at a minimum is in compliance with the OSHA respiratory protection program standard. This program should include a written program, medical evaluation, fit-testing, cartridge change protocol, training, and record keeping.

- Ensure that all sizes of respirators and cartridges are always available.

- Require the mandatory use of respirators in work areas with high risk of cobalt-associated lung disease (**grinding, pressing, shaping, and zinc**). Continue to use respirators until the excess disease risk is eliminated.

- Require the mandatory use of respirators in work areas where current cobalt air levels exceed the NIOSH REL (charging, reprocessing, screening, spray dry, and zinc) and for all cleaning activities. Continue to use respirators until cobalt air levels are reduced (through the implementation of engineering controls).

- While the mixing process remains non-mechanized, chargers should use respiratory protection that provides protection to the level of the NIOSH REL. Because company environmental sampling demonstrated an exposure as high as 0.8 mg cobalt/m^3, the minimum required respirator protection factor for this work area is 16 (16X). This protection level is provided by full-facepiece negative pressure air purifying respirators (50X), powered air purifying respirators (PAPRs) (50X), and (air line) pressure demand respirators (1000X).

- Require that workers in screening, reprocessing, and Zinc B use non-powered half-facepiece air purifying respirators (10X) or respirators with a higher protection level.

3.   Skin Protection:

- Ensure that workers are trained on the proper use of gloves (for example the donning of gloves before putting on work boots) and that all sizes of non-latex gloves are always available. Require the use of these gloves by workers in **grinding, pressing, shaping,** and zinc (where an elevated risk of cobalt-associated lung disease has been identified)

4.   Medical Surveillance:

a.   *Spirometry and chest radiograph*
    (1)   Perform a baseline spirometry test and posteroanterior chest x-ray on all newly hired workers. Have a physician evaluate new workers with pre-existing lung disease or abnormal pre-placement spirometry or chest x-ray, to determine whether work exposures place them at increased risk for progression of their lung disease. Spirometry tests need to be of high quality in order to compare results over time. Chest x-rays need to be interpreted by a B-reader in order to identify lung damage from priordust exposure (asbestos, silica, coal dust, and hard metal, among others).

(2) Perform spirometry tests annually and chest x-rays every three years on production workers. Chest x-rays should be interpreted by a B-reader.

(3) Designate a safety person in each plant and encourage production workers to report respiratory symptoms to this person.

(4) Ensure that workers who are either symptomatic or who have an abnormal chest x-ray or abnormal (or borderline abnormal) spirometry test results are medically evaluated by a lung doctor (pulmonologist).

(5) Prevent further exposure of any worker found to have work-related lung disease.

(6) Use screening findings to establish effectiveness of interventions by looking at therates of new cases of lung disease in the high risk groups of **grinders, pressers, shapers, and zinc workers**.

b.   *Cobalt blood testing*

(1) Repeat cobalt blood tests on workers who had elevated levels during the March-May 2003 testing period. Tests should be performed following long work absences prior to the worker returning to work and repeated end of the shift, end of the work week.

(2) Perform periodic cobalt blood tests on workers exposed to cobalt air levels in excess of the NIOSH REL and workers exposed to high peakcobalt levels (such as with cleaning operations). When we return, we will perform cobalt blood tests on workers in those work areas wherethere is an increased risk of lung disease (**grinding, pressing, shaping, and zinc**) in order to determine whether periodic cobalt blood testing should be performed on these workers also.

We appreciate all the help that you and your staff provided to facilitate NIOSH's medical survey at your plant. We hope our findings and recommendations will be helpful to you and your workers. In addition the information gained from these surveys will contribute to what is known regarding the risk for lung disease from cobalt exposure in hard metal manufacturing plants and will help NIOSH protect workers in this industry.

In accordance with the Code of Federal Regulations, Title 42, Part 85, copies of this letter must be posted by management in a prominent place accessible to the employees for a period of 30 calendar days.

Sincerely,

Nancy M. Sahakian, M.D., M.P.H.

Daniel Yereb, M.S.
Respiratory Disease Hazard Evaluation and
        Technical Assistance Program
Field Studies Branch
Division of Respiratory Disease Studies

cc:
Dink Barron
Darryl Baker
Jack Smith
Confidential Employee Requestors
Dr. Robert Johnson
OSHA Region 4
Richard Hartle (HETAB)

References

1. American Thoracic Society [1995]. Standardization of spirometry: 1994 update. Am J Resp Crit Care Med 152:1107-1136.

2. Hankinson JL, Odencrantz JR, Fedan KB [1999]. Spirometric reference values from a sample of the general U.S. population. Am J Resp Crit Care Med 159:179-187.

3. CDC [1996]. Third National Health and Nutrition Examination Survey, 1988-1994, NHANES III Examination Date File [CD-ROM]. Hyattsville, Maryland: U.S. Department of Health and Human Services, Public Health Service, Centers for Disease Control and Prevention. (Public use data file documentations No. 76300).

4. American Thoracic Society [1991]. Lung function testing: selection of reference values and interpretive strategies. Am Rev Resp Dis 144:1202-1218.

5. Miller A, Thornton J, Warshaw R et al. [1983]. Single breath diffusing capacity in a representative sample of the population of Michigan, a large industrial state. Am Rev Respir Dis 127:270-277.

6. Venables K, Farrer N, Sharp L. et al. [1993]. Respiratory symptoms questionnaire for asthma epidemiology: validity and reproducibility. Thorax 48:214-219.

7. Kusaka Y, Yokoyama K, Sera Y, et al. [1986]. Respiratory diseases in hard metal workers: an occupational hygiene study in a factory. Br J Ind Med 43:474-485.

Table 1. Metalworking fluid (MWF) analysis, cobalt and nickel content in micrograms cobalt per gram material (µg/g), endotoxin concentration in endotoxin units per milliliter fluid (EU/ml), culturable fungi and bacteria concentrations in colony forming units per milliliter fluid (CFU/ml), Grant plant, July 7, 2003

Sample Type	Cobalt Content (µg/g)	Nickel Content (µg/g)	Endotoxin Concentration (EU/ml)	Fungi	Bacteria	Mycobacteria
Unused Rich Grind™ MWF	(1)	ND	< 0.5	No growth	No growth	No growth
In-use liquid MWF from centerless grinder	(1)	ND	200	No growth	Staphylococcus 1700 CFU/ml	No growth
Liquid sludge in MWF filter system	74	2	NA	NA	NA	NA
Solid sludge in MWF filter system	6600	82	NA	NA	NA	NA

ND, not detectable; NA, not analyzed; limits of detection (LOD) and quantification (LOQ) for cobalt are 0.8 and 3 µg/g, respectively; LOD and LOQ for nickel are 1 and 4 µg/g, respectively; LOD for endotoxin is 0.005 EU/ml (LOQ is not available); LOD for fungal and bacterial growth is 100 CFU/ml; parentheses indicate semiquantitative values which are between the LOD and LOQ.

Table 2. Company cobalt air levels in milligrams cobalt per cubic meter air (mg cobalt/m³)

Plant	Work Process	N	Range (mg cobalt/ m³)	Date
Grant	Pressing	1	0.01	September 2001
		2	0.02-0.04	February 1993
		7	<0.01-0.03	March 1988
		4	0.05-0.32	June 1985
Grant	Tray Preparation	1	<0.01	March 1988
Grant	Shaping/Round Cell	1	0.01	September 2001
		1	0.06	May 2000
		3	0.001-0.06	June 1999
		3	0.03-0.26	February 1993
Grant	Grinding *	1	0.04	September 2001
		1	0.002	April 1999
		3	<0.01-0.11	March 1988
		2	0.08-0.16	January 1985
Grant	Sandblasting	1	0.02	March 1988
		2	0.09	January 1985
Grant	Sintering	1	<0.01	March 1988
Grant	Furnace operator	1	0.009	January 1985
Gurley	Charging/Blending⁻	2	0.12-0.80	April 2003
		5	0.06-0.84	August 2001
		2	0.10-0.32	March 2000
		5	0.06-18.6	March 1999
		2	14.52-18.63	February 1999
		1	0.28	August 1998
		1	0.11	April 1993
		5	<0.01-0.08	March 1988
		1	0.01	February 1986
		1	0.01	November 1985
		2	0.32-0.38	January 1985
Gurley	Reprocessing⁻	1	0.27	April 2003
Gurley	Mill	1	0.01	March 1999
		1	0.01	February 1999
		1	0.03	April 1993
		2	<0.01-0.02	March 1988
Gurley	Spray Dry⁻	2	0.04-0.62	April 1993
		5	<0.01-0.06	March 1988
		1	0.03	February 1986
		1	0.02	November 1985
		1	0.01	January 1985
Gurley	Screening⁻	2	0.16-.030	April 2003
		3	0.04-0.44	August 2001
		2	0.04-0.44	August 1998
		1	0.01	February 1986
		1	0.03	November 1985
Huntsville	Zinc A	1	0.02	August 2002
		2	0.11-0.33	November 2000
Huntsville	Zinc B⁻	4	0.03-0.15	July 2003
		1	0.26	August 2002
		2	0.36-0.76	November 2000
Huntsville	APT	2	0.02-0.04	August 2002
		2	0.003-0.05	November 2000

* prior to 1999, the grinding operation was located in the Gurley plant; areas where recent cobalt air measurements have exceeded NIOSH recommended exposure limit of 0.05 mg cobalt/m³ are in bold/⁻

Table 3. Cobalt blood sample levels in micrograms per liter blood (µg/L) for Gurley plant workers, 1998 to 2003.

Parameter	December 1998 (N=23)	February 1999 (N=24)	June 1999 (N=25)	November 1999 (N=23)	March 2000 (N=6)	March to May 2003 (N=23)
Mean (µg/L)	11.2	8.2	7.8	9.9	13.0	18.6
Median (µg/L)	7.1	6.8	5.3	4.5	7.2	9.9
Range (µg/L)	(0.5-47.3)	(1.5-32.7)	(1.3-40.5)	(0.5-58.7)	(0.5-32.2)	(0.5-119.6)
Standard Deviation	11.7	7.6	8.4	14.6	14.6	27.3

Biological Exposure Index (BEI) is 1 µg/L in an end of shift, end of work week blood sample; BEIs are developed by the American Conference of Governmental Industrial Hygienists to indicate exposure levels which exceed currently recommended exposure limits.

Table 4. Demographics of participants, September 2003, Metalworking Products

Demographics	Grant plant (N=97)	Gurley plant (N=37)	Huntsville plant (N=31)	All participants (N=165)
Age (years)				
- Mean	44	45	41	44
- Median	44	43	39	44
- Range	(25-64)	(29-71)	(26-59)	(25-71)
Gender				
- Males	53%	89%	100%	70%
- Females	47%	11%	0%	30%
Smoking status				
- Smokers (current & former smokers)	50%	62%	52%	53%
- Never smokers	50%	38%	48%	47%
Pack-years (for smokers)				
- Mean	22.3	28.0	20.6	23.5
- Median	18.1	23.0	11.5	20.2
- Range	(0.4-120)	(1.5-114)	(0.5-71)	(0.4-120)
Tenure (years)				
- Mean	12	12	12	12
- Median	10	10	8	10
- Range	(1-37)	(1-31)	(4-32)	(1-37)

Table 5. Prevalence rates (percent) of reported symptoms, physician diagnoses, and spirometry abnormalities among participants, September 2003, Metalworking Products

Symptoms/Physician Diagnoses/Spirometry Abnormalities	Grant (N=97)	Gurley (N=37)	Huntsville (N=31)	Total (N=165)
	N (%)	N (%)	N (%)	N (%)
Respiratory Symptoms				
Any breathing troubles	33 (34)	11(30)	12 (39)	56 (34)
Shortness of breath with hurrying on level ground or walking up a slight hill	39 (40)	17 (46)	7 (23)	63 (38)
Shortness of breath walking with people same age	20 (21)	5 (14)	4 (13)	29 (18)
Any shortness of breath (onset after hire)	22 (23)	14 (38)	7 (23)	43 (26)
Usual cough	24 (25)	5 (14)	11 (35)	40 (24)
Usual cough (onset after hire)	14 (14)	3 (8)	10 (32)	27 (16)
Chronic cough	17 (18)	3 (8)	7 (23)	27 (16)
Ever wheezed	45 (46)	24 (65)	12 (39)	81 (49)
Ever wheezed (onset after hire)	25 (26)	11 (30)	7 (23)	43 (26)
Wheeze aside from a cold	27 (28)	10 (27)	8 (26)	45 (27)
Nasal irritation	61 (63)	21 (57)	20 (65)	102 (62)
Non-Respiratory Symptoms				
Fever, chills, or night sweats	38 (40)*	11 (30)	11 (35)	60 (37)*
Unusual fatigue	35 (36)	14 (38)	13 (42)	62 (38)
Eye irritation	48 (49)	17 (46)	12 (39)	77 (47)
Skin irritation	33 (34)	16 (43)	10 (32)	59 (36)
Physician Diagnoses				
Episode(s) of bronchitis since hire	36 (37)	6 (16)	9 (29)	51 (31)
Chronic bronchitis since hire	10 (10)	2 (5)	1 (3)	13 (8)
Post-hire asthma	7 (7)	3 (8)	0 (0)	10 (6)
Spirometry Abnormalities†				
Airways obstruction	9 (9)	2 (6)	1 (3)	12 (7)
Restriction	2 (2)	0 (0)	1 (3)	3 (2)

* one person did not answer this question; † 2 participants from Grant and 1 participant from Gurley did not have a spirometry test performed

Table 6. Individual workers with restriction, borderline restriction, or low lung diffusing capacity for carbon monoxide (DLCO) with forced vital capacity, body mass index, and symptoms, Metalworking Products, September 2003

Worker	Restriction	FVC % predicted	DLCO % predicted	TLC % predicted	BMI	Symptoms
A‡	Moderate	54.9*	71.7	69.7*	22.0†	Current smoker. Usual cough and phlegm production; both improved away from work. Wheeze; improved away from work. Short of breath after walking a few minutes on level ground.
B‡	Mild	78.5*	78.1	78.0*	26.2†	Lifetime nonsmoker. Usual cough and phlegm; both not improved away from work. Wheeze.
C‡	Mild	74.4*	Not done	Not done	18.5†	Lifetime nonsmoker. Usual cough.
D‡	Borderline	78.1*	102.9	79.5*	27.0†	Former smoker. No symptoms.
E‡	Borderline	80.4*	90.5	77.4*	21.7†	Lifetime nonsmoker. No symptoms.
F	Borderline	80.9*	Not done	Not done	17.7	Former smoker. No symptoms.
G	No	101.6	62.8*	98.5	17.6	Current smoker. Wheeze; improved away from work.
H	No	100.1	72.0*	104.6	18.0	Current smoker. Usual phlegm; improved away from work. Wheeze; same away from work.

FVC, forced vital capacity; DLCO, lung diffusing capacity for carbon monoxide; TLC, total lung capacity; BMI, body mass index
* below lower limit of normal; † BMI greater than or equal to 18.5 and less than 30.0; ‡ cases that were considered to have suspected interstitial lung disease

Table 7. Respiratory symptoms and physician-diagnosed asthma and chronic bronchitis among current workforce compared to expected numbers from the NHANES III survey, expressed as prevalence rate ratios (with 95% confidence intervals), adjusted for smoking status, age, gender, and race, September 2003, Metalworking Products

Category	Number	Shortness of breath on hurrying on level ground or walking up a slight hill	Chronic cough (cough on most days)	Chronic bronchitis	Wheeze or whistling in the last 12 months	Asthma (ever diagnosed)
Grant	97	1.9* (1.4-2.6)*	1.9* (1.2-3.0)*	2.0* (1.1-3.6)*	1.9* (1.4-2.7)*	2.1* (1.3-3.5)*
Gurley	37	1.9* (1.1-3.2)*	0.8 (0.27-2.37)	2.3 (0.90-5.95)	1.9* (1.1-3.3)*	2.5* (1.2-5.1)*
Huntsville	31	1.4 (0.7-2.8)	2.7* (1.3-5.6)*	2.0 (0.55-7.37)	1.8 (1.0-3.42)	1.3 (0.4-3.8)
Entire Workforce	161	1.9* (1.5-2.5)*	1.8* (1.2-2.6)*	2.1* (1.3-3.3)*	1.9* (1.5-2.5)*	2.0* (1.4-3.0)*

Statistically significant rate ratios are in bold/*; a Poisson distribution was assumed in the calculation of the 95% confidence intervals

Table 8. Airways obstruction on spirometry among current workforce compared to expected numbers from the NHANES III survey, expressed as prevalence ratios (with 95% confidence intervals), adjusted for smoking status, age, gender, and race, September 2003, Metalworking Products

Category	Current & former smokers N	Current & former smokers # Obs	Current & former smokers # Exp	Current & former smokers Ratio Obs/Exp (95% CI)	Never smokers N	Never smokers # Obs	Never smokers # Exp	Never smokers Ratio Obs/Exp (95% CI)	All participants N	All participants # Obs	All participants # Exp	All participants Ratio Obs/Exp (95% CI)
White Males												
17-39 yrs old	22	1	1.13	0.9 (0.2-5.0)	14	2	0.24	**8.5 (2.3-30.4)***	36	3	1.27	2.2 (0.7-6.4)
40-69 yrs old	34	3	3.76	0.8 (0.3-2.4)	20	0	0.60	0 (0.0-6.4)	54	3	4.4	0.7 (0.2-2.0)
Total	56	4	4.9	0.8 (0.3-2.1)	34	2	0.83	2.4 (0.7-8.8)	90	6	5.73	1.0 (0.5-2.3)
White Females												
17-39 yrs old	0	0	0	-	6	0	0.18	0 (0.0-21.3)	6	0	0.18	0 (0.0-21.3)
40-69 yrs old	22	4	3.4	1.2 (0.5-3.1)	13	2	0.33	**6.0 (1.7-22.1)***	35	6	3.69	1.6 (0.8-3.6)
Total	22	4	3.4	1.2 (0.5-3.1)	19	2	0.52	**3.9 (1.1-14.0)***	41	6	3.88	1.5 (0.7-3.4)
Whites Total	78	8	8.25	1.0 (0.5-1.9)	53	4	1.35	**3.0 (1.2-7.6)***	131	12	9.6	1.2 (0.7-2.2)
Blacks Total	6	0	0.37	0 (0.0-10.4)	21	0	0.63	0 (0.0-6.1)	27	0	1.0	0 (0.0-3.8)
Whites and Blacks	84	8	8.62	0.9 (0.5-1.8)	74	4	2.0	2.0 (0.8-5.2)	158	12	10.6	1.1 (0.7-2.0)

N, number; # Obs, number observed; # Exp, number expected; Obs/Exp, number observed ÷ number expected; CI, confidence interval; statistically significant prevalence ratios are in bold/*; a Poisson distribution was assumed in the calculation of the 95% confidence intervals; excludes Hispanics and Asians

Table 9. Airways obstruction on spirometry among current workforce by plant compared to expected numbers from the NHANES III survey, expressed as prevalence ratios (with 95% confidence intervals), controlled for smoking status, age, gender, and race, September 2003, Metalworking Products

Category	Current and former smokers N	Current and former smokers # Obs	Current and former smokers # Exp	Current and former smokers Ratio Obs/ Exp (95% CI)	Never smokers N	Never smokers # Obs	Never smokers # Exp	Never smokers Ratio Obs/ Exp (95% CI)	All N	All # Obs	All # Exp	All Ratio Obs/ Exp (95% CI)
Grant												
Whites	46	6	5.20	1.2 (0.5-2.5)	37	3	0.98	3.1 (1.0-9.0)*	83	9	6.2	1.5 (0.7-2.8)
Blacks	0	0	0	-	8	0	0.18	0 (0.0-21.3)	8	0	0.18	0 (0.0-21.3)
All	46	6	5.20	1.2 (0.5-2.5)	45	3	1.15	2.6 (0.9-7.7)	91	9	6.35	1.4 (0.8-2.7)
Gurley												
Whites	20	1	2.03	0.5 (0.1-2.8)	12	1	0.29	3.4 (0.6-20.0)	32	2	2.32	0.9 (0.2-3.1)
Blacks	2	0	0.10	0 (0.0-38.4)	2	0	0.07	0 (0.0-54.9)	4	0	0.17	0 (0.0-22.6)
All	22	1	2.13	0.5 (0.1-2.8)	14	1	0.36	2.8 (0.4-12.9)	36	2	2.49	0.8 (0.22-2.9)
Huntsville												
Whites	12	1	1.03	1.0 (0.2-5 5)	4	0	0.08	0 (0.0-48.0)	16	1	1 11	0.9 (0.2-5.1)
Blacks	4	0	0.27	0 (0.0-14.2)	11	0	0.37	0 (0.0-10.4)	15	0	0.64	0 (0.0-6.0)
All	16	1	1.30	0.8 (0.1-4.4)	15	0	0.45	0 (0.0-8.5)	31	1	1.75	0.6 (0.20-3.2)

N, number; # Obs, number observed; # Exp, number expected; Obs/Exp, number observed ÷ number expected; CI, confidence interval; * statistically significant rate ratios are in bold with single asterisk; a Poisson distribution was assumed in the calculation of the 95% confidence intervals; excludes Hispanics and Asians; due to rounding, confidence interval which includes 1.0 is statistically significant

Table 10. Numbers of workers with suspected interstitial lung disease (whose symptoms began in indicated work areas) as a proportion of workers who ever worked in those work areas, September 2003, Metalworking Products

Work area	Number of workers with suspected interstitial lung disease* whose symptoms began in the indicated work areas	Numbers of workers with suspected interstitial lung disease (whose symptoms began in indicated work areas) as a proportion of workers who ever worked in those work areas
Pressing	2	2/53 (4%)**
Grinding	3	3/36 (8%)**
Zinc	1	1/22 (5%)
Sintering	1	1/18 (6%)
Total	7	--

* Suspected interstitial lung disease is defined as restriction, borderline restriction, or low lung diffusing capacity for carbon monoxide with the following qualifiers: 1) cases were included only if the Body Mass Index (BMI) was greater than or equal to 18.5 and less than 30 and the total lung capacity (if known) was below the lower limit of normal; 2) cases of borderline restriction were included only if FVC was below the lower limit of normal. 7 workers were identified with suspected interstitial lung disease (5 participants and 2 index cases); index cases were included in numerators and denominators;
** prevalence rates for identified high risk areas are in bold with a double asterisk

Table 11. Numbers of workers with suspected post-hire asthma (whose symptoms began in indicated work areas) as a proportion of workers who ever worked in those work areas, September 2003, Metalworking Products

Work area	Number of workers with suspected post-hire asthma* whose symptoms began in the indicated work areas	Numbers of workers with suspected post-hire asthma (whose symptoms began in indicated work areas) as a proportion of workers who ever worked in those work areas
Pressing/Tray Preparation	10	10/54 (19%)**
Sintering	2	2/18 (11%)
Shaping/Round Cell	7	7/35 (20%)**
Grinding	2	2/34 (6%)
Shipping	1	1/29 (3%)
Product Testing	1	1/15 (7%)
Charging/Blending/Reprocessing	1	1/14 (7%)
Screener	1	1/8 (13%)
Mill/Spray Dry	2	2/21 (10%)
APT	1	1/18 (6%)
Zinc	5	5/22 (23%)**
Maintenance	2	2/11 (18%)
Other	3	--
Total	38	--

* Suspected post-hire asthma is defined as post-hire onset of asthma, 3 or more Venables' asthma symptoms, use of asthma medication, or obstruction on spirometry (workers with pre-hire asthma were excluded). 48 workers were identified with suspected post-hire asthma (47 participants and 1 index case), 10 of these workers who did not have symptom onset dates were excluded; index case was included in one numerator and appropriate denominators; prevalence rates for identified high risk areas are in bold with double asterisk

Table 12. Prevalence rates (percent) of respiratory symptoms, asthma diagnosis, and spirometry test abnormalities in workers who <u>ever</u> worked in certain work areas compared to workers who never worked in those work areas, September 2003, Metalworking Products

Health Outcome	Pressing Ever (N=54) (%)	Pressing Never (N=111) (%)	Shaping Ever (N=36) (%)	Shaping Never (N=129) (%)	Grinding Ever (N=34) (%)	Grinding Never N=(131) (%)	Sandblasting Ever (N=14) (%)	Sandblasting Never (N=151) (%)	Product Testing Ever (N=15) (%)	Product Testing Never (N=150) (%)
Usual cough	30	22	14	27	29	23	36	23	27	24
Cough most days	26	12	14	17	21	15	14	17	13	17
Bronchitis since hire	50*	22	33	30	41	28	64*	28*	47	29
Chronic bronchitis diagnosis	15	8	3	13	15	9	7	11	20	9
Short of breath walking when with others same age	26**	14	17	18	32*	14*	29	17	33	16
Short of breath when hurrying on level ground or walking up a slight hill	41	37	39	38	53**	34	43	38	53	37
Ever wheezed	54	47	47	50	62	46	79*	46*	60	48
Wheeze in last 12 months	37	31	31	33	45	29	57**	30	33	33
Woken up with wheeze within the last 4 weeks	24	13	19	16	26	14	29	15	27	15
Wheeze better away from work	11	13	6	14	15	11	14	12	7	13
Asthma diagnosis (ever)	15	17	14	17	21	15	43*	14*	20	16
Asthma diagnosis (current)	13	10	8	12	15	10	36*	9*	20	10
Obstruction +	11	6	20*	4*	3	9	0	8	20**	6
Restriction +	2	2	0	2	3	2	7	1	0	2
Abnormal spirometry +	13	7	20*	6*	6	10	7	9	20	8
Suspected post-hire asthma +	38	25	43**	25	35	27	36	28	27	29

* Statistically significant (p < 0.05) comparisons are in bold with single asterisk; ** marginally significant (p < 0.10) comparisons; + 3 participants did not have a spirometry test performed; suspected post-hire asthma is defined as post-hire onset of asthma, 3 or more Venables' asthma symptoms, use of asthma medication, or obstruction on spirometry (workers with known pre-hire asthma were excluded); Chi-square and Fisher's exact test were used

Table 14. Odds ratio comparisons (and 95% confidence intervals) of health-related outcomes in workers who <u>ever</u> worked in certain work areas compared to workers who never worked in these work areas, controlled for age, gender, and pack-years of smoking, September 2003, Metalworking Products

Plant	Work Area +	Usual Cough	Bronchitis since hire	Short of breath when walking with others same age	Short of breath when walking up a slight hill	Wheeze (ever)	Woken up with wheeze within last 4 weeks	Asthma diagnosis (current)
Grant	Ever Pressing	1.4 (0.6-3.4)	2.8* (1.2-6.5)	2.0 (0.8-5.9)	1.0 (0.4-2.3)	1.1 (0.5-2.5)	2.0 (0.7-5.4)	0.6 (0.2-2.1)
Grant	Ever Shaping	0.4** (0.1-1.1)	1.0 (0.5-2.4)	0.9 (0.3-2.4)	1.0 (0.4-2.2)	0.7 (0.3-1.6)	1.2 (0.5-3.2)	0.6 (0.2-2.4)
Grant	Ever Grinding	1.4 (0.6-3.4)	1.8 (0.8-4.1)	3.0* (1.2-7.3)	2.1** (0.9-4.6)	2.1** (0.9-4.9)	2.4** (1.0-6.0)	1.4 (0.5-4.6)
Grant	Ever Sandblasting	1.7 (0.5-5.9)	3.5* (1.0-11.6)	1.7 (0.5-6.0)	1.2 (0.4-3.8)	5.2* (1.2-22.0)	1.9 (0.5-6.9)	4.4* (1.1-16.0)
Grant	Ever Product Testing	1.3 (0.3-4.9)	1.6 (0.5-5.3)	2.4 (0.7-8.7)	2.2 (0.7-7.3)	2.5 (0.7-8.8)	2.0 (0.5-7.8)	1.4 (0.3-6.4)
Gurley	Ever Charging	0.4 (0.1-2.1)	0.7 (0.2-2.9)	0.9 (0.2-4.5)	2.1 (0.6-7.0)	3.8** (0.9-15.7)	1.0 (0.2-4.9)	++
Gurley	Ever Mill	0.7 (0.1-6.2)	0.6 (0.1-5.1)	++	2.1 (0.4-10.1)	0.6 (0.1-3.6)	0.9 (0.1-9.1)	++
Gurley	Ever Spray Dry	0.4 (0.1-2.0)	1.1 (0.3-3.8)	1.5 (0.4-5.9)	3.9* (1.2-12.9)	5.0* (1.2-20.0)	0.9 (0.2-4.5)	++
Huntsville	Ever Zinc	2.0 (0.7-5.9)	1.3 (0.5-3.8)	0.9 (0.2-3.4)	0.4 (0.1-1.4)	0.8 (0.3-2.2)	1.0 (0.3-3.8)	0.6 (0.1-5.1)
Huntsville	Ever APT	1.8 (0.6-5.7)	2.2 (0.7-6.8)	1.2 (0.3-4.7)	0.5 (0.1-1.6)	0.5 (0.2-1.5)	0.6 (0.1-3.0)	0.7 (0.1-6.7)
	Ever Maintenance	2.9 (0.7-11.8)	0.3 (0.0-2.4)	1.3 (0.2-6.6)	0.9 (0.2-3.6)	1.2 (0.3-4.7)	1.6 (0.3-8.3)	3.0 (0.5-17.4)

+ Workers who ever worked in these work areas (work areas grouped by plant for ease of identification); ++ we were unable to calculate these odds ratios because no workers in these work groups had these symptoms or diagnoses; * statistically significant ($p < 0.05$) comparisons are in bold with single asterisk; ** marginally significant ($p < 0.10$) comparisons are in bold with double asterisk; due to rounding, confidence interval with a lower limit of 1.0 was statistically significant

Table 15. Odds ratio comparisons of suspected post-hire asthma in workers who <u>ever</u> worked in certain work areas compared to workers who never worked in these work areas, controlled for age, gender, and pack-years of smoking, September 2003, Metalworking Products

Work Area	Suspected post-hire asthma
Pressing	2.0 (0.8-4.7)
Shaping	2.2 (1.0-4.8)*
Grinding	1.4 (0.6-3.2)
Sandblasting	1.3 (0.4-4.5)
Product Testing	0.8 (0.2-3.1)
Charging	1.0 (0.3-3.6)
Mill	0.6 (0.3-9.0)
Spray Dry	0.9 (0.3-3.4)
Zinc	1.4 (0.5-4.1)
APT	0.7 (0.2-2.6)
Maintenance	1.7 (0.4-6.7)

There were no statistically significant ($p < 0.05$) comparisons; * marginally significant ($p < 0.10$) comparisons; 3 participants did not have a spirometry test performed; suspected post-hire asthma is defined as post-hire onset of asthma, 3 or more Venables' asthma symptoms, use of asthma medication, or obstruction on spirometry (workers with pre-hire asthma were excluded)

Table 16. Linear regression model for FEV1/FVC ratio and percent predicted FEV1 and FVC in workers who <u>ever</u> worked in certain work areas compared to workers who never worked in these work areas, controlled for age, gender, height, weight, and pack-years of smoking for FEV1/FVC and controlled for weight and pack-years of smoking for percent predicted FEV1 and FVC, September 2003, Metalworking Products

Plant	Work Area +	% predicted FEV1 Parameter estimate	% predicted FEV1 P value	% predicted FVC Parameter estimate	% predicted FVC P value	FEV1/FVC Parameter estimate	FEV1/FVC P value
Grant	Ever pressing	-2.07	0.37	-1.89	0.39	-0.06	0.97
Grant	Ever shaping	-3.69	0.16	-0.09	0.97	-3.18*	0.02*
Grant	Ever grinding	-1.62	0.55	-0.17	0.95	-1.19	0.38
Grant	Ever sandblasting	-9.96*	0.01*	-4.33	0.23	-4.60*	0.02*
Grant	Ever product testing	-5.21	0.16	-5.90**	0.09	-0.73	0.72
Gurley	Ever charging	-1.37	0.74	-2.11	0.58	0.49	0.82
Gurley	Ever mill/spray dry	-2.23	0.50	-1.95	0.52	-0.50	0.77
Huntsville	Ever zinc	2.72	0.39	3.40	0.25	0.44	0.79
Huntsville	Ever APT	4.15	0.23	0.09	0.98	4.39*++	0.02*
Grant/Gurley	Ever maintenance	-0.18	0.97	-0.12	0.98	-1.21	0.59

Predicted FEV1 and FVC are based on average lung volumes from asymptomatic never-smokers of the same age, gender, and height as the individual worker; * statistically significant (p < 0.05) comparisons are in bold with single asterisk; ** marginally significant (p < 0.10) comparisons; + workers who ever worked in these work areas, unrelated to which plant they currently are working (work areas grouped by plant for ease of identification as to where these work areas are currently located); parameter estimate is the unit change in FEV1/FVC ratio and in percent predicted FEV1 and FVC if ever worked in indicated work area, compared to workers who never worked in these work areas; ++ FEV1/FVC was increased in workers who had ever worked in APT.

Table 17. Prevalence rates (percent) of health outcomes in workers who <u>currently</u> work in certain work areas compared to workers who do not currently working in those work areas, September 2003, Metalworking Products

Health Outcome	Pressing Current (N=19)	Pressing Not Current (N=146)	Shaping Current (N=17)	Shaping Not Current (N=148)	Grinding Current (N=12)	Grinding Not Current (N=153)	Product Testing Current (N=8)	Product Testing Not Current (N=157)
Usual cough	26	24	12	26	25	24	38	23
Cough most days	21	16	12	17	17	16	25	16
Bronchitis since hire	42	30	18	32	17	32	38	31
Chronic bronchitis diagnosis	16	10	0	12	8	11	25	10
Short of breath when walking with others same age	21	17	18	18	25	17	50	38
Short of breath when hurrying on level ground or walking up a slight hill	37	38	41	38	50	37	50	38
Ever wheezed	32	51	47	49	17*	52*	63	48
Wheeze in last 12 months	16**	35	41	32	17	34	38	32
Woken up with wheeze within the last 4 weeks	16	16	29	15	8	17	25	16
Wheeze better away from work	11	12	12	12	8	12	0	13
Asthma diagnosis (ever)	11	17	12	17	17	16	25	16
Asthma diagnosis (current)	11	11	12	11	8	11	25	10
Obstruction +	0	8	19**	6	0	8	25	6
Restriction +	5	1	0	2	0	2	0	2
Abnormal spirometry +	5	10	19	8	0	10	25	8
Suspected post-hire asthma +	21	30	50**	27	17	30	25	29

* Statistically significant (p < 0.05) comparisons are in bold;
** Marginally significant (p < 0.10) comparisons;
\+ 3 participants did not have a spirometry test performed;
suspected post-hire asthma is defined as post-hire onset of asthma, 3 or more Venables' asthma symptoms, use of asthma medication, or obstruction on spirometry (workers with known pre-hire asthma were excluded); current workers in sandblasting were excluded due to small cell numbers.

Table 18. Prevalence rates (percent) of respiratory symptoms and spirometry test abnormalities in workers who <u>currently</u> work in certain work areas, compared to workers who do not work in those work areas, September 2003, Metalworking Products

	Mill/Spray Dry Current (N=7)	Mill/Spray Dry Not Current (N=158)	Zinc Current (N=16)	Zinc Not Current (N=149)	APT Current (N=15)	APT Not Current (N=150)	Grant/ Gurley Maintenance Current (N=9)	Grant/ Gurley Maintenance Not Current (N=156)
Usual cough	0	25	44*	22	27	24	22	24
Cough most days	0	17	25	15	20	16	22	16
Bronchitis since hire	14	32	25	32	33	31	0*	33
Chronic bronchitis diagnosis	0	11	13	10	0	11	11	10
Short of breath walking when with others same age	14	18	19	17	7	19	22	17
Short of breath when hurrying on level ground or walking up a slight hill	29	39	31	39	13*	41	33	38
Ever wheezed	14	51	44	49	33	51	33	50
Wheeze in last 12 months	0*	34	38	32	20	34	33	33
Woken up with wheeze within the last 4 weeks	0	17	19	16	7	17	22	16
Wheeze better away from work	0	13	13	12	13	12	33*	11
Asthma diagnosis (ever)	0	17	13	17	7	17	22	16
Asthma diagnosis (current)	0	11	6	11	7	11	22	10
Obstruction**	14	7	0	8	7	7	0	8
Restriction**	0	2	6	1	0	2	0	2
Abnormal spirometry**	14	9	6	10	7	10	0	10
Suspected post-hire asthma**	14	30	38	28	13	31	22	29

There were no statistically significant (p < 0.05) comparisons;
* marginally significant (p < 0.10) comparisons;
** 3 participants did not have a spirometry test performed;
suspected post-hire asthma is defined as post-hire onset of asthma, 3 or more Venables' asthma symptoms, use of asthma medication, or obstruction on spirometry (workers with known pre-hire asthma were excluded); current workers in charging were excluded due to small cell numbers

Table 19. Odds ratio comparisons (and 95% confidence intervals) of suspected post-hire asthma in workers who <u>currently</u> work in certain work areas compared to workers who do not currently work in these work areas, controlled for age, gender, and pack-years of smoking, September 2003, Metalworking Products

Current work area	Suspected post-hire asthma
Pressing	0.6 (0.2-2.0)
Shaping	2.8 (0.9-8.1)*
Grinding	0.5 (0.1-2.6)
Product Testing	0.7 (0.1-4.1)
Mill/Spray Dry	0.6 (0.1-5.6)
Zinc	1.9 (0.6-6.2)
APT	0.4 (0.1-1.7)
Maintenance	0.9 (0.2-4.9)

There were no statistically significant (p < 0.05) comparisons; * marginally significant (p < 0.10) comparisons; 3 participants did not have a spirometry test performed; current sandblasters and chargers were excluded due to small cell numbers; suspected post-hire asthma is defined as post-hire onset of asthma, 3 or more Venables' asthma symptoms, use of asthma medication, or obstruction on spirometry (workers with pre-hire asthma were excluded)

FIGURES

Prevalence rates (percent) of usual cough, physician-diagnosed bronchitis since hire, shortness of breath when walking with others the same age (SOB), ever having wheezed, current physician-diagnosed asthma, airways obstruction on spirometry, and any spirometry abnormality in workers who <u>previously</u> worked and who <u>currently</u> work in certain work areas, September 2003, Metalworking Products (Figures 1-3.)

Figure 1. Grinders

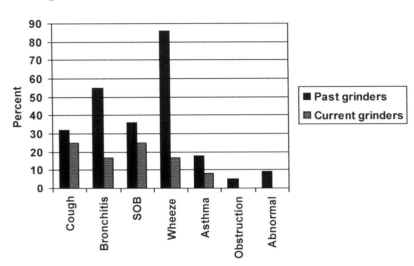

Figure 2. Pressers

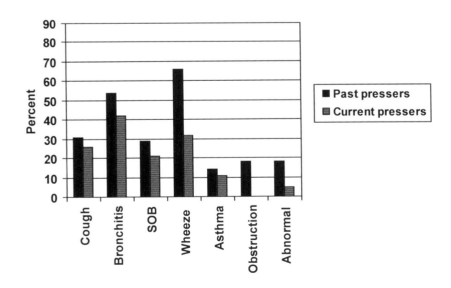

Figure 3. Shapers

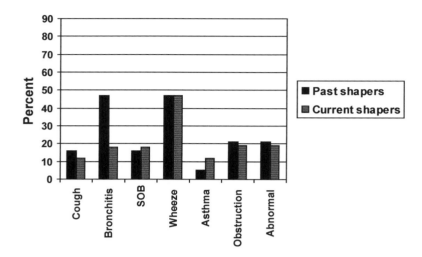

APPENDIX A: BACKGROUND INFORMATION

Background Information on Cobalt

Cobalt can be absorbed by the lungs, gastrointestinal tract, and skin. Based on studies using cobalt oxide, approximately 30% of the cobalt that is inhaled is absorbed. Lung absorption is greatly increased in the presence of tungsten carbide.[1] Based on studies using cobalt chloride, approximately 5% to 20% of ingested cobalt is absorbed. Skin absorption occurs with prolonged skin contact with cobalt dust or cobalt-contaminated MWF. Absorption is probably much higher with exposure to contaminated MWF than with cobalt dust. In a human experiment, a subject who held his hand in a mixture of cobalt and tungsten carbide powder for 90 minutes, demonstrated a 10-fold increase in urinary cobalt levels (his urinary cobalt level increased from 0.2 μg cobalt/L to 20 μg cobalt/L.[2] Cobalt is rapidly and primarily excreted in the urine for the first few days following an exposure to cobalt. However, the remainder of retained cobalt is more slowly excreted over a number of years.[3] Urine cobalt levels obtained prior to shift at the beginning of the work week reflect long-term exposure, whereas end of the shift, end of the work week urinary levels indicate cumulative exposures from the week. In a study of three hard metal manufacturing factories, average worker urine cobalt levels prior to a 24-, 31-, and 38-day factory shut-down (summer holiday) were 112, 62, and 41 μg cobalt /L, respectively. Average worker urine cobalt levels immediately prior to return and at the end of shift of the first week back at work in these three factories were 25, 5, and 4; and 74, 48, 30 μg cobalt /L, respectively.[2] Percent declines in urine cobalt levels due to the approximately one month vacations were 87/112 (78%), 57/62 (92%), and 37/41(90%), respectively.

Cobalt exposure has been associated with upper airway irritation, cough, poor lung function,[4,5] occupational asthma, interstitial lung disease, heart muscle damage (cardiomyopathy), and allergic contact dermatitis. Individual susceptibility may be a major factor in determining which workers develop asthma and a scarring lung disease called hard metal pneumoconiosis. Workers with average exposures lower than 0.1 milligram (mg) cobalt/cubic meter (m^3) of air have developed hard metal pneumoconiosis and, in at least one case, this disease occurred with an average exposure of 0.003 mg cobalt/m^3.[6] An immune-mediated etiology has been proposed for both cobalt asthma and hard metal pneumoconiosis based on the following findings: 1) presence of cobalt antibodies in some workers with cobalt asthma;[7] and 2) recurrence of giant cell pneumonitis in a transplanted lung in one worker.[8] Based on spirometry test results, less than 1% of all hard metal workers have evidence of hard metal pneumoconiosis. When chest x-rays are used, this increases to 3.8%.[9] Airways obstruction among non-smokers,[9] cobalt asthma,[10] and work-related wheeze[9] prevalence rates among hard metal workers have been estimated at 5%, 5.6%, and 10.9%, respectively.

A minimum of several months of exposure to cobalt is usually required before a worker will develop cobalt asthma. Age and atopy (i.e. history of eczema, hayfever, or asthma) are risk factors.[11] Once cobalt asthma develops, symptoms usually occur after 4 to 8 hours of work exposure. In one study, the risk of work-related wheeze doubles with higher current cobalt exposures (0.05-0.1 mg cobalt/m^3 compared to < 0.05 mg cobalt/m^3).[6]

Hard metal pneumoconiosis occurs in workers exposed to both cobalt and tungsten carbide. Common early symptoms include dry cough with minimal amount of sputum and shortness of breath on exertion. The disease may develop after as little as 2 years from the time of first exposure, but usually 10 to12 years is required.[12] Exposure for the entire time period is not necessary. As the disease progresses lung function tests become abnormal (restriction on spirometry and decreased lung diffusing capacity). The disease is usually not reversible, even when there is no further exposure. Animals exposed to a cobalt air level of 0.1 mg cobalt/m^3 have developed early stages of lung scarring.

If a lung biopsy is performed on a worker with interstitial lung disease and large cells with many nuclei (giant cells) are seen in the air sacs (alveoli) of the lung, the condition is referred to as giant cell pneumonitis.[13] Giant cell pneumonitis has been seen in grinders, powder mixers, and shapers.[14]

Several cases of cardiomyopathy have been diagnosed in workers with elevated cobalt levels in heart tissue or blood.[15-17] Two studies in hard metal workers demonstrated an association between cobalt exposure and poor heart function (left ventricular ejection fraction).[18,19] Animal studies have confirmed this association.[20-22] An allergic skin rash may result from skin exposure to cobalt. Other effects of cobalt exposure include increased number of red blood cells and thyroid enlargement.

Background Information on Tungsten

Tungsten carbide does not cause injury in animals exposed to tungsten carbide alone.[13] However, in laboratory studies, uptake of cobalt by immune system cells (macrophages) is enhanced in the presence of tungsten carbide.[23]

Background Information on Metalworking Fluids (MWFs)

Exposure to MWFs is associated with respiratory symptoms, decreased lung function,[24,25] asthma,[26-29] and hypersensitivity pneumonitis (HP).[30,31] Hypersensitivity pneumonitis may cause either respiratory and/or non-respiratory symptoms. Respiratory symptoms consist of cough and shortness of breath on exertion. Non-respiratory symptoms include fever, chills, fatigue, decreased appetite, and weight loss. Lung scarring may result if workers continue to be exposed. When this occurs, lung function tests typically show a pattern of restriction and decreased lung diffusing capacity. Important exposures include the components of the MWF, additives (e.g. biocides), metals, and microbial contamination.

Outbreaks of HP in workers exposed to MWF have been thought to be due to microbial contamination of the MWF by mycobacteria, gram-positive bacteria, and/or fungi. In several instances, high numbers of *Mycobacterium chelonae* were present in water-based MWFs.

MWF-related asthma may be the result of aggravation of pre-existing asthma or MWF may cause asthma to develop (MWF asthma). MWF components (ethanolamine, colophony, pine oil, tall oil), additives (formaldehyde, chlorine), and contaminants (chromium, nickel, cobalt, tungsten carbide, bacteria, fungi, and endotoxin) have been associated with MWF-related asthma. The usual latency period for MWF asthma is 12 years with a range from under 1 year to up to 41 years.[32]

References

1. Lasfargues G et al. [1992] Comparative study of the acute lung toxicity of pure cobalt powder and cobalt-tungsten carbide mixture in rat. Toxicol Appl Pharmacol 112:41-50.

2. Scansetti G, Botta GC, Spinelli P et al. [1994]. Absorption and excretion of cobalt in the hard metal industry. Sci Total Environ 150:141-144.

3. Elinder CG, Friberg L. Cobalt. In: Friberg L, Norbers G, Vouk V, eds. Handbook on the Toxicology of Metals. 2nd ed. Vol II. Amsterdam (Belgium): Elsevier Science Publishers, 1986.

4. Nemery B, Casier P, Roosels D et al. [1992]. Survey of cobalt exposure and respiratory health in diamond polishers. Am Rev Respir Dis 145:610-616.

5. Kusaka Y, Ichikawa Y, Shirakawa T et al. [1986]. Effect of hard metal dust on ventilatory function. BMJ 43:486-489.

6. Sprince NL, Oliver LC, Eisen EA et al. [1988]. Cobalt exposure and lung disease in tungsten carbide production. Am Rev Respir Dis 138:1220-1226.

7. Shirakawa T, Kusaka Y, Fujimura N et al. [1989]. Occupational asthma from cobalt sensitivity in workers exposed to hard metal dust. Chest 95:29-37.

8. Frost AE, Keller CA, Brown RW et al. [1993]. Giant cell interstitial pneumonitis. Am Rev Respir Dis 148:1401-1404.

9. Sprince NL, Chamberlin RI, Hales CA et al. [1984] Respiratory disease in tungsten carbide production workers. Chest 86(4): 549-557.

10. Kusaka Y, Yokoyama K, Sera Y, et al. [1986]. Respiratory diseases in hard metal workers: an occupational hygiene study in a factory. Br J Ind Med 43:474-485.

11. Kusaka Y, Iki M, Kumagai S et al. [1996]. Epidemiological study of hard metal asthma. Occup Environ Med 53:188-193.

12. Barceloux D. [1999]. Cobalt. Clinical Toxicology 37(2):201-216.

13. Cugell DW, Morgan KC, Perkins DG et al. [1990]. The respiratory effects of cobalt. Arch Intern Med 150:177-183.

14. Ohori NP, Sciurba FC, Owens GR et al. [1989]. Giant-cell interstitial pneumonia and hard-metal pneumoconiosis. Am J Surg Pathol 13(7): 581-587.

15. Jarvis JQ, Hammond E, Meier R et al. [1992]. Cobalt cardiomyopathy: a report of two cases from mineral assay laboratories and a review of the literature. J Occup Env Med 34:620-626.

16. Barborik M, Dusek J. [1972]. Cardiomyopathy accompanying industrial cobalt exposure. Br Heart J 34:113-116.

17. Kennedy A, King R, Dornan JD. [1981]. Fatal cardiac disease associated with industrial exposure to cobalt. Lancet 1(8217):412-414.

18. Horowitz SF, Fischbein A, Matza D, et al. [1988]. Evaluation of right left ventricular function in hard metal workers. British Journal of Industrial Medicine 1988:742-746.

19. D'Adda F, Borleri D, Migliori M, et al. [1994]. Cardiac function study in hard metal workers. Sci Total Environ 150:179-186.

20. Mohiuddin SM, Taskar PK, Rheault M, et al. [1970]. Experimental cobalt cardiomyopathy. Am Heart J 80(4):532-543.

21. Speijers GJA, Krajnc EI, Berkvens JM, et al. [1982]. Acute oral toxicity of inorganic cobalt compounds in rats. Food Chem Toxicol 20:311-314.

22. Morvai V, Szakmary E, Tatrai E, et al. [1993]. The effects of simultaneous alcohol and cobalt. Acta Physiol Hung 81 (3):253-61.

23. Lison D, Lauwerys R [1990]. In vitro cytotoxic effects of cobalt-containing dusts on mouse peritoneal and rat alveolar macrophages. Environ Res 52:187-198.

24. Robins T, Seixas N, Franzblau A et al. [1997]. Acute respiratory effects on workers exposed to metalworking fluid aerosols in an automotive transmission plant. Am J Ind Med 31:510-524.

25. Eisen E, Smith T, Kriebel D et al. [2001]. Respiratory health of automobile workers and exposures to metal-working fluid aerosols: lung spirometry. Am J Ind Med 39:443-453.

26. Chan-Yeung M, Malo J-L [1995]. Compendium I: table of the major inducers of occupational asthma. In: Bernstein IL, Chan-Yeung M, Malo J-L, Bernstein DI, eds. Asthma in the workplace. New York, NY: Marcel-Dekker, Inc., pp. 595-623.

27. Savonius B, Keskinen H, Tuppurainene M et al. [1994]. Occupational asthma caused by ethanolamines. Allergy 49:877-881.

28. Rosenman K, Reilly M, Kalinowski D [1997]. Work-related asthma and respiratory symptoms among workers exposed to metal-working fluids. Am J Ind Med 32:325-331.

29. Kreibel D, Sama S, Woskie S et al. [1997]. A field investigation of the acute respiratory effects of metal working fluids. I: Effects of aerosol exposures. Am J Ind Med 31:756-766.

30. Kreiss K, Cox-Ganser J [1997]. Metalworking fluid-associated hypersensitivity pneumonitis: a workshop summary. Am J Ind Med 32:423-432.

31. Hodgson M, Bracker A, Yang C et al. [2001]. Hypersensitivity pneumonitis in a metal-working environment. Am J Ind Med 39:616-628.

32. Robertson As, Weir DC, Burge PS. [1988]. Occupational asthma due to oil mists. Thorax 43(3):200-205.

APPENDIX B: EVALUATION CRITERIA

Cobalt

The Occupational Safety and Health Administration (OSHA) Permissible Exposure Limit (PEL)[1] for cobalt (metal, dust, and fume) as a time-weighted average (TWA) over an 8-hour shift for a 40-hour work week is 0.1 mg cobalt/m^3. The American Conference of Governmental Industrial Hygienists (ACGIH) Threshold Limit Value (TLV)[2] for cobalt (elemental and inorganic compounds) as a TWA over an 8-hour shift for a 40-hour workweek is 0.02 mg cobalt/m^3. The National Institute for Occupational Safety and Health (NIOSH) Recommended Exposure Limit (REL)[3] for cobalt (metal, dust, and fume) as a TWA over a 10-hour shift for a 40 hour workweek is 0.05 mg cobalt/m^3. NIOSH recommends that manufacturers and users of all cobalt compounds perform industrial hygiene surveys at a minimum of every 3 years.[4]

The ACGIH Biological Exposure Indices (BEIs)[2] for cobalt are 1 μg cobalt/L in the blood and 15 μg cobalt/L in urine. Test time should be at the end of shift at end of work week for both blood and urine tests. Cobalt blood levels in workers exposed to soluble cobalt compounds (metal, salts, and hard metals), but not in workers exposed to insoluble cobalt compounds (cobalt oxide), correspond to the level of recent exposure.[5] NIOSH recommends pre-placement and periodic examinations for workers exposed to cobalt. Examinations should include a medical history and physical examination (with special attention to the lung, skin, and thyroid gland and, if there is a potential for high level exposure, the cardiac and hematologic systems).[4]

Metal Working Fluids (MWFs)

NIOSH recommends a MWF aerosol occupational exposure limit of 0.4 mg/m^3 (thoracic particulate mass) as a 10-hour TWA.[6] This corresponds to approximately 0.5 mg/m^3 for total particulate mass. OSHA and ACGIH have not set occupational exposure limits for MWF. No occupational exposure limits exist for the amount of endotoxin, bacterial, or suspended cobalt allowable in MWFs. Researchers suggest that well-maintained MWFs have bacterial contamination less than 10^6 colony forming units (CFU)/mL fluid. Typical bacterial counts are 10^5 to 10^7 CFU/mL fluid. Cobalt in MWF may have a greater toxicity than cobalt in the form of a dry powder. MWF cobalt levels can increase to 200 μg/g (approximately 200 mg/L) in some MWFs within the first few weeks of use.[7]

References

1. CFR [1999]. 29CFR 1910.1000 Code of Federal Regulations. Washington, DC: U.S. Government Printing Office, Office of the Federal Register.

2. ACGIH [2003]. 2003 TLVs and BEIs; Threshold Limit Values for Chemical Substances and Physical Agents. Cincinnati, OH: American Conference of Governmental Industrial Hygienists.

3. NIOSH [2003]. Pocket guide to chemical hazards. Cincinnati, OH: U.S. Department of Health and Human Services, Public Health Service, Centers for Disease Control and Prevention, National Institute for Occupational Safety and Health, DHHS (NIOSH) publication No. 97-140.

4. DHHS (NIOSH). Criteria for Controlling Occupational Exposure to Cobalt. Publication No. 82-107. 1981.

5. Lison E, Buchet JP, Swennen B et al. [1994]. Biological monitoring of workers exposed to cobalt metal, salt, oxides, and hard metal dust. Occup Environ Med 51:447-450.

6. DHHS (NIOSH). Criteria for a Recommended Standard, Occupational Exposure to Metalworking Fluids. Publication No. 98-102. 1998.

7. Sjogren I, Hillerdal G, Andersson A et al. [1980]. Hard metal lung disease: importance of cobalt in coolants. Thorax 35:653-659.

DEPARTMENT OF HEALTH & HUMAN SERVICES

Phone: (304) 285-5751
Fax: (304) 285-5820

Public Health Service

Centers for Disease Control
and Prevention (CDC)
National Institute for Occupational
Safety and Health (NIOSH)
1095 Willowdale Road
Morgantown, WV 26505-2888

March 2, 2005
HETA 2003-0257
Interim Letter II

Mr. Steve Robuck
Director of Safety and Environment
Metalworking Products
1 Teledyne Place
La Vergne, Tennessee 37086

Dear Mr. Robuck:

The purpose of this letter is to report the progress of National Institute for Occupational Safety and Health (NIOSH) industrial hygiene surveys at the Alldyne Powder Technologies plants located in Huntsville and Gurley, Alabama and the Firth Sterling plant located in Grant, Alabama. NIOSH surveyed these plants in July 2003, May 2004, October 2004, and November 2004 in response to a confidential employee request concerning respiratory health effects and exposure to cobalt, nickel, chromium, tungsten carbide, and metalworking fluids.

The purpose, types of samples collected, and available results for each industrial hygiene survey are summarized below. A concluding discussion and recommendations follow the summaries of the four surveys.

Sincerely,

Nancy M. Sahakian, M.D., M.P.H.

Aleksandr Stefaniak, Ph.D.
Respiratory Disease Hazard Evaluation and
Technical Assistance Program
Field Studies Branch
Division of Respiratory Disease Studies

cc:
Confidential Requesters

July 7 – 8, 2003

Survey goal:

Perform a walk-through survey of the Alldyne Powder Technologies plants located in Huntsville and Gurley, Alabama and the Firth Sterling plant located in Grant, Alabama to understand the production process and collect preliminary information.

Samples collected:

As summarized in the Interim Letter 1 (dated February 20, 2004) previously sent to you, bulk samples of unused RichGrind™ metalworking fluid (MWF), in-use MWF from a centerless grinder, liquid sludge in the MWF filter system, and solid sludge in the MWF filter system were collected during this survey.

All bulk samples were analyzed for cobalt and nickel content by a laboratory accredited for metals analysis by the American Industrial Hygiene Association (AIHA) Industrial Hygiene Laboratory Accreditation Program (IHLAP). A portion of the bulk samples of unused and in-use MWF were analyzed by a laboratory accredited for microbiological analysis by the AIHA Environmental Microbiology Laboratory Accreditation Program (EMLAP) to determine levels of endotoxin (a component of gram-negative bacteria), and culturable fungi, bacteria, and mycobacteria. The analytical limits of detection (LOD) and quantification (LOQ) for cobalt were 0.8 and 3 µg/g, respectively; the LOD and LOQ for nickel were 1 and 4 µg/g, respectively. The LOD for endotoxin was 0.005 endotoxin units per milliliter (EU/ml) (LOQ was not available) and the LOD for fungal and bacterial growth was 100 colony forming units per milliliter (CFU/ml) (LOQ was not available).

Results:

As summarized in Interim Letter 1 (dated February 20, 2004) previously sent to you, levels of cobalt or nickel in the samples of unused and in-use MWF were ≤ 1 µg/g. Levels of cobalt or nickel in the samples of liquid sludge and solid sludge did not exceed 6600 µg/g. Endotoxin and culturable fungi, bacteria, or microbacteria were not detected in the sample of unused MWF. In the sample of in-use MWF from a centerless grinder, 200 EU/ml were detected. In this same sample culturable fungi or mycobateria were not detected, but 1700 CFU/ml of culturable bacteria was measured.

May 20 – 27, 2004

Survey goal:

Characterize the amount, size distribution, and number concentration of airborne particles at various steps in the hard metal production processes utilized at the Alldyne Powder Technologies plants located in Huntsville and Gurley, Alabama and the Firth Sterling plant located in Grant, Alabama.

Samples collected:

Micro-orifice uniform deposit impactor (MOUDI)

Seventeen samples of airborne particles were collected in seven different work areas (see Table I) using micro-orifice uniform deposit impactor (MOUDI) samplers (Model 110, MSP Corporation, Shoreview, MN). The aerodynamic diameter cut points for the MOUDI sampler were >18 µm (pre-filter), 10 µm (stage 1), 5.6 µm (stage 2), 3.2 µm (stage 3), 1.8 µm (stage 4), 1.0 µm (stage 5), 0.56 µm (Stage 6), 0.32 µm (stage 7), 0.18 µm (stage 8), 0.10 µm (stage 9), 0.056 µm (stage 10), and <0.056 (final filter). Fifteen of the 17 samples were collected on polyvinyl chloride (PVC) substrate and two of the 17 samples were collected on mixed cellulose ester (MCE) substrate. All substrates were sprayed with silicone to prevent particle bounce during sampling. All PVC substrates were pre- and post-weighed at NIOSH to determine the mass of particulate matter collected on the substrates. All substrates were submitted for analysis of cobalt, chromium, and nickel content in accordance with NIOSH Method 7300 by a laboratory accredited for metals analysis by the AIHA IHLAP. The LOD and LOQ for cobalt were 0.2 and 0.6 μg/filter, respectively; the LOD and LOQ for chromium were 0.3 and 1 μg/filter, respectively; and, the LOD and LOQ for nickel were 0.4 and 1 μg/filter, respectively. Analyses of data from the MOUDI samples included an estimate of total particle mass concentration, total particle size distribution, total element mass concentration, element size distribution, and element mass fraction information as a function of particle size.

Marple cascade impactor

Eleven samples of airborne particles were collected in seven different work areas (see Tables II and III) using Marple series 290 8-stage cascade impactor samplers. Five of the eleven cascade impactor samples were positioned in the personal breathing zone of employees during the course of their normal work activities. The remaining six cascade impactor samples were collected at a stationary location in a work area during specific process activities. The aerodynamic diameter cut points for the cascade impactor sampler were >21.3 μm (stage 1), 14.8 μm (stage 2), 9.8 μm (stage 3), 6.0 μm (stage 4), 3.5 μm (stage 5), 1.55 μm (stage 6), 0.93 μm (stage 7), 0.52 μm (stage 8), and <0.52 (final filter). All 11 samples were collected on PVC substrate that was sprayed with silicone to prevent particle bounce during sampling.

All substrates were analyzed for cobalt, chromium, and nickel content in accordance with NIOSH Method 7300 by a laboratory accredited for metals analysis by the AIHA IHLAP. The LOD and LOQ for cobalt were 0.3 and 1 μg/filter, respectively; the LOD and LOQ for chromium were 0.7 and 2 μg/filter, respectively; and, the LOD and LOQ for nickel were 0.9 and 3 μg/filter, respectively. Analyses of data from the Marple impactor samples included an estimate of total element mass concentration and element size distribution. For analysis of element size distribution data, a value reported by the analytical laboratory was considered a real number if it was between the LOD and LOQ. The LOD was substituted for a value reported as <LOD provided at least 85% of the mass on all substrates in a sample was contributed by measured values (i.e., values above the LOQ). Note that an alternative approach for censored data is to substitute a value of one-half the LOD for a value reported as <LOD, but this substitution would not have an appreciable effect on the reported results.

37-mm open- and close-faced filter cassette

Twenty six half-shift or full-shift samples of airborne particles were collected in 12 different work areas (see Tables IV and V) using 37-mm cassette samplers. Eighteen of the 26 cassette samples were positioned in the personal breathing zone of employees during the course of their normal work activities. The remaining eight cassette samples were collected at stationary locations in work areas during specific process activities. Close- and open-faced cassette samples were collected on MCE substrate. Note that close-faced sampling is standard practice for cobalt; however, open-faced cassette samples were collected to ensure even distribution of particles on the substrate, regardless of size, during sampling. One personal cassette sample was voided because the cassette fell on the ground for an unknown period of time during sampling.

All substrates were analyzed for cobalt, chromium, and nickel content in accordance with NIOSH Method 7300 by a laboratory accredited for metals analysis by the AIHA IHLAP. The LOD and LOQ for cobalt were 0.02 and 0.07 μg/filter, respectively; the LOD and LOQ for chromium were 0.06 and 0.2 μg/filter, respectively; and, the LOD and LOQ for nickel were 0.04 and 0.1 μg/filter, respectively.

GRIMM particle size and number concentration

Fourteen samples of airborne particle size distribution and number concentration were determined in seven different work areas using optical particle counters (Model 1.108, GRIMM Technologies Inc., Douglasville, GA). Optical particle count samples were collected at stationary locations in work areas during specific process activities. The GRIMM particle counter units cover the physical size range 0.3 µm to >20 µm in 15 channels: >0.3 µm, >0.4 µm, >0.5 µm, >0.65 µm, >0.8 µm, >1.0 µm, >1.6 µm, >2.0 µm, >3 µm, >4 µm, >5 µm, >7.5 µm, >10 µm, >15 µm, and >20 µm. To ensure adequate counting statistics, two GRIMM units were operated in tandem at each work area in the fast-sampling-time mode (collection of data every second). One unit covered channels 1 through 8: >0.3 µm, >0.4 µm, >0.5 µm, >0.65 µm, >0.8 µm, >1.0 µm, >1.6 µm, and >2.0 µm and the second unit covered channels 8 through 15: >2.0 µm, >3 µm, >4 µm, >5 µm, >7.5 µm, >10 µm, >15 µm, and >20 µm. Note that channel eight was overlapped by both sampling units.

Results

Note that all results reported for the May 2004 survey are preliminary results and a summary of completed final results will be reported in a future letter.

Micro-orifice uniform deposit impactor (MOUDI)

Total cobalt and nickel concentrations determined using MOUDI samplers are summarized in Table I. The level of cobalt in air ranged from <LOD (Pressing) to 1321 µg/m^3 (Charging) and nickel levels were generally low as evidenced by the LOD being exceeded in just two of the 17 samples. Chromium levels were similar to background levels in substrate for all samples.

Figure 1 is a histogram showing the measured particle cobalt mass distribution for a sample collected during the loading of crucibles in Zinc A (while a crusher was in operation). The y-axis of the plot is sample mass collected on an impactor stage normalized for the aerodynamic particle size interval of the stage and the x-axis of the plot is aerodynamic diameter. The shape of the histogram is representative of the histograms plotted for cobalt and nickel at the remaining six work areas and indicates that the data are log-normally distributed. The mass median aerodynamic diameter (MMAD) and geometric standard deviation (GSD) of cobalt and nickel particles are also included in Table I. Aerodynamic diameter is the diameter of a spherical particle with density 1 g/cm^3 that has the equivalent settling velocity as the particle under study. The MMAD is the aerodynamic diameter above which 50% of the particles have greater mass and below which 50% of the particles have less mass. In a log-normal distribution, 68% of the particles fall within the size range MMAD/GSD to MMAD×GSD and 95% of particles fall within the size range MMAD/GSD^2 to MMAD×GSD^2. With the exception of grinding, the MMAD was generally greater than 10 µm in most work areas. Note that estimates of total particle concentration, total particle size distribution, and cobalt particle size distribution were not completed for all samples at the time this letter was written.

Marple cascade impactor

Total cobalt, chromium, and nickel concentrations measured in the personal breathing zone of employees using Marple impactor samplers are summarized in Table II. The level of cobalt in air ranged from 11 (Shaping) to 311 µg/m^3 (Milling at Gurley), chromium levels were generally semi-quantitative (i.e., between the LOD and LOQ), and airborne nickel levels ranged from <LOD (Screening, Shaping, Tray Prep) to 104 µg/m^3 (Charging).

The MMAD and GSD of cobalt and nickel particles are included in Table II. For all work areas sampled, calculated MMAD were greater than 10 µm.

Total cobalt concentrations measured at stationary locations in different work areas using Marple impactor samplers are summarized in Table III. The level of cobalt in air ranged from <LOD (Sandblasting) to 139 $\mu g/m^3$ (Spokane crusher in Zinc B). Nickel and chromium levels in all samples were <LOD.

The MMAD and GSD of cobalt particles measured in area samples are also included in Table III. With the exception of tray prep, MMAD were greater than 10 μm for all work areas in which cobalt was measured.

37-mm open- and close-faced filter cassette

Total cobalt, chromium, and nickel concentrations measured in the personal breathing zones of employees using close- and open-faced 37-mm cassette samplers are summarized in Table IV. Levels of cobalt ranged from 1.6 (Shipping at Grant) to 815 $\mu g/m^3$ (Charging), chromium levels ranged from <LOD (Zinc B) to 2.9 $\mu g/m^3$ (Milling), and airborne nickel levels ranged from 0.2 (Extrusion) to 805 $\mu g/m^3$ (Charging).

Total cobalt, chromium, and nickel concentrations measured at stationary locations in different work areas using close- and open-faced 37-mm cassette samplers are summarized in Table V. The level of cobalt in air ranged from 0.7 (Sandblasting) to 556 $\mu g/m^3$ (Zinc A). Chromium levels in air did not exceed approximately 6 $\mu g/m^3$ in any of the work areas sampled, and airborne nickel levels were below 3.5 $\mu g/m^3$.

GRIMM particle size and number concentration

The fourteen optical particle counter measurements were recorded at stationary locations in Charging, Screening, Blending, Grinding, Tray Prep, Zinc A, and Zinc B. Efforts are ongoing to combine the count data from the two units used to collect each sample and merge the data from the overlapped channel (>2 μm).

October 25 – November 2, 2004

Survey goal:

Estimate personal breathing zone full-shift exposure to cobalt, chromium, nickel, tungsten, and MWF using total dust and particle size-selective samplers in pre-identified work areas throughout the Alldyne Powder Technologies plants located in Huntsville and Gurley, Alabama and the Firth Sterling plant located in Grant, Alabama.

Samples collected:

Marple cascade impactor

One hundred eight (108) samples of airborne particles were collected in 27 different work areas using Marple series 290 8-stage cascade impactor samplers positioned in the personal breathing zones of employees during the course of their normal work activities. The aerodynamic diameter cut points for the cascade impactor sampler were >21.3 μm (stage 1), 14.8 μm (stage 2), 9.8 μm (stage 3), 6.0 μm (stage 4), 3.5 μm (stage 5), 1.55 μm (stage 6), 0.93 μm (stage 7), 0.52 μm (stage 8), and <0.52 (final filter). All samples were collected on pre-weighed PVC substrate that was sprayed with silicone to prevent particle bounce during sampling.

All PVC substrates were post-weighed at NIOSH to determine the mass of particulate matter collected on the substrates.

37-mm close-faced filter cassette

Two hundred fifty two (252) samples of airborne particles were collected in the same 27 work areas as above, but using 37-mm cassette samplers. All close-faced cassette samples were collected on pre-weighed PVC substrate positioned in the personal breathing zones of employees during the course of their normal work activities. One sample was discarded because the air sampling pump faulted during collection, yielding a net of 251 samples.

All PVC substrates were submitted for determination of total dust in accordance with NIOSH Method 0500, and cobalt, chromium, and nickel content in accordance with NIOSH Method 7300, and tungsten content in accordance with NIOSH Method 7074 by a laboratory accredited for metals analysis by the AIHA IHLAP. The LOD for total dust was 0.02 mg (LOQ was not available). At the time this letter was written, samples were being analyzed for cobalt, chromium, nickel, and tungsten content.

37-mm close-faced filter cassette for MWF

Sixteen (16) samples of airborne particles were collected in the grinding area at the Grant, AL plant using 37-mm cassette samplers. Eight (8) of the 16 close-faced cassette samples were collected on pre-weighed polytetrafluoroethylene (PTFE) substrate positioned in the personal breathing zones of employees during the course of their normal work activities. The remaining eight cassette samples were collected at different stationary locations in the grinding work area.

All PTFE substrates were submitted for determination of total dust and MWF by gravimetric analysis in accordance with NIOSH Method 5524. The LOD for total dust was 0.01 mg and the LOQ was 0.04 mg. The LOD for MWF was 0.01 mg and the LOQ was 0.03 mg.

Results

Marple cascade impactor

At the time this letter was written, filter post-sampling weight results were being reviewed and used to develop a strategy to submit samples for determination of cobalt, chromium, nickel, and tungsten content in accordance with NIOSH standard methods as noted above.

37-mm close-faced filter cassette

Total dust levels for the cassette samples are summarized by work area in Table VI. Dust levels ranged from 21.7 $\mu g/m^3$ (Powder laboratory) to 10, 859.2 $\mu g/m^3$ (Reprocessing at Gurley). The dustiest work areas tended to be the areas where bulk material handling and comminution processes were performed (*e.g.*, Zinc reclamation, Reprocessing, Charging, and Screening). The least dusty areas tended to be areas where solid final product was handled and where engineering controls currently exist (Sandblasting, Product Testing, and Shipping at Grant). Total dust levels were <LOD for three of the 251 cassette samples (one sample each in the Powder Laboratory, Shaping, and Milling).

37-mm close-faced filter cassette for MWF

Total dust level, MWF level, and the fraction of dust mass accounted by MWF for the personal breathing zone and area PTFE cassette samples are summarized Table VII. With the exception of one personal sample, total dust levels did not exceed 0.5 mg/m³ in any of the samples. One employee spray painted during his/her shift and had a total dust exposure of 3.47 mg/m³. For all personal and area samples, MWF concentrations were generally below 0.4 mg/m³. Note that the MWF exposure concentration for the employee who spray painted was similar to levels measured for other employees and on the area samples indicating that the elevated total dust exposure was probably due to spray paint overspray. The mass fraction of total dust that was accounted for by MWF ranged from 0.09 to 0.88.

Figure 2 illustrates the relationship between MWF concentration and total dust concentration for personal breathing zone samples and for area samples. The plot of personal breathing zone sampling results does not include the sample from employee who spray painted during his/her shift. In general, levels of MWF were positively related to levels of dustiness in the grinding work area as indicated by the positive R^2 values given in the plots (personal samples $R^2 = 0.89$; area samples $R^2 = 0.98$). An R^2 value is an estimate of the relationship between two variables and can range from -1 (exact negative linear relationship) to 1 (exact positive linear relationship).

November 7 – 12, 2004

Survey goal:

Conduct a dermal exposure assessment to determine concentrations of cobalt on surfaces in work areas, estimate the masses of cobalt on workers' hands, and estimate the transfer of cobalt from workers' hands to their necks throughout the Alldyne Powder Technologies plants located in Huntsville and Gurley, Alabama and the Firth Sterling plant located in Grant, Alabama. A secondary goal of the survey was to collect particle size-selective samples on filters to test the hypotheses that airborne particle physicochemical properties vary 1) as a function of production process, *i.e.* become more heterogeneous as raw materials are processed into final product, and 2) vary as a function of particle size within production processes.

Samples collected:

Dermal exposure assessment

Surface wipe sampling

A total of 156 surface wipe samples were collected (six surfaces within each of 26 pre-designated work areas selected for wipe sampling). Note that the work areas selected for wipe sampling were generally the same as the work areas in which air samples were collected during the October 2004 survey. One notable exception was the inclusion of administrative employees in the November survey. Each sample was collected from a surface routinely contacted by employees using a 10-cm x 10-cm disposable template in accordance with NIOSH Method 9100 and a moistened substrate (ASTM Method E1792).

All substrates were submitted for determination of cobalt, chromium, and nickel content in accordance with NIOSH Method 7300, and tungsten content in accordance with NIOSH Method 7074 by a laboratory accredited for metals analysis by the AIHA IHLAP.

Dermal wipe sampling

Prior to the start of each work shift employees in production work areas (n = 26), administrative staff that enter the production areas (n = 13), and administrative staff that do not enter production areas (n = 2) provided dermal swipe samples of their hands and neck using a moistened substrate. At a pre-determined time during the work shift, but not less than 3.5 hours after their shift started, dermal wipe samples of hands and neck were again collected from each employee. A total of 114 dermal wipe samples of hands and 114 dermal wipe samples of necks were collected during the survey.

All substrates were submitted for determination of cobalt, chromium, and nickel content in accordance with NIOSH Method 7300, and tungsten content in accordance with NIOSH Method 7074 by a laboratory accredited for metals analysis by the AIHA IHLAP.

Micro-orifice uniform deposit impactor (MOUDI)

Seventeen samples of airborne particles were collected in 17 different work areas using MOUDI samplers (Model 110, MSP Corporation, Shoreview, MN). The aerodynamic diameter cut points for the MOUDI sampler were >18 µm (pre-filter), 10 µm (stage 1), 5.6 µm (stage 2), 3.2 µm (stage 3), 1.8 µm (stage 4), 1.0 µm (stage 5), 0.56 µm (Stage 6), 0.32 µm (stage 7), 0.18 µm (stage 8), 0.10 µm (stage 9), 0.056 µm (stage 10), and <0.056 (final filter). All samples were collected on MCE substrate. To prevent particle bounce during sampling and to minimize the opportunity of contaminating the chemistry of collected particles, only the pre-filter of each sample substrate was sprayed with silicone.

Planned analyses of substrate include transmission electron microscopy (TEM) to assess particle morphology (shape and size) and energy dispersive x-ray spectrometry (XEDS) to assess particle elemental chemistry. At the time this letter was written, substrates were not yet analyzed.

Results

Dermal exposure assessment

At the time this letter was written, surface wipe and dermal wipe samples were submitted to the analytical laboratory and were in the queue for analysis of cobalt, chromium, nickel, and tungsten levels.

Micro-orifice uniform deposit impactor (MOUDI)

At the time this letter was written, substrates were not yet analyzed.

Discussion

Metal Working Fluids (MWF)

As summarized in the Interim Letter 1 (dated February 20, 2004) previously sent to you, levels of cobalt measured in bulk samples (collected July 2003) of unused RichGrind™ MWF and in-use MWF from a centerless grinder were low. The form of cobalt detected in these bulk samples (dissolved or undissolved particles) is unknown. However, according to the product manufacturer, RichGrind™ MWF is specifically formulated to minimize dissolution of cobalt particles entrapped in the MWF. Levels of endotoxin and culturable fungi and bacteria (including mycobacteria) in these bulk samples were generally low and or not detectable. Note that no safe level (legal or recommended) currently exists for endotoxin or culturable fungi or bacteria in MWF.

All personal breathing zone and area cassette sample measurements collected in October 2004 were below 0.4 mg MWF/m^3 of air. NIOSH recommends exposure to MWF be limited to 0.5 mg MWF/m^3 total particulate mass as a time-weighted average (TWA) concentration for up to 10 hr/day during a 40-hour workweek (NIOSH Criteria for a Recommended Standard: Occupational Exposure to Metalworking Fluids, January 1998). Note that endotoxin and culturable fungi and bacterial levels were not assessed for samples collected during our October 2004 survey.

As demonstrated in Figure 2, levels of airborne MWF were positively associated with airborne total dust. This finding suggests that engineering, good housekeeping, and good work practice efforts in the grinding area to control dust levels should concurrently decrease MWF exposure levels.

Particle mass distribution

Preliminary analyses of particle mass distribution data (Tables I to III, Figure 1) indicate that cobalt and nickel aerosol particles generated during most work activities surveyed were non-respirable (*i.e.*, greater than 10 µm in aerodynamic diameter), with the exception of aerosol generated during grinding activities. In general, the MMAD decreases as the mechanical and thermal energy imparted on the material increases. The observed large particle mass distributions were consistent with low-energy powder handling activities such as those performed during Zinc reclamation (*e.g.*, crushing), Blending, Milling, Screening, Pressing, and Shaping. The observed small particle mass distributions were consistent with a higher-energy activity such as in Grinding.

Cobalt

As shown in Tables I to V, airborne cobalt levels exceeded the U.S. Occupational Safety and Health Administration (OSHA) permissible exposure limit (PEL) of 100 µg/m^3 in Zinc A, Zinc B, Charging, Milling, and Spray Drying. The NIOSH recommended exposure limit (REL) for cobalt (50 µg/m^3) was exceeded in the same areas, but also in Screening. The American Conference of Governmental Industrial Hygienists (ACGIH) threshold limit value (TLV) for cobalt (20 µg/m^3) was exceeded in the same areas as listed in which the PEL and REL was exceeded, but also in Tray Prep, Extrusion, Pressing, and Shaping.

Multiple area samples were collected in Zinc A and Zinc B while specific activities were performed (Table I). From these data, it appears that specific activities may contribute disproportionately to measured exposure levels. For example, in Zinc A crucible loading generated higher levels of cobalt dust relative to operation of the cake crusher. In Zinc B, operation of the ball mill, big Spokane crusher, and blender generated higher levels of cobalt dust relative to operation of the little Spokane crusher.

Chromium

Airborne chromium levels were well below the PEL, REL, and TLV in all work areas surveyed.

Nickel

Levels of airborne nickel were below the PEL, REL, and TLV in all work areas surveyed, except Charging and Milling, where the NIOSH REL for nickel (15 µg/m^3) was exceeded.

Recommendations

As described in detail in the document "Criteria for a Recommended Standard: Occupational Exposure to Metalworking Fluids" (NIOSH, 1998) [copy enclosed], the following recommendations are made with respect to MWF:

- Routine monitoring of inhalation and skin MWF exposures of affected employees
  - At least annually and whenever any major process change takes place
    - Inhalation exposure should be sampled in the personal breathing zone
    - Skin exposure should be qualitatively evaluated
- Employee training
  - As part of your existing employee training program, train employees on the potential adverse health effects associated with exposure to MWF, how to detect potential hazardous situations (*e.g.*, appearance of bacteria overgrowth and degradation of MWF), and appropriate work practices (*e.g.*, minimizing skin contact with MWF)
- Engineering
  - Minimize the generation of MWF mists through appropriate operation and control of the MWF delivery system (see for example, *Mist Control Considerations for the Design, Installation, and Use of Machine Tools Using Metalworking Fluids*, American National Standards Institute

Technical Report B11 TR 2-1997)
- For control of exposure, utilize the industrial hygiene hierarchy of controls (ranked in order of most preferred to least preferred control method): elimination> substitution> engineering>work practices> personal protective equipment
- Work practices
  - Augment your current MWF inspection protocol as appropriate to include a written MWF management plan that specifies procedures for maintenance of fluid chemistry (*e.g.*, pH, temperature, viscosity, storage, mixing and diluting MWF concentrate, preparing additives such as biocides and a cobalt agglomerator, and monitoring tramp oil contamination) and maintenance of the fluid filtration and delivery systems (*e.g.*, fluid level in sump tank)
  - Employees in grinding should stand at a reasonable distance away from grinding machines during operation. Distance between the operator and the machine should be optimized to permit employees to oversee machine processes while minimizing the amount of MWF in the breathing zone
- Protective clothing and equipment
  - Appropriate protective clothing should be worn when working with MWF (note that nitrile is thought to afford the most chemical resistance to MWF)
  - If MWF exposure exceeds $0.5 - 5.0$ mg MWF/m^3 use an air-purifying, half-mask respirator equipped with any P-or R-series particulate filter (P95, P99, P100, R95, R99, and R100)
  - If MWF exposure exceeds $5.0 - 12.5$ mg MWF/m^3 use a powered air-purifying respirator equipped with a hood or helmet and a high efficiency particulate air (HEPA) filter
- Personal Hygiene
  - Employees should periodically wash MWF-contaminated skin with mild soap and water and dry with clean towels
  - Employees should be reminded to refrain from placing their bare skin repeatedly into MWF
  - The use of a barrier cream to protect skin from MWF is not recommended. Barrier creams are not universally protective from MWF.

Building on our recommendations from Interim Letter 1 (dated February 20, 2004) previously sent to you, the following recommendations are made concerning exposure to cobalt at all three plants:

- Routinely monitor inhalation exposure to metals
  - At least annually and whenever any major process change takes place
    - Inhalation exposure should be sampled in the personal breathing zone
- Engineering
  - In work areas with elevated cobalt exposures, reduce cobalt exposure levels to below the current OSHA PEL (or to a lower professionally recognized level)
    - Utilize the industrial hygiene hierarchy of controls (ranked in order of most preferred to least preferred control method): elimination> substitution> engineering>work practices> personal protective equipment
  - To aid in identification of specific work activities that may contribute disproportionately to metal exposure in a work area:
    - Dissect each job in a work area of elevated exposure into step-by-step activities (utilize employee input)
    - Use a portable real-time particle counter to identify the activities of a job that generate more aerosol than other activities

- Work practices
  - Dedicate equipment (*e.g.*, hand tools) to specific work areas to prevent cobalt contamination migration from an area of higher cobalt to an area of lower cobalt contamination
  - Provide a high-efficiency particulate air (HEPA) filtered vacuum in the pressing area for employees to clean their machines and work area. Use of a HEPA filtered vacuum will minimize transfer of cobalt from surfaces to air and unprotected areas of the skin when cleaning
  - Employees in grinding stand at a reasonable distance away from grinding machines during operation. Distance between the operator and the machine will permit employees to oversee machine processes while minimizing the amount of cobalt in the breathing zone
  - Ensure and routinely check the integrity of the sandblasting glove box air hoses and gloves
  - Implement a skin protection program to minimize contamination of skin with metal powders
    - Use a non-latex material for gloves and other barriers.
- Personal protective clothing and equipment
  - Use a non-latex glove material (*e.g.*, nitrile) with over gloves made of a resilient material when performing activities that require durable protection from substantial cobalt skin exposure
  - Appropriate respiratory protection should be worn by properly trained personnel when job activities could result in metal aerosol exposure levels above the pertinent OSHA PEL (or a lower feasible professionally recognized level) that could not be controlled to an acceptable level by engineering and work practice controls
    - Respiratory protection may not perform as intended if it is not donned, used and maintained properly. As such, the use of personal protective equipment is not recommended as a primary means of reducing exposure levels on a long term basis
- Personal Hygiene
  - Employees should periodically wash metal-contaminated skin with mild soap and water and dry with clean towels
    - Especially before eating, smoking, or using the bathroom
  - Employees should be reminded to refrain from placing their bare skin repeatedly into metal powders
  - Shower soon after work
  - Improve cleanliness of non-production areas
    - Thoroughly clean and maintain lunch rooms and identify as "Clean Areas"
    - Minimize migration of cobalt from production to non-production areas

Table I. Total element concentration and mass median aerodynamic diameter of area samples collected using MOUDI impactors (May 2004)

Plant	Work Area	Sample	Total concentration (μg/m³)*	Total concentration (μg/m³)*	Total concentration (μg/m³)*	MMAD, μm (GSD)**	MMAD, μm (GSD)**	MMAD, μm (GSD)**
			Particle	Cobalt	Nickel	Particle	Cobalt	Nickel
Huntsville	Zinc A (crucible loading)	K	--	191.9	ND	--	29.2 (6.2)	NA
Huntsville	Zinc A (cake crusher)	L	--	27.4	ND	--	--	NA
Huntsville	Zinc B (Big Spokane)	M	--	77.4	ND	--	27.0 (5.9)	NA
Huntsville	Zinc B (Little Spokane)	Q	--	21.4	ND	--	24.1 (6.3)	NA
Huntsville	Zinc B (Ball mill)	O	--	132.2	ND	--	41.7 (5.4)	NA
Gurley	Charging	D	--	70.5	ND	--	10.8 (3.9)	NA
Gurley	Charging	C	--	1321.1	ND	--	19.3 (3.9)	NA
Gurley	Charging	A	--	145.2	ND	--	7.0 (2.8)	4.9 (11.2)
Gurley	Charging	PP	--	91.5	9.7	--	12.7 (3.7)	NA
Gurley	Spray drying	N	--	9.5	ND	--	7.2 (2.8)	NA
Gurley	Screening	B	--	81.2	ND	--	11 2 (4.2)	NA
Gurley	Screening	KK	--	8.2	2.1	--	12.3 (5.6)	23.6 (10.6)
Grant	Pressing	P	--	ND	ND	--	NA	NA
Grant	Pressing	G	--	13.0	ND	--	--	NA
Grant	Grinding	I	--	1.2	ND	--	5.9 (8.4)	NA
Grant	Grinding	H	--	0.9	ND	--	5.5 (10.3)	NA
Grant	Grinding	R	--	0.7	ND	--	6.2 (6.9)	NA

NA = Not applicable
ND = Below the analytical limit of detection (LOD)
* Total concentration = sum of element mass on each impactor stage substrate for a given sample divided by air volume sampled
** MMAD = mass median aerodynamic diameter; GSD = geometric standard deviation
~Value not calculated (data analysis ongoing)

Table II. Total element concentration and mass median aerodynamic diameter of personal breathing zone samples collected using Marple series 290 8-stage cascade impactors (May 2004)

Plant	Work Area	Sample	Total concentration $(\mu g/m^3)^*$ Cobalt	Total concentration $(\mu g/m^3)^*$ Chromium	Total concentration $(\mu g/m^3)^*$ Nickel	MMAD, μm (GSD)** Cobalt	MMAD, μm (GSD)** Chromium	MMAD, μm (GSD)** Nickel
Gurley	Charging	V	143.4	0.5***	104.1	14.1 (2.4)	--	13.8 (2.4)
Gurley	Milling	U	311.1	8.1	58.6	16.3 (2.5)	--	17.0 (2.8)
Gurley	Screening	W	48.6	ND	ND	19.1 (3.3)	NA	NA
Grant	Shaping	T	11.3	ND	ND	18.3 (4.7)	NA	NA
Grant	Tray Prep	S	46.4	4.2***	ND	13.5 (3.1)	--	NA

~ Value not calculated (data analysis ongoing)
ND = Below the analytical limit of detection (LOD)
NA = Not applicable
* Total concentration = sum of element mass on each impactor stage substrate for a given sample divided by air volume sampled
** MMAD = mass median aerodynamic diameter; GSD = geometric standard deviation
*** Semi-quantitative

Table III. Total cobalt concentration and mass median aerodynamic diameter for area samples collected using Marple series 290 8-stage cascade impactors (May 2004)

Plant	Work Area	Sample	Total concentration ($\mu g/m^3$)[*]	MMAD, μm (GSD)[**]
Huntsville	Zinc B (Spokane)	N	139.4	13.8 (2.7)
Huntsville	Zinc B (Ball mill)	M	133.6	17.7 (2.9)
Huntsville	Zinc B (Blender)	L	109.5	12.1 (2.5)
Grant	Tray Prep	P	8.8	8.7 (3.5)
Grant	Sandblasting	Q	ND	NA
Grant	Shaping	R	2.1[***]	NA

NA = Not applicable
ND = Below the analytical limit of detection (LOD)
   [*] Total concentration = sum of element mass on each impactor stage substrate for a given sample divided by air volume sampled
   [**] MMAD = mass median aerodynamic diameter; GSD = geometric standard deviation
   [***] Semi-quantitative

Table IV. Total element concentration for samples collected in the personal breathing zone using close- and open-faced 37-mm filter cassettes (May 2004)

µg/m³	µg/m³	µg/m³	µg/m³	µg/m³	µg/m³
Plant	Work Area	Cassette	Cobalt	Chromium	Nickel
Huntsville	Zinc B	Closed-faced	43.2	<LOD	0.4
Huntsville	Zinc B	Closed-faced	57.2	0.7	0.4
Huntsville	Zinc B	Closed-faced	82.8	0.8	0.3
Huntsville	Zinc B	Closed-faced	107.8	1.1	1.0
Gurley	Charging	Closed-faced	89.0	0.2	107.2
Gurley	Charging	Closed-faced	815.4	0.8	804.7
Gurley	Milling	Closed-faced	318.7	2.9	66.6
Gurley	Spray Drying	Open-faced	110.4	0.7	2.6
Grant	Extrusion	Closed-faced	34.6	0.8	0.2
Grant	Pressing	Closed-faced	37.5	1.0	0.7
Grant	Pressing	Closed-faced	17.1	1.0	0.3
Grant	Shaping	Closed-faced	9.5	0.0	0.3
Grant	Shaping	Closed-faced	33.1	0.4	0.6
Grant	Grinding	Open-faced	1.8	0.5	0.7
Grant	Grinding	Open-faced	2.3	0.5	0.3
Grant	Shipping	Open-faced	1.6	0.5	0.3
Grant	Tray Prep	Closed-faced	39.3	1.6	1.7
		OSHA PEL	100.0	1000.0	1000.0
		NIOSH PEL	50.0	500.0	15.0
		ACGIH TLV	20.0	500.0	1500.0

Table V. Total element concentration for area samples collected using close- and open-faced 37-mm filter cassettes (May 2004)

µg/m³	µg/m³	µ/m³	µg/m³	µg/m³	µg/m³
Huntsville	Zinc A	Close-faced	556.2	6.3	3.5
Huntsville	Zinc B	Open-faced	65.4	0.6	0.3
Huntsville	Zinc B	Close-faced	54.2	0.1	0.2
Huntsville	Zinc B	Close-faced	183.8	1.0	0.3
Huntsville	Zinc B	Close-Faced	61.1	1.0	0.3
Grant	Shaping	Open-faced	4.3	0.7	0.2
Grant	Sandblasting	Open-faced	0.7	0.5	<0.07
Grant	Tray Prep	Open-faced	6.9	0.2	0.2
		OSHA PEL	100.0	1000.0	1000.0
		NIOSH REL	50.0	500.0	15.0
		ACGIH TLV	20.0	500.0	1500.0

Table VI. Total dust level summarized by work area for samples collected in the personal breathing zone using close-faced 37-mm filter cassettes (October 2004)

Plant	Work Area*	No. Samples	Dust (µg/m³) Average ± St Dev	Dust (µg/m³) Minimum	Dust (µg/m³) Maximum
Huntsville	APT Plant	30	2475.7 ± 2199.9	336.0	8682.5
Huntsville	Zinc A	5	1538.0 ± 964.6	178.2	2486.9
Huntsville	Zinc B	9	1547.6 ± 1012.5	176.5	2923.4
Huntsville	Zinc A and B	9	1377.0 ± 820.0	37.0	2510.0
Huntsville	Powder Laboratory	18	119.7 ± 116.9	21.7	427.3
Gurley	Inventory Control	2	98.4 ± 24.1	81.4	115.5
Gurley	Reprocessing	2	7261.7 ± 5087.6	3664.3	10859.2
Gurley	Charging	11	2069.9 ± 1655.9	173.4	5071.0
Gurley	Milling	10	623.3 ± 419.7	216.5	1538.5
Gurley	Spray Drying	16	907.4 ± 642.2	184.5	2473.1
Gurley	Screening	7	1866.0 ± 1272.5	741.1	4282.4
Gurley	Shipping	2	237.2 ± 12.8	228.2	246.3
Gurley	Leadman	6	239.7 ± 90.1	178.6	383.8
Gurley	Maintenance	4	463.3 ± 497.3	30.2	1165.5
Gurley	Utility	3	860.8 ± 1058.9	231.5	2083.3
Gurley	Custodian	2	717.7 ± 662.2	249.5	1186.0
Grant	Powder Inventory	5	152.9 ± 101.8	72.8	328.1
Grant	Pressing	13	436.5 ± 192.5	215.4	777.3
Grant	Extrusion	5	448.5 ± 529.8	85.2	1364.8
Grant	Round Cell	7	200.9 ± 58.3	114.2	263.8
Grant	Shaping	20	544.5 ± 830.1	87.3	3255.8
Grant	Breakdown	1	975.9	--	--
Grant	Grinding	15	543.4 ± 709.6	108.8	2820.0
Grant	Sandblasting	9	262.9 ± 198.0	102.5	705.0
Grant	Product Testing	15	149.2 ± 47.1	65.0	224.3
Grant	Shipping	16	228.9 ± 180.6	65.8	803.6
Grant	Maintenance	10	310.6 ± 242.7	111.5	886.8

* Location that employee reported working on the day sample was collected

Table VII. Total dust level, MWF level, and the fraction of dust mass accounted by MWF ($f_{MWF/Dust}$) for the personal breathing zone and area PTFE cassette samples collected in grinding area (October 2004)

Plant	Work Area	Sample	Total dust ($\mu g/m^3$)	MWF ($\mu g/m^3$)	$f_{MWF/Dust}$
Grant	Grinding	Personal	201.9	78.4	0.39
Grant	Grinding	Personal	411.0	285.4	0.69
Grant	Grinding	Personal	147.4	36.3	0.25
Grant	Grinding	Personal	185.2	83.3	0.45
Grant	Grinding	Personal	317.3	120.4	0.38
Grant	Grinding	Personal	350.1	240.7	0.69
Grant	Grinding	Personal[*]	3470.7	303.7	0.09
Grant	Grinding	Personal	162.7	75.9	0.47
Grant	Grinding	Area	114.4	88.0	0.77
Grant	Grinding	Area	136.9	74.8	0.55
Grant	Grinding	Area	125.0	106.5	0.85
Grant	Grinding	Area	393.5	347.2	0.88
Grant	Grinding	Area	91.9	71.8	0.78
Grant	Grinding	Area	493.7	417.7	0.85
Grant	Grinding	Area	145.9	67.6	0.46
Grant	Grinding	Area	106.9	73.9	0.69

[*] Employee spray painted during first half of shift

Figure 1. Measured particle cobalt mass distribution for MOUDI sample K collected while crucibles were loaded in Zinc A (May 2004). The y-axis of the plot is the mass fraction of sample collected on an impactor stage relative to the total mass collected on all stages of the sampler normalized for the aerodynamic particle size interval of the stage. The x-axis of the plot is aerodynamic diameter (diameter of a spherical particle with density 1 g/cm³ that has the equivalent settling velocity as the particle under study). The shape of the histogram indicates that the data are log-normally distributed.

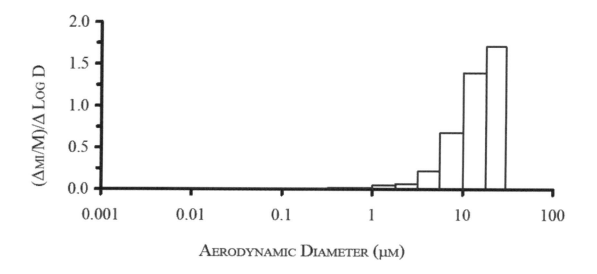

Figure 2. Relationship between levels of MWF and levels of total dust for personal breathing zone sample and area samples collected in the Grinding area at Grant, AL (October 2004). Levels of MWF were positively related to levels of dustiness in the grinding work area as indicated by the positive R^2 values given in the plots. An R^2 value is an estimate of the relationship between two variables and can range from -1 (exact negative linear relationship) to 1 (exact positive linear relationship).

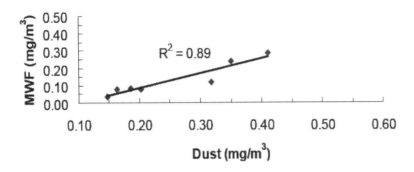

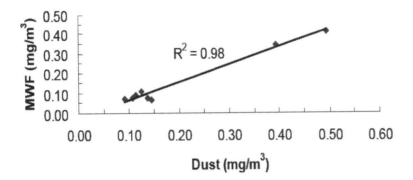

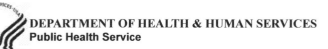

DEPARTMENT OF HEALTH & HUMAN SERVICES
Public Health Service

Phone: (304) 285-5751
Fax: (304) 285-5820

Centers for Disease Control
and Prevention (CDC)
National Institute for Occupational
Safety and Health (NIOSH)
1095 Willowdale Road
Morgantown, WV 26505-2888

March 25, 2005
HETA 2003-0257
Revision of Interim Letter I

Mr. Steve Robuck
Director of Safety and Environment
Metalworking Products
1 Teledyne Place
La Vergne, Tennessee 37086

Dear Mr. Robuck:

In September 2003 the National Institute for Occupational Safety and Health (NIOSH) performed a medical survey of Metalworking Products employees of the Grant, Gurley, and Huntsville, Alabama plants. This survey included a questionnaire, chest x-ray, spirometry test (breathing test), bronchodilator trial (a test that indicates whether airways obstruction is reversible), and diffusing lung capacity for carbon monoxide (DLCO) (a test designed to measure how well the lungs exchange gases). In February 2004 you were sent an interim letter with our preliminary findings. Since then, we have made the following changes. We have modified our suspected work-related asthma case definition to exclude cases with obstruction or borderline obstruction who either had no reversibility with a bronchodilator or who failed to complete a bronchodilator trial and who did not have any other suspected work-related asthma inclusion criteria. We have excluded one former worker diagnosed by a physician with hard metal disease because we did not have access to this worker's total lung capacity (TLC) results. We have also corrected miscalculated basal metabolic indices (BMIs). This letter includes the results of our reanalysis. Differences in suspected case numbers are provided in Table 1.

METHODS

Plant lists of employee names, addresses, and work histories were used to identify employees from the three plants with potential cobalt exposure. For Grant and Gurley, this included employees who currently or previously worked in either production or engineering jobs; and for Huntsville, this included employees who currently worked in either the reclamation (zinc) or ammonia paratungstate (APT) departments. We mailed invitations to 235 employees with potential cobalt exposure, asking them to participate in a medical survey.

Medical Survey

From September 9-20, 2003, we tested workers during regularly scheduled 15-minute work breaks, lunch breaks, before or after work, and on non-work days. The testing schedule was designed to include workers from all shifts. Testing before or after work and on non-work days included: administration of a medical questionnaire; chest x-ray; a baseline spirometry test; and, if the spirometry test was abnormal, administration of a medication (bronchodilator) to help open the airways, repeat spirometry test, and DLCO. TLC was estimated from DLCO test results. Abbreviated testing was used on workers scheduled during 15-minute work breaks and lunch breaks. This testing included a short written questionnaire (completed at home), chest x-ray, and a baseline spirometry test.

The methods of performance and interpretation for chest x-ray, spirometry, bronchodilator trial, and DLCO are unchanged from our first interim letter.

Suspected Hard Metal Disease and Work-Related Asthma Definitions

We defined suspected hard metal disease as:

- Low DLCO with either obstruction, borderline obstruction, restriction, or borderline restriction and a TLC below 80% of predicted

  OR

- Restrictive or borderline restriction with Body Mass Index (BMI) greater than or equal to 18.5 and less than 30 and with TLC below 80% of predicted (TLC could only be calculated in those with a DLCO test)

  OR

- Chest x-ray with a profusion score of 1/0 or greater

Since we did not offer DLCO to participants with normal spirometry tests, an abnormal DLCO in the presence of normal spirometry result would not have been detected. BMI is calculated as: weight in kilograms ÷ (height in meters)^2. We have recalculated BMI calculations, which were miscalculated in our previous interim letter.

We defined suspected work-related asthma as:

- Post-hire onset, current, physician-diagnosed asthma

  OR

- Three of more current asthma symptoms with post-hire wheeze or shortness of breath

  OR

- Current use of asthma medication with post-hire wheeze or shortness of breath

  OR

- Reversible obstruction with post-hire wheeze or shortness of breath

Work Area Categories

The charging, blending, and reprocessing work areas were combined into one work area called "charging"; round cell and shaping work areas were combined into one work area referred to as "shaping". Because of job exposure differences, utility breakdown employees were not included in the "product testing" work area. Non-cobalt containing work areas (such as the production of tungsten carbide), work areas with few employees, as well as utility breakdown employees were combined into an "other" work area. A complete list of work areas is included in Table 4.

Health Conditions Associated with Formerly or Currently Working in a Work Area

Odds ratios contrast the likelihood of a specific event occurring in one group compared to another. We calculated odds ratios for certain health conditions to occur in workers who formerly and currently worked in specific work areas compared to workers who had never worked in that area. Odds ratios took into account age, gender, and pack-years of smoking.

Case Review Analysis

We used reported symptom and/or asthma onset-dates to identify work areas possibly associated with the development of hard metal disease and work-related asthma. We included two former workers (one with suspected hard metal disease and one with suspected work-related asthma) in this analysis.

Work Areas Associated with Suspected Hard Metal Disease

We identified work areas where suspected hard metal disease cases either first developed symptoms of cough and/or shortness of breath and/or were diagnosed with suspected hard metal disease. Since hard metal disease is rare, we considered any suspected occurrence to identify work areas at possible higher risk for the development of this disease.

Suspected Work-Related Asthma Incidence Rates

For each suspected work-related asthma case, we identified the work area where they reportedly first developed symptoms of wheeze or shortness of breath and/or their asthma began. Suspected cases who were working in two work areas, were counted as cases for both work areas.

An incidence rate is the number of new cases that occur in a population during a defined period of time. We calculated work area specific suspected work-related asthma incidence rates by dividing the number of suspected cases that reportedly occurred in specific work areas by the workforce time at risk. Only employees who were at risk for developing suspected work-related asthma were included. Excluded work experiences were: 1) work experiences after the date of disease onset; 2) work experiences of employees with pre-hire asthma, pre-hire wheeze and/or shortness of breath, and/or unknown dates of disease or symptom onset; and 3) work experiences of employees with airways obstruction or borderline obstruction who did not receive a bronchodilator trial and who did not meet our suspected work-related asthma case definition. Time at risk, expressed as person-years, is calculated by summing up the time employees worked in a specific work area. Work areas with incidence rates within the upper third (tertile) for all work areas and which did not have excessively small denominators (less than 50 person-years) and numerators (less than 2 employees), were identified as at possible higher risk for the development of asthma.

We compared the total number of suspected work-related asthma cases that occurred in the last 5 years

(September 1998 to September 2003) to the number of cases that occurred prior to September 1998, in order to evaluate the effect of possible workplace environmental changes due to improved engineering controls and personal protective equipment use.

Health Outcome Prevalence and Prevalence Ratios

We calculated workforce prevalence of restriction, suspected hard metal disease, airways obstruction, ever-diagnosed and current asthma, post-hire asthma, and suspected work-related asthma. Prevalences of respiratory symptoms, ever-diagnosed asthma, current asthma, and airways obstruction were compared to National Health and Nutrition Examination Survey III (NHANES III)[2] rates, adjusting for smoking status, age, gender, and race. Behavioral Risk Factor Surveillance System (BRFSS) is a state-based telephone survey of residents 18 years of age or older. Prevalences of ever-diagnosed and current asthma were also compared to 2003 Alabama (BRFSS)[3] results, controlling for gender.

Physician-Diagnosed Asthma Incidence Rate Ratios

We calculated the workforce physician-diagnosed asthma incidence rate by dividing the total number of post-hire asthma cases by the total workforce tenure up to the date of our September 2003 survey. We excluded from workforce tenure, tenure of employees with pre-hire asthma or asthma with no known date of onset and tenure of post-hire asthma cases subsequent to their diagnosis date.

We used population statistics from the 1970 U.S. Census to calculate a hypothetical rate of the total workforce incidence rate, directly standardized for age and gender. We compared this calculated rate to an NHANES expected rate of 2.1 physician-diagnosed asthma cases per 1000 person-years.[4] We used 1970 U.S. Census population statistics as the basis for our standardization because this was the reference population used in the NHANES study.

Post-Hire/Pre-Hire Adult-Onset Asthma Incidence Rate Ratio

We defined adult-onset asthma as asthma diagnosed in an individual 16 years of age or older. Case numbers and person-time at risk for pre-hire and post-hire periods were used to calculate respective adult-onset asthma incidence rates. We excluded the entire person-time for asthma cases with no known diagnosis date and person-time subsequent to diagnosis for asthma cases with a known diagnosis date. Post-hire and pre-hire adult asthma incidence rates were then compared.

Statistical Tests

Logistic regression was used to calculate odds ratios. A Poisson distribution was used to determine confidence intervals for prevalence and incidence rate ratios. We chose the probability value of 0.05 as the criterion for statistical significance. Dates that did not specify the month were assigned the month of July for calculations.

RESULTS

Demographic Data and Participation Rates

One hundred seventy one of 249 (69%) "invited" plant employees participated in the survey. "Invited" refers to employees who were mailed invitations as well as 14 employees who inadvertently were not mailed one. Most employees (68%) were male (Table 2). The median age was 44 years. Employees were almost equally divided among those who had never smoked cigarettes and those who had ever (currently or previously) smoked. Of the 171 participants, 3 did not complete a questionnaire, 3 did not complete a spirometry test, and 4 did not complete a chest x-ray (Table 3). Of the 31 with abnormal spirometry, 24 completed both a bronchodilator trial and DLCO.

Health Conditions Associated with Formerly and Currently Working in a Work Area

Employees who formerly or ever worked in milling, spray drying, grinding, and sandblasting were 3.8 to 9.5 times (statistically significant) more likely to have shortness of breath, ever wheezed, and suspected work-related asthma compared to employees who had never worked in these areas (Table 4). Other odds ratios were elevated but did not meet statistical significance because of wide confidence intervals and small numbers. However, these results were given for completeness. Health outcome odds ratios were 5 or more times greater in former compared to current workers in milling, powder laboratory, grinding, and APT, possibly indicating a migration of workers away from symptom-provoking work areas. Former grinders were statistically more likely to have 3 health conditions (shortness of breath, ever have wheezed, and suspected work-related asthma) compared to employees who had never worked in grinding. Among the 8 former grinders with suspected work-related asthma, only one was working in grinding at the time that symptoms of wheeze or shortness of breath developed and 6 others had worked in grinding a median of 8 years prior to developing symptoms.

Case Review Analysis

Work Areas Associated with Suspected Hard Metal Disease

We identified 3 cases of suspected hard metal disease that reportedly developed symptoms and/or disease while working in pressing, sintering, and grinding.

Suspected Work-Related Asthma Incidence Rates

Suspected work-related asthma incidence rates in screening, maintenance (Gurley), pressing, sandblasting, product testing, and shipping (Grant) were within the upper tertile for all work areas (Table 5). However, screening and sandblasting work area incidence rates had very small numerators and denominators, so that we could not asses risk in these two work areas.

Health Outcome Prevalence and Prevalence Ratios

Hard Metal Disease

None of the employees had a chest x-ray with a profusion score of 1/0 or greater. Suspected hard metal disease was present in 2 of 168 (1%) current employees who had restriction or borderline restriction, a TLC less than 80%, and a normal range BMI. Restriction or borderline restriction was present in 4 other current employees. However, 2 of these employees did not have an estimated TLC and 2 other employees did not have a normal range BMI. DLCO (which was performed only if a participant had an abnormal spirometry test result) was below the lower limit of normal in 2 employees. Both of these employees had an estimated TLC greater than 80% predicted.

Airways Obstruction and Asthma

Post-hire asthma and suspected work-related asthma were present in 7% (11 of 168) and 17% (28 of 168) of the current workforce, respectively. There were 12 cases of suspected work-related asthma cases that occurred prior to September 1998 compared to 16 cases that occurred on or after September 1998.

Airways obstruction was present in 12 of 168 (7%) employees. Airways obstruction was 2.8 times more prevalent in white non-smokers than expected based on NHANES III data. White male never-smokers aged 17 to 39 had 8.5 times more airways obstruction; and white female never-smokers aged 40 to 69 had 4.9 times more airways obstruction compared to NHANES III participants. These prevalence ratios were statistically significant.

The estimated workforce prevalences of ever-diagnosed asthma and current asthma were 16.4% (28 of 171 employees) and 10.5% (18 of 171 employees), respectively. Ever-diagnosed and currently diagnosed asthma were both 2.1 times more prevalent in the total workforce than expected based on NHANES III data, when controlled for race, age, gender, and smoking status (Table 6). Ever-diagnosed asthma and current asthma were, respectively, 1.49 and 1.61 times more prevalent than predicted by the 2003 Alabama BRFSS data. NHANES and BRFSS asthma prevalence ratios were statistically significant.

Symptoms

Shortness of breath when hurrying on level ground or walking up a slight hill, cough on most days, chronic bronchitis, and wheeze or whistling in the last 12 months were 1.7 to 2.1 times more frequent in the workforce than predicted by NHANES III (Table 6).

Physician-Diagnosed Asthma Incidence Rate Ratio

The <u>standardized</u> physician-diagnosed post-hire asthma incidence rate was 5.8 cases per 1000 person-years. When compared to the standardized NHANES asthma incidence rate of 2.1 cases per 1000 person-years, the incidence rate ratio was 2.8 with a confidence interval of 1.2 to 6.2. This indicates that the rate of post-hire onset asthma in this workforce is statistically greater than would be predicted, based on a national study.

Post-Hire/Pre-Hire Adult-Onset Asthma Incidence Rate Ratio

The pre-hire adult-onset asthma incidence rate was 2.1 cases per 1000 person-years, identical to that estimated by the NHANES study. In contrast, the post-hire adult-onset asthma incidence rate was 5.5 cases per 1000 person-years or 2.6 times higher. This post-hire/pre-hire incidence rate ratio had a confidence interval of 1.23 to 6.23, indicating a statistically higher incidence rate in the post-hire compared to the pre-hire period.

DISCUSSION AND CONCLUSIONS

There is a high asthma burden in this workforce. Compared to national data, there was a greater than 2-fold excess in ever-diagnosed asthma and current asthma; and about a 3-fold excess in post-hire onset asthma in employees. Compared to Alabama state prevalences, there was about a 1.5-fold excess of ever-diagnosed asthma and current asthma. Because the NHANES III participation rate was 86%, whereas the Alabama 2003 BRFSS participation rate was only 50%, the NHANES asthma rates are likely to be less biased by self-selection of participants.

Logistic regression was one of two separate analyses performed to identify possible higher risk work areas. This analysis compared the presence of health conditions in workers who ever (previously and/or currently) worked in certain work areas to workers who never worked in these same work areas. The suspected work-related asthma odds ratio in former grinders was elevated, with most having worked in grinding prior to developing this health condition. A possible explanation is that these grinders became sensitized due to exposures while in grinding but many additional years of exposure was needed for them to develop apparent wheezing and/or shortness of breath. Case review analyses considered work areas where cases of suspected disease reportedly developed their symptoms and/or disease. Because the case review analysis provided a much better temporal association between work area and disease, we relied on this analysis to define possible higher risk work areas. However, work areas suggested to be at risk by the logistic regression analysis may also be suspect of higher risk.

Based on three workers with suspected hard metal disease who developed symptoms and/or disease in pressing, sintering, and grinding, these same work areas were identified as possible higher risk areas for the development of this disease.

The incidence rate analysis identifies screening, maintenance (Gurley), pressing, sandblasting, product testing, and shipping (Grant) as having suspected work-related asthma incidence rates within the upper tertile for all work areas. When we excluded screening and sandblasting because of small numerators and person-year denominators, the resulting possible higher risk work areas for the development of asthma were maintenance (Gurley), pressing, product testing, and shipping (Grant).

One limitation of our analyses is that the use of symptom and/or disease onset dates relies on workers correctly remembering these dates. Error in the dates reported could result in an inaccurate assignment of work areas where suspected disease purportedly began. Another limitation is our presumption that the work area where symptoms and/or disease began is responsible for the suspected disease. This is particularly problematic for hard metal disease, which can take a number of years to develop. If the work exposure truly responsible for disease was prior to the onset of symptoms, we could misidentify responsible work exposures. Work-related asthma, unlike hard metal disease, frequently develops after very short periods of exposure. So, using symptom and/or disease onset dates to identify possible higher risk work areas, is more likely to be accurate for work-related asthma than for hard metal disease. Another limitation is the small number of identified suspected cases and the small individual work area person-time values which may have reduced our ability to identify all higher risk work areas.

Another limitation of our analysis is that symptomatic employees may have left the workforce. In this case, our estimated incidence rate for asthma in this workforce would be lower than an incidence rate calculated on current and former employees. Employees may have transferred out of work areas where their symptoms began to other work areas where they are less symptomatic. We tried to address this limitation by calculating health outcome odds ratios separately for employees who formerly and currently worked in work areas. Health outcome odds ratios were 5 or more times higher for employees who formerly worked in 4 work areas, compared to employees who currently worked in these work areas. Environmental changes and improvements in personal protective equipment use or employee migration could cause these differences. Because the number of cases of suspected work-related asthma that developed within 5 years of the medical survey was about equal to the number of cases that developed prior to this period, employee migration may better explain these differences.

We would like to thank Metalworking Products for their help during our September 2003 and our January/ February 2005 medical surveys.

In accordance with the Code of Federal Regulations, Title 42, Part 85, copies of this letter must be posted by management in a prominent place accessible to employees for a period of 30 calendar days.

Sincerely,

Nancy Sahakian, M.D., M.P.H., LCDR USPHS
Respiratory Disease Hazard Evaluation and
Technical Assistance Program
Field Studies Branch
Division of Respiratory Disease Studies

cc:
Daryl Baker
Larry Hollingsworth
Junior Pugh
Confidential Employee Requestors
HETAB file (HETA 2003-0257)

REFERENCES

1. Venables K, Farrer N, Sharp L. et al. [1993]. Respiratory symptoms questionnaire for asthma epidemiology: validity and reproducibility. Thorax 48:214-219.

2. CDC [1996]. Third National Health and Nutrition Examination Survey, 1988-1994, NHANES III Laboratory Data File [CD-ROM]. Hyattsville, MD: U.S. Department of Health and Human Services, Public Health Service, Centers for Disease Control and Prevention. (Public use data file documentation No. 76300).

3. Division of Adult and Community Health, National Center for Chronic Disease Prevention and Health Promotion, Centers for Disease Control and Prevention, Behavioral Risk Factor Surveillance System Online Prevalence Data, 1995-2003.

4. McWhorter W, Polis M, Kaslow R. [1989]. Occurrence, predictors, and consequences of adult asthma in NHANES I and follow-up survey. Am Rev Respir Dis 139:721-724.

Table 1. February 2004 and current suspected work-related asthma and suspected hard metal disease case numbers in current participants and three former workers, September 2003, Metalworking Products

Suspected Cases	February 2004 Analysis	Current Analysis
Work-related asthma	38	29
Hard metal disease	7	3

Table 2. Demographics of invited participants (N=171), September 2003, Metalworking Products

Demographics	Invited Participants
Age (years)	
- Median	44
- Range	25-71
Gender	
- Males	68.4%
- Females	31.6%
Smoking status	
- Current smokers	29.2%
- Former smokers	23.4%
- Never smokers	47.4%
Pack-years (for ever-smokers)	
- Median	20.4
- Range	0.4-120
Tenure (years)	
- Median	9.5
- Range	0.2-37
Race or Ethnic group	
- White	81.6%
- Black	16.1%
- Hispanic	1.8%
- Asian	0.6%

Table 3. Number of Participants Who Completed Medical Survey Components, September 2003, Metalworking Products

Questionnaire	Chest X-Ray	Spirometry	Normal Spirometry	Abnormal Spirometry
171	167	168	137	31 - 24 completed bronchodilator trial - 24 completed DLCO

Table 4. Odds ratios of health conditions in employees who formerly and currently worked in certain work areas compared to employees who never worked in these work areas, controlled for age, gender, and pack-years of smoking, September 2003, Metalworking Products

Work Areas Ever Worked In	Current or Former Employees	Cough (on most days)	Shortness of Breath when hurrying on level ground or walking up a slight hill	Shortness of Breath when walking on level ground with others the same age	Wheeze (ever)	Suspected Work-Related Asthma
Charging	Former	**	1.3	0.7	4.5	4.2
	Current	1.5	6.9	1.3	3.4	**
Milling	Former	0.6	9.0*	2.6	3.7	1.3
	Current	**	0.8	**	**	**
Spray Drying	Former and Current	0.4	4.1*	1.5	5.2*	1.2
Screening	Former	1.1	1.7	4.0	2.9	4.5
	Current	1.4	3.8	**	**	6.4
Powder Laboratory	Former	6.5	**	8.5	**	8.8
	Current	**	0.91	0.8	4.7	1.1
Shipping (Gurley)	Former	**	2.6	4.3	1.5	0.9
	Current	**	1.1	**	6.2	1.5
Maintenance (Gurley)	Former	8.0	**	**	**	**
	Current	6.1	1.8	7.1	1.6	4.2
Pressing	Former	1.6	1.3	2.6	1.7	2.5
	Current	1.5	1.1	1.8	0.4	0.8
Shaping	Former	0.5	0.9	0.9	0.7	1.1
	Current	0.3	1.2	1.0	0.7	1.7
Sintering	Former	1.5	1.0	1.3	2.1	0.5
	Current	1.0	0.9	0.7	2.7	1.1
Grinding	Former	1.6	2.2	3.8*	9.5*	4.5*
	Current	1.4	2.4	2.3	0.3	0.6
Sandblasting	Former and Current	1.8	1.3	1.8	4.5*	3.0
Product Testing	Former	0.7	2.9	2.2	1.9	1.8
	Current	1.8	1.4	2.4	1.4	1.4
Shipping (Grant)	Former	0.9	0.9	1.3	2.2	1.1
	Current	0.8	0.4	0.4	2.3	0.5
Maintenance (Grant)	Former and Current	0.8	0.3	**	0.6	**
Reclamation	Former	**	**	**	0.5	**
	Current	4.0	0.7	1.4	1.0	2.1
APT	Former	7.5	3.9	12.1	1.7	6.3
	Current	1.3	0.3	0.4	0.4	0.3

* statistically significant (p<0.05) odds ratios;
** unable to calculate odds ratios because of inadequate data;
"reclamation" refers to Zinc A and B; N = 171 for usual cough and shortness of breath health conditions; N = 141 for suspected work-related asthma (30 workers were excluded because they had suspected asthma but were unable to provide diagnosis and/or symptom onset dates; the onset of their symptoms or asthma diagnosis predated their hire date; or they had airways obstruction or borderline obstruction without other suspected work-related asthma case inclusion criteria and they failed to complete a bronchodilator trial).

Table 5. Suspected work-related asthma incidence rates by work area (N=143), September 2003, Metalworking Products

Work Area	Number of Cases	Person-Years	Incidence Rates (cases per 1000 person-years)
Charging	1	50	20.0
Milling/Spray Drying	1	98	10.2
Screening* ++	1	11	90.9
Powder Laboratory	0	35	0
Shipping (Gurley)	0	37	0
Maintenance (Gurley)* +	2	32	62.5
Pressing* +	8	255	31.4
Shaping	2	113	17.7
Sintering	2	78	25.6
Grinding	1	184	5.4
Sandblasting* ++	1	10	100.0
Product Testing* +	2	61	32.8
Shipping (Grant)* +	2	76	26.3
Maintenance (Grant)	0	96	0
Reclamation	3	156	19.2
APT	0	70	0
Other	5	286	17.5
All Work Areas	29	1648	Median: 19.2 Upper Tertile: 26.3 Upper Quartile: 31.4

* incidence rate of suspected work-related asthma within upper tertile for all work-areas; reclamation refers to Zinc A and B;
+ suspected higher-risk areas for work-related asthma;
++ risk level could not be assessed due to small case numerators and small person-year denominators; two former employees with suspected occupational lung disease were included in numerators and denominators; two cases of suspected work-related asthma were assigned to two work-areas.

Table 6. Prevalence ratios for health outcomes among employees compared to expected numbers from the NHANES III Survey, adjusted for smoking status, age, gender, and race, September 2003, Metalworking Products

Worker Category	Number	Shortness of breath when hurrying on level ground or walking up a slight hill	Usual cough (cough on most days)	Chronic bronchitis	Wheeze or whistling in the last 12 months	Asthma (ever diagnosed)	Asthma (diagnosed and current)
Gurley Plant	36	2.3*	0.8	2.4	1.8*	2.2	2.3
Grant Plant	100	1.7*	1.7*	2.1*	2.0*	2.2*	2.3*
Huntsville Plant	31	1.4	2.7*	2.0	1.8	1.3	1.3
Entire Workforce	167	1.8*	1.7*	2.1*	1.9*	2.1*	2.1*

*statistically significant (p< 0.05) prevalence ratios. Workers of unknown or Asian race were excluded.

DEPARTMENT OF HEALTH & HUMAN SERVICES

Public Health Service

Phone: (304) 285-5751
Fax: (304) 285-5820

Centers for Disease Control
and Prevention (CDC)
National Institute for Occupational
Safety and Health (NIOSH)
1095 Willowdale Road
Morgantown, WV 26505-2888

June 17, 2005
HETA 2003-0257

Mr. Steve Robuck, P.E. Director of Safety and Environment
Metalworking Products
#1 Teledyne Place
LaVergne, Tennessee 37086

Dear Mr. Robuck:

The purpose of this letter is to report the progress of a National Institute for Occupational Safety and Health (NIOSH) industrial hygiene survey for airborne tungsten oxide whiskers (i.e., fibers) and cobalt at Alldyne Powder Technologies plants located in Huntsville and Gurley, Alabama and the Firth Sterling Plant located in Grant, Alabama. NIOSH personnel surveyed these plants from October 25 to November 12, 2004. The preliminary industrial hygiene assessment described in the attached document was conducted as part of the industrial hygiene assessment for the Health Hazard Evaluation (HHE). The purpose, types of samples collected, and preliminary results for 12 of 69 samples are summarized in the attached interim letter. A concluding discussion follows the summary of the survey results.

To date, we have not received laboratory results for all of the samples collected. Due to analytical expenses, we would like to use the preliminary results presented in this letter to apply for additional extramural funding from the National Toxicology Program to complete the analysis of the remaining 57 samples. Before applying for this funding, we would appreciate your expedited review of the attached report for trade secret information. If we are successful in obtaining funding, we will report the results from the remaining samples in subsequent letters or reports. If you have questions, please feel free to contact us.

Sincerely,

Nancy Sahakian, M.D., M.P.H.
Respiratory Disease Hazard Evaluation and
Technical Assistance Program
Field Studies Branch
Division of Respiratory Disease Studies

HETA 2003-0257: Allegheny Technologies – Interim Letter III Page 2

John McKernan, MSc, CIH
Division of Surveillance Hazard Evaluation and Field
Studies

cc: Confidential Requestors

Background

In processing tungsten (W) containing ores to obtain useful forms of tungsten, tungsten manufacturing processes commonly create WOX (tungsten oxide) compounds as products of chemical reactions. Results from studies within the Swedish hard metal industry have shown that calcination and reduction of tungsten compounds, including ammonium paratungstate, result in the formation of airborne WOX fibers (Sahle 1992; Sahle, Laszlo et al. 1994; Leanderson and Sahle 1995; Sahle, Krantz et al. 1996). WOX fiber sampling investigations in the US hard-metal industry have not been conducted previously.

Currently there are no validated collection methods, standard analytical methods, exposure standards or professional recommendations for airborne WOX fibers. Additionally, it is unknown if there are human health effects related to exposure to airborne WOX fibers. However, one laboratory study that involved exposing human lung cells to WOX fibers and crocidolite (asbestos) fibers showed that greater cell damage resulted when lung cells were exposed to WOx compared to the crocidolite fibers (Leanderson and Sahle 1995).

Purpose

Perform a walk-through survey of the Alldyne Powder Technologies plants located in Huntsville and Gurley, Alabama and the Firth Sterling plant located in Grant, Alabama to understand the production process and collect preliminary information. Conduct personal breathing-zone (PBZ) and area monitoring to collect airborne particles, examine their shape (morphology), and determine if airborne particle groups (agglomerates) were present at various steps in the hard metal production processes at the Alldyne Powder Technologies plants located in Huntsville and Gurley, Alabama and the Firth Sterling plant located in Grant, Alabama.

Methods

Sampling Methodology

From preliminary walk-through investigations of the facilities and available published data from the industry, 12 hard metal production processes were identified (see Table I). In this preliminary exposure assessment, NIOSH personnel used a sampling strategy that would potentially produce a broad range of fiber exposures. This included collecting personal breathing zone (PBZ) and area air samples for WOX fibers. Sampling included the collection of 7 personal breathing zone and 62 area samples for airborne WOX fibers.

Because no validated method for collecting air samples of WOX fibers exists, samples were collected in accordance with NIOSH Method 7402: Asbestos by TEM (NIOSH 2003). Personal breathing zone (PBZ) and area air samples were collected on 25 millimeter (mm) diameter conductive cassettes preloaded with mixed cellulose ester (MCE) 0.45 micrometer ($\mu m = 1 \times 10^6$ m) pore-size membrane filters (SKC Inc., Eighty Four, PA). Air sampling was conducted through the use of battery operated pumps calibrated at 2 liters per minute (LPM) using a standard flow calibration device (BIOS International Corp., Butler, NJ).

In general, samples were collected over a full shift (e.g., 7 to 8 hours). Area samples were collected near the processes being conducted by workers. The type and number of samples collected in each of the production processes included in the preliminary exposure assessment are provided in Table I.

Sample Analysis

Preliminary analysis was conducted for 12 area samples collected near processes that NIOSH personnel believed, based on expert judgment, have the greatest potential for fiber generation and/or release.

The MCE filters were removed from the sample cassettes and prepared for analysis using the direct transfer method as outlined in NIOSH Method 7402. After preparation, each sample was individually loaded into the transmission electron microscope (TEM) for analysis. Fiber counting and analysis of particle shape were conducted using the TEM (Philips, Model 420, Eindhoven, Netherlands). Elemental content of the fibers was determined through the use of an energy dispersive x-ray (EDX) spectrometer (PGT-EDAX, Model Avalon, Rocky Hill, NJ) connected to the TEM. This instrument can detect elements with atomic numbers greater than 11 (sodium). In our analysis, we were interested in reporting the presence of elemental tungsten and cobalt if it was detected as part of the fiber, or if it was in the form of particles on or around the fiber. The recommended limit of detection (LOD) of the method is 0.01 fibers per cubic centimeter of air (f/cc) for atmospheres free of interferences. The recommended quantitative working range of the method is 0.01 to 0.5 f/cc per 1,000 L air sample (NIOSH 2003). The NIOSH "A" counting rule (NIOSH 2003) was modified and used to count the fibers on the sample. Modifications included counting fibers with lengths > 0.5, > 5 and > 15 μm. Additionally, an overall average fiber diameter was estimated based on the 12 analyzed samples. Micrographs (photographs taken through the TEM viewfinder) of various fiber shapes and sizes were collected during the analysis.

Preliminary Results

Preliminary results from the 12 area samples analyzed are provided in Table II. Airborne WOX fiber concentrations ranged from < 0.01 to 0.268 f/cc in the following processes: calcination, reduction, carburizing, charging, screening, sintering and spray drying. Spray drying, sintering, and screening processes produced the lowest concentrations (all < 0.01) and the calcination process for tungsten oxide (e.g., 'blue' oxide, $WO2.70$ or $WO2.85$) produced the highest. EDX analysis showed that all fibers counted contained tungsten. In processes where hard-metal binders were added (e.g., charging, screening, sintering and spray drying) cobalt was also detected both on and near the WOX fibers on the filter. The cobalt particles appeared to be randomly distributed on the surface of the filter. Cobalt particles did not appear to preferentially attach to the fibers observed; that is a proportionate number of cobalt particles were detected attached and unattached to the fibers counted. As expected, processes involved in reducing tungsten compounds to elemental tungsten (e.g., calcination and reduction) and the process intended to create tungsten carbide (e.g., carburizing) were free of cobalt contamination.

Figure 1 is a micrograph from the preliminary TEM-EDX analysis of a typical WOX fiber from one area sample collected near the 'blue' calcination process. It is notable in Figure 1 that these airborne WOX fibers were long (> 5 μm) and have diameters < 1 μm. Preliminary results indicate that overall average airborne fiber diameters are < 0.25 μm. Fibers with these dimensions are categorized as respirable (ACGIH 2004). This term applies to particles that deposit in the respiratory airways and lung when inhaled.

Summary Discussion

During a meeting on October 25, 2005, in which Steve Robuck, Jim Doherty, Dan Yereb, John McKernan, and a maintenance worker at the Gurley facility were present, the issue of determining the size and shape of airborne particles that are associated with your processes was raised. The sampling results from this preliminary assessment provide information on one shape (fibers) detected in the air samples collected. Information on the size of the fibers detected is also provided. Data from this limited preliminary analysis indicate that the dimensions of the airborne WOX fibers detected are overall < 5 μm long by < 0.25 μm in diameter.

Another issue that management expressed interest in was whether airborne particle groups (agglomerates) were present. The preliminary data and micrographs of the airborne WOX fibers show that particles appeared to be randomly distributed on the surface of the filter. In the case of cobalt particles, they did not appear to preferentially attach to the fibers observed; that is a proportionate number of cobalt particles were detected attached and unattached to the fibers counted. Figure 1 provides an illustration of the way that most of the fibers were found.

Conclusions

The preliminary results provided here show that there is wide variability in the number and concentration of airborne WOX fibers from your refining and production processes. Results also indicate that a number of processes release of airborne WOX fibers and cobalt. From these preliminary data, it appears that high-temperature processes designed to reduce ammonium paratungstate (complex tungsten compound) to simple tungsten compounds in ambient air produce the greatest number of WOX fibers. These processes include calcination and reduction. Cobalt was detected in area air samples collected from processes subsequent to the charging process (e.g., charging, screening, sintering and spray drying).

Recommendations

A description of airborne particle shape, size and concentration from the remaining samples collected at your facilities will be reported when available. Currently, we do not recommend additional changes beyond those included in the interim letter you received dated March 30 of this year.

References

ACGIH (2004). <u>Threshold Limit Values for Chemical Substances and Physical Agents and Biological Exposure Indicies</u>. Cincinnati, American Conference of Governmental Industrial Hygienists.

Leanderson, P. and W. Sahle (1995). "Formation of Hydroxyl Radicals and Toxicity of Tungsten Oxide Fibers." <u>Toxic. in Vitro</u> 9(2): 175-183.

NIOSH (2003). <u>NIOSH Manual of Analytical Methods (NMAM)</u>. Cincinnati, OH, National Institute for Occupational Safety and Health.

Sahle, W. (1992). "Possible Role of Tungsten Oxide Whiskers in Hard-Metal Pneumoconiosis." <u>Chest</u> 102: 1310.

Sahle, W., S. Krantz, et al. (1996). "Preliminary Data on Hard Metal Workers Exposure to Tungsten Oxide Fibers." <u>Sci. Total Environ.</u> 191: 153-167.

Sahle, W., I. Laszlo, et al. (1994). "Airborne Tungsten Oxide Whiskers in a Hard-Metal Industry. Preliminary Findings." <u>Ann. Occup. Hyg.</u> 38(1): 37-44.

Table I: Number of Air Samples for Tungsten Oxide Fibers, by Production Process

Process	Sample Type	N
Ammonium paratungstate (APT) production	A	1
Calcination	A	7
Crushing	A	2
Reduction	A	10
	P	1
Ball mill	A	2
	P	1
Carburizing	A	5
	P	1
Charging	A	3
	P	1
Reprocessing	A	1
	P	1
Spray drying	A	5
	P	1
Screening	A	11
	P	1
Pressing/Molding	A	7
Sintering	A	8

A = Area air sample; P = Personal air sample

Table II: Preliminary Results for Airborne Tungsten Oxide Fiber Concentrations

Process	Fibers Counted	Fibers >0.5 um	Fibers >5 um	Fibers >15 um	Fiber Concentration (f/mm2)	Sample Volume (cc)	Airborne Concentration (f/cc)*	Cobalt Detected
Calcination (Blue)	93	93	16	1	395	567420	0.268	No
Calcination (Yellow)	34	34	9	ND	72	577210	0.048	No
Reduction	19	19	1	ND	35	540540	0.025	No
Reduction	12	12	ND	ND	20	502740	0.015	No
Carburizing	17	17	5	2	29	732160	0.015	No
Carburizing	6	6	1	ND	10	709020	0.005	No
Charging	17	17	1	ND	30	960795	0.012	Yes
Screening	6	6	ND	ND	10	1049180	0.004	Yes
Screening	ND**	ND	ND	ND	<0.01	1043420	0.007	Yes
Sintering	5	5	1	ND	8	785960	0.004	Yes
Spray drying	5	5	ND	ND	7	990150	0.003	Yes
# of Fibers	214	214	34	3				

ND = Not detectable
* From NMAM 7402, the quantitative working range is 0.01 - 0.5 f/cc calculated using the number of fibers > 0.5 um, with a preferable fiber concentration range of 100 to 1300 f/mm2
** 0.01/($\sqrt{2}$) was used to determine airborne concentration; See NMAM 7402 NOTE: 12 filter samples were submitted, one could not be analyzed due to overloading (area sample near APT dryer)

Figure 1: Airborne Tungsten Oxide Fibers from 'Blue' Calcination Process

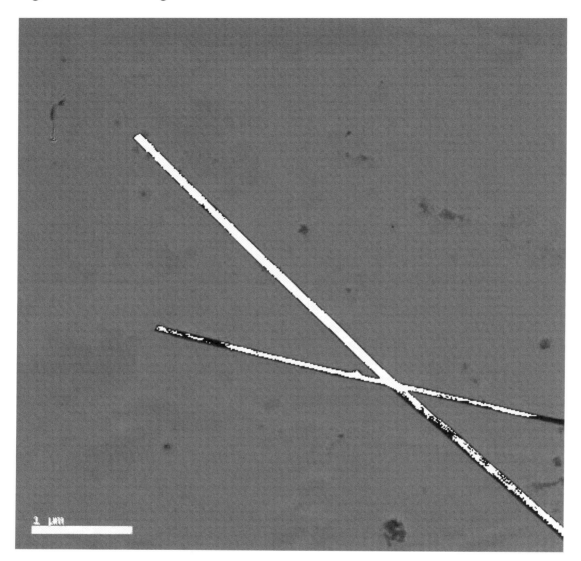

DEPARTMENT OF HEALTH & HUMAN SERVICES

Phone: (304) 285-5751
  Fax: (304) 285-5820

Public Health Service

Centers for Disease Control
  and Prevention (CDC)
National Institute for Occupational
Safety and Health (NIOSH)
1095 Willowdale Road
Morgantown, WV 26505-2888

August 15, 2005
HETA 2003-0257
Interim Letter IV

Mr. Steve Robuck, P.E.
Director of Safety and Environment
Metalworking Products
#1 Teledyne Place
LaVergne, Tennessee 37086

Dear Mr. Robuck:

We are sending you the interim report on tungsten fiver sampling at your company that was produced by a
National Institute for Occupational Safety and Health (NIOSH) industrial hygienist. The data presented in
this report were collected from air sampling conducted at the Alldyne Powder Technologies plants located in
Huntsville and Gurley, Alabama and the Firth Sterling Plant located in Grant, Alabama.

From October 26 to November 4, 2005 62 area samples and 7 personal breathing zone samples for airborne
tungsten fivers were collected at the three plants. Twelve of these samples have been analyzed and the results of
those samples are presented in the enclosed interim report.

NIOSH will be applying to another federal agency for funding to analyze the remaining samples. If funded, the
results of those samples will be provided to Allegheny Technology, Inc., the workers, and the Health Hazard
Evaluation requestors.

In accordance with the Code of Federal Regulations, Title 42, Part 85, copies of this letter must be posted by
management in a prominent place accessible to employees for a period of 30 calendar days.

Sincerely,

Nancy Sahakian, M.D., M.P.H.
Lieutenant Commander, USPHS
Respiratory Disease Hazard Evaluation and
  Technical Assistance Program
Field Studies Branch
Division of Respiratory Disease Studies

HETA 2003-0257 - Metalworking Products   Page 2

cc:
Daryl Baker
Larry Hollingsworth
Junior Pugh
Confidential Employee Requestors
HETAB file (2003-0257)

enclosure

Presence of Tungsten Oxide Fibers in Hard-Metal Processes

John McKernan, MSPH, CIH
National Institute for Occupational Safety and Health
Division of Surveillance, Hazard Evaluations and Field Studies
Industry-wide Studies Branch
Phone: 513-841-4212
Email: JMcKernan@cdc.gov

August 15, 2005

Purpose

To date, the existence of tungsten oxide fibers in the hard-metal industry (or any other tungsten-using industry) has not been evaluated in the United States. The purpose of this research project was to 1) perform a walk-through survey at the Alldyne Powder Technologies plants located in Huntsville and Gurley, Alabama and the Firth Sterling plant located in Grant, Alabama to understand the production processes and collect preliminary information; 2) conduct general area and personal breathing-zone (PBZ) air sampling to collect filter samples of airborne particles at various steps in the hard metal production processes; and 3) analyze the filter samples to determine the shape (morphology) and chemical composition of airborne particles collected in the three plants to determine if tungsten oxide fibers exist in the workplace atmosphere.

Background

To make tungsten metal (W), tungsten-containing material (*e.g.*, ore, reclaimed material in the form of ammonia paratungstate) is oxidized to form tungsten trioxide (WO_3). WO_3 is heated under an inert atmosphere and reduced to W. During calcination to form WO_3 and during reduction of WO_3, a series of lower tungsten oxide (referred to as WO_x in this report) compounds can be formed as byproducts of incomplete chemical reactions. Studies within the Swedish hard metal industry have shown that calcination of ammonium paratungstate and reduction of tungsten-containing compounds can generate WO_x compounds in the form of airborne fibers (Sahle, 1992; Sahle et al., 1994; Leanderson and Sahle, 1995; Sahle et al., 1996).

It is unknown if there are any potential adverse health effects related to human exposure to airborne WO_x fibers; however, one laboratory study conducted *in vitro* observed greater damage to human lung cells that were exposed to tungsten oxide fibers compared to human lung cells that were exposed to crocidolite asbestos fibers (Leanderson and Sahle 1995).

Methods

A specific validated method for collection and analysis of airborne WO_x fibers is lacking. As a result, all air samples were collected in accordance with National Institute for Occupational Safety and Health (NIOSH) Methods 7400 and 7402: Asbestos and other Fibers by Phase Contrast and Transmission Electron Microscopy (NIOSH 2003), which are standard methods for sampling and analysis of airborne asbestos-containing fibers.

Sampling Strategy

From the preliminary walk-through investigations of the facilities and available published data from the Swedish hard metal industry, 16 production processes with the potential to produce a broad range of fiber exposures were identified for air sampling (see Table I). Both general area samples and personal breathing zone (PBZ) samples for airborne WO_x fibers were collected. Sixty-two area samples were collected at stationary locations in work areas to capture potential WO_x fiber generation during specific process activities. Seven PBZ samples were collected to capture potential WO_x fiber exposures during the course of normal employee work activities.

Sample Collection

Area and PBZ air samples were collected on 25 millimeter diameter electrically-conductive cassettes preloaded with mixed cellulose ester (MCE) 0.45 micrometer (μm) pore-size membrane filters (SKC Inc., Eighty Four, PA). The purpose of the electrically-conductive cassette was to ensure uniform deposition of fibers on the filter substrate. Air was drawn through the cassettes with battery operated pumps calibrated at 2 liters per minute (LPM) using a standard flow calibration device (BIOS International Corp., Butler, NJ).

In general, samples were collected over a full shift (e.g., 7 to 8 hours). The type and number (area or PBZ) of samples collected in each of the 16 production areas are provided in Table I.

Sample Analysis

Twelve area samples (out of the 69 total air samples) were selected for the preliminary analysis. Those selected represented processes that were determined by industrial hygienists to be the most likely to produce positive results (i.e., greatest potential to generate fibers).

Each MCE filter was removed from its sample cassette and prepared for analysis using the direct transfer method outlined in NIOSH Method 7402. After preparation, each sample was individually loaded into a transmission electron microscope (TEM) (Philips, Model 420, Eindhoven, Netherlands) for analysis.

Fibers were defined as particles having an aspect ratio of at least 3:1; that is, the fiber length was at least three times greater than the diameter. A modified version of the NIOSH counting rule "A" was used to count fibers on the sample. The "A" rule prescribes counting all particles that lie entirely in the field of view and have length >5 μm, diameter >0.25 μm, and aspect ratio (length to width) ≥3:1 (NIOSH, 2003). The modification to the "A" counting rule included counting fibers with lengths >0.5, >5, and >15 μm. These size cuts were based on fiber size distribution data previously reported by Sahle et al., and take into account the size of fibers that can be effectively cleared from the lung by lung macrophage cells. For counting purposes, the size cuts are cumulative sizes, *e.g.*, a 7 μm fiber was counted as >0.5 and >5 μm. The recommended limit of detection (LOD) of NIOSH Method 7402 is 0.01 fibers per cubic centimeter of air (f/cm^3) for atmospheres free of interferences. The recommended quantitative working range of the method is 0.01 to 0.5 f/cm^3 per 1,000 L air sample (NIOSH 2003).

The elemental composition of fibers and particles were determined using an energy dispersive x-ray (EDX) spectrometer (PGT-EDAX, Model Avalon, Rocky Hill, NJ) connected to the TEM. This EDX detector can identify elements having atomic numbers greater than 11 (sodium).

Preliminary Results

Fibers composed of WO_x (see elemental composition data below) were present in quantifiable levels on 6 of 12 air samples that were analyzed (Table II). The concentration of airborne fibers ranged from <LOD (Carburizing, Spray drying, Screening, and Sintering) to 0.268 (Calcining of "blue" tungsten oxide at Huntsville) f/cm^3.

Overall, preliminary results indicate that average airborne fiber diameters are < 0.25 μm, and fiber lengths are < 5 μm. Figure 1 is a micrograph from an area sample collected near the 'blue' calcining process at the Huntsville facility. Although the fibers pictured are atypically long, their diameters are < 0.25 μm. The micrograph provides a very good illustration of the way most fibers were found on the samples. In general, the fibers were not in bundles, and were not agglomerated with other non-fibrous particles.

Using EDX analysis, it was determined that all fibers counted were composed of tungsten. For the samples collected at processes where hard-metal binders were present (*i.e.*, Charging, Screening, Spray drying, and Sintering), the number of cobalt-containing particles that were attached to WO_x fibers was similar to the number of cobalt-containing particles that were not attached to WO_x fibers. This result indicated that cobalt-containing particles were not attached preferentially to WO_x fibers. Cobalt was not detected on filter samples collected in work areas where tungsten oxides were reduced to W (*i.e.*, calcining and reduction) or in work areas where tungsten carbide was formulated (*i.e.*, carburizing plant).

Summary

The preliminary results indicate that WO_x fibers exist in the workplace air at concentrations up to 0.268 f/cm^3. Currently, the potential adverse health effects related to human exposure to WO_x fibers are unknown. Among the samples analyzed, those collected from high-temperature processes involved in the oxidation of ammonium paratungstate to tungsten oxide and the reduction of tungsten oxide to tungsten metal contained the highest number concentration of WO_x fibers. In general, WO_x fibers were < 5 μm in length by < 0.25 μm in diameter. Cobalt was detected in air samples collected from processes subsequent to and including Charging (*i.e.*, Spray drying, Screening, and Sintering). WO_x fibers were not preferentially agglomerated to cobalt particles.

Recommendations

Formation of WO_x fibers may be the result of incomplete oxidation of ammonia paratungstate or aerosolization of these fibers during reduction of WO_3 to tungsten metal. To be prudent, NIOSH recommends that engineering studies be undertaken to better understand the production process conditions (time, temperature, and oxygen content) under which WO_x fibers are formed. Adjustment of any or all of these operating conditions may eliminate the formation of WO_x fibers. In the interim, high efficiency particulate (HEPA) respirator use is prudent for workers exposed to fibers, since health effects of tungsten oxide fibers are unknown.

References

Leanderson, P. and W. Sahle (1995). "Formation of Hydroxyl Radicals and Toxicity of Tungsten Oxide Fibers." Toxic. in Vitro 9(2): 175-183.

NIOSH (2003). NIOSH Manual of Analytical Methods (NMAM). Cincinnati, OH, National Institute for Occupational Safety and Health.

Sahle, W. (1992). "Possible Role of Tungsten Oxide Whiskers in Hard-Metal Pneumoconiosis." Chest 102: 1310.

Sahle, W., et al. (1994). "Airborne Tungsten Oxide Whiskers in a Hard-Metal Industry. Preliminary Findings." Ann. Occup. Hyg. 38(1): 37-44.

Sahle, W., et al. (1996). "Preliminary Data on Hard Metal Workers Exposure to Tungsten Oxide Fibers." Sci. Total Environ. 191: 153-167.

Table I. Type and Number of Air Samples for Tungsten Oxide Fibers, by Plant and Production Process

Plant	Process	Sample Type	Sample N
Huntsville	Ammonium paratungstate production	A = area	1
		P = personal	0
Huntsville	Calcining (blue & yellow)	A	7
		P	0
Huntsville	Reduction	A	10
		P	1
Huntsville	Carburizing	A	5
		P	1
Huntsville	Reclamation (ball mill)	A	2
		P	0
Huntsville	Reclamation (barrel dry)	A	1
		P	0
Huntsville	Reclamation (crushing)	A	1
		P	0
Huntsville	Reclamation (screening)	A	2
		P	0
Gurley	Ball mill	A	0
		P	1
Gurley	Charging	A	3
		P	1
Gurley	Reprocessing (crushing)	A	1
		P	1
Gurley	Reprocessing	A	3
		P	0
Gurley	Screening	A	6
		P	1
Gurley	Spray drying	A	5
		P	1
Grant	Pressing/Molding	A	7
		P	0
Grant	Sintering	A	8
		P	0

A = Area air sample collected at stationary locations in work areas to capture potential WO_x fiber generation during specific process activities
P = Personal breathing zone air sample collected to capture potential WO_x fiber exposures during the course of normal employee work activities

Table II. Preliminary Results for Airborne Tungsten Oxide Fiber Concentrations

Process	Fiber Count Total	Fiber Count >0.5μm	Fiber Count >5 μm	Fiber Count >15 μm	Concentration Filter (f/mm²)	Concentration Total Airborne (f/cm³)*	Cobalt?
Calcining (blue)	93	93	16	1	395	0.268	NO
Calcining (yellow)	34	34	9	ND	72	0.048	NO
Reduction	19	19	1	ND	35	0.025	NO
Reduction	12	12	ND	ND	20	0.015	NO
Carburizing	17	17	5	2	29	0.015	NO
Carburizing	6	6	1	ND	10	<LOD	NO
Spray drying	5	5	ND	ND	7	<LOD	
Charging	17	17	1	ND	30	0.012	Yes
Screening	6	6	ND	ND	10	<LOD	Yes
Screening	ND**	ND	ND	ND	<0.01	<LOD	Yes
Sintering	5	5	1	ND	8	<LOD	Yes
Total	214	214	34	3			

ND = not detected
LOD = limit of detection
* The quantitative working range of this technique is 0.01 to 0.5 f/cm³ as calculated using the number of fibers with length >0.5 μm and with a preferable fiber concentration range of 100 to 1200 f/mm²
** Airborne fiber concentration calculated using the limit of detection (0.01 f/cm³) divided by √2 (NIOSH, 2003)
Note: 12 filter samples were submitted for analysis but 1 sample could not be analyzed because the filter was overloaded with material (area sample collected near APT dryer)

Figure 1: Airborne Tungsten Oxide Fibers from 'Blue' Calcination Process

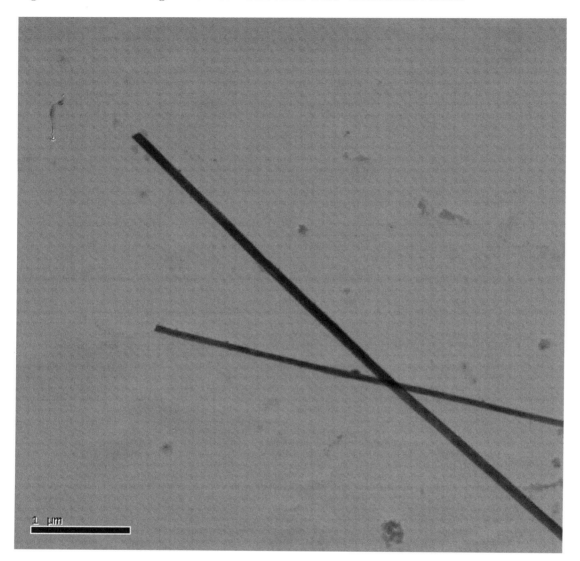

DEPARTMENT OF HEALTH & HUMAN SERVICES

Public Health Service

Phone: (304) 285-5751
Fax: (304) 285-5820

Centers for Disease Control
and Prevention (CDC)
National Institute for Occupational
Safety and Health (NIOSH)
1095 Willowdale Road
Morgantown, WV 26505-2888

August 30, 2005
HETA 2003-0257
Interim Letter V

Mr. Steve Robuck
Director of Safety and Environment
Metalworking Products
1 Teledyne Place
La Vergne, Tennessee 37086

Dear Mr. Robuck:

The purpose of this interim letter is to report the final results of two National Institute for Occupational Safety and Health (NIOSH) industrial hygiene surveys at the Alldyne Powder Technologies plants located in Huntsville and Gurley, Alabama and the Firth Sterling plant located in Grant, Alabama. NIOSH surveyed these plants in July 2003 and May 2004 in response to a confidential employee request concerning respiratory health effects and exposure to cobalt, nickel, chromium, tungsten carbide, and metalworking fluids.

The purpose, types of samples collected, and results for each industrial hygiene survey are summarized in this letter. A concluding discussion and recommendations follow the summaries of these two surveys.

Sincerely,

Nancy M. Sahakian, M.D., M.P.H.

Aleksandr Stefaniak, Ph.D., C.I.H.
Respiratory Disease Hazard Evaluation and
Technical Assistance Program
Field Studies Branch
Division of Respiratory Disease Studies

cc:
Confidential Requesters
OSHA Region 4
HETAB files

July 7 – 8, 2003 Survey

The goal of the July 7-8, 2003 survey was to perform a walk-through of the Alldyne Powder Technologies plants located in Huntsville and Gurley, Alabama and the Firth Sterling plant located in Grant, Alabama to understand the production process and collect preliminary information.

Samples collected

As summarized in the Interim Letter I (dated February 20, 2004) previously sent to you, bulk samples of unused RichGrind™ metalworking fluid (MWF), in-use MWF from a centerless grinder, liquid sludge in the MWF filter system, and solid sludge in the MWF filter system were collected.

All bulk samples were analyzed for cobalt and nickel content by a laboratory accredited for metals analysis by the American Industrial Hygiene Association (AIHA) Industrial Hygiene Laboratory Accreditation Program (IHLAP). The analytical limits of detection (LOD) and quantification (LOQ) for cobalt were 0.8 and 3 µg/g, respectively; the LOD and LOQ for nickel were 1 and 4 µg/g, respectively. A portion of the bulk samples of unused and in-use MWF were analyzed by a laboratory accredited for microbiological analysis by the AIHA Environmental Microbiology Laboratory Accreditation Program (EMLAP) to determine levels of endotoxin (a component of gram-negative bacteria), and culturable fungi, bacteria, and mycobacteria. The LOD for endotoxin was 0.005 endotoxin units per milliliter (EU/ml) (LOQ was not available) and the LOD for fungal and bacterial growth was 100 colony forming units per milliliter (CFU/ml) (LOQ was not available).

Results

Levels of cobalt and nickel in the samples of unused and in-use MWF were ≤ 1 µg/g. Levels of cobalt and nickel in the samples of liquid sludge and solid sludge were < 6600 µg/g. Endotoxin and culturable fungi, bacteria, or microbacteria were not detected in the sample of unused MWF. In the sample of in-use MWF from a centerless grinder, 200 EU/ml were detected. In this same sample, culturable fungi or mycobateria were not detected, but 1700 CFU/ml of culturable bacteria was measured.

May 20 – 27, 2004 Survey

The goal of this survey was to characterize the amount, size distribution, and number concentration of airborne particles at various operations in the hard metal production processes utilized at the Alldyne Powder Technologies plants located in Huntsville and Gurley, Alabama and the Firth Sterling plant located in Grant, Alabama.

Samples collected

Bulk powders

Bulk samples of powders (see Table I) were obtained for a range of process feed materials (e.g., tungsten, tungsten carbide, and chromium carbide) and for a range of process steps (e.g., Chamfer grind dust, Shaper dust, and dust from the Spokane Crusher). Density (g/cm³) was determined for triplicate measurements of each powder using a helium pycnometer (Multipycnometer, Quantachrome, Boynton Beach, FL). Measured values were compared to published handbook values. Knowledge of the particle densities and physical particle size distributions of feed stock and process powders provides insight into the observed airborne particle size distributions measured aerodynamically by cascade impaction and measured optically by the GRIMM particle counter.

Micro-orifice uniform deposit impactor (MOUDI)

Seventeen samples of airborne particles were collected in seven different work areas using micro-orifice uniform deposit impactor (MOUDI) samplers (Model 110, MSP Corporation, Shoreview, MN). The MOUDI sampler collects airborne particles based on their size. The aerodynamic diameter cut points for the MOUDI sampler were >18 μm (inlet stage), 10 μm (stage 1), 5.6 μm (stage 2), 3.2 μm (stage 3), 1.8 μm (stage 4), 1.0 μm (stage 5), 0.56 μm (stage 6), 0.32 μm (stage 7), 0.18 μm (stage 8), 0.10 μm (stage 9), 0.056 μm (stage 10), and <0.056 (final filter). Fifteen of the 17 samples were collected on polyvinyl chloride (PVC) substrate and two of the 17 samples were collected on mixed cellulose ester (MCE) substrate. PVC substrates are weight-stable and this media was used for most samples to gravimetrically determine the total mass of airborne particulate collected on each substrate. The weight of MCE substrates is unstable so this substrate media was used for a few samples to determine only the elements on the substrates. All impactor substrates except the final filters were sprayed with silicone to prevent particle bounce during sampling.

The total mass of airborne particulate collected on each PVC substrate was determined gravimetrically at NIOSH using a calibrated weighing balance (Model UMX2, Metler Toledo Inc.) stationed in a temperature and humidity controlled chamber. All substrates (PVC and MCE) were submitted for analysis of cobalt, chromium, and nickel content in accordance with NIOSH Method 7300: Inductively Coupled Plasma-Atomic Emission Spectroscopy by a laboratory accredited for metals analysis by the AIHA IHLAP. The LOD and LOQ for cobalt were 0.2 and 0.6 μg/filter, respectively; the LOD and LOQ for chromium were 0.3 and 1 μg/filter, respectively; and, the LOD and LOQ for nickel were 0.4 and 1 μg/filter, respectively.

Reduction of analytical data from the MOUDI samples included an estimate of total particle concentration, total element concentration, total particle size distribution, element size distribution, and element mass fraction information as a function of particle size. For the gravimetric determinations of total particle mass, on occasion a substrate weighed less after sampling than before sampling. The most likely cause for the apparent loss of weight from a substrate is residual silicon spray sticking to the substrate holder when the substrate was removed after sampling for weighing. In the event that a loss in filter weight was recorded, a value of zero was substituted for the purposes of data reduction. (Note that it was possible to have a quantifiable mass of cobalt, chromium, or nickel on a substrate for which the total particle mass was negative because elemental mass and total particle mass were determined using two different techniques.) For analysis of element size distribution data, a value reported by the analytical laboratory was considered a real number if it was between the LOD and LOQ. To calculate concentration and an estimate of particle size, the LOD was substituted for a value reported as <LOD provided at least 85% of the mass on all substrates in a sample was contributed by measured values (*i.e.*, values above the LOQ). Note that an alternative approach for censored data is to substitute a value of one-half the LOD for a value reported as <LOD, but this substitution would not have an appreciable effect on the reported results.

Marple cascade impactor

Eleven samples of airborne particles were collected in seven different work areas using Marple series 290 8-stage cascade impactor samplers (MSP Corporation, Shoreview, MN). Five of the eleven cascade impactor samples were worn in the personal breathing zone of employees during the course of their normal work activities. The remaining six cascade impactor samples were collected at a stationary location in a work area during specific process activities. The aerodynamic diameter cut points for the cascade impactor sampler were >21.3 μm (stage 1), 14.8 μm (stage 2), 9.8 μm (stage 3), 6.0 μm (stage 4), 3.5 μm (stage 5), 1.55 μm (stage 6), 0.93 μm (stage 7), 0.52 μm (stage 8), and <0.52 μm (final filter). All 11 samples were collected on PVC substrate that was sprayed with silicone to prevent particle bounce during sampling.

All cascade impactor substrates were analyzed for cobalt, chromium, and nickel content in accordance with

NIOSH Method 7300 by a laboratory accredited for metals analysis by the AIHA IHLAP. (Gravimetric determination of the mass of airborne particles collected on the substrate was not performed for the cascade impactor samples because the 2.0 L/min flow rate for the impactor is not sufficient to collect large enough airborne particle masses for weighing.) The LOD and LOQ for cobalt were 0.3 and 1 μg/filter, respectively; the LOD and LOQ for chromium were 0.7 and 2 μg/filter, respectively; and, the LOD and LOQ for nickel were 0.9 and 3 μg/filter, respectively. Analyses of data from the Marple impactor samples included an estimate of total element mass concentration and element size distribution. As with the MOUDI samples, for analysis of element size distribution data, a value reported by the analytical laboratory was considered a real number if it was between the LOD and LOQ. To calculate concentration and an estimate of particle size, the LOD was substituted for a value reported as <LOD provided at least 85% of the mass on all substrates in a sample was contributed by measured values (*i.e.*, values above the LOQ). Note that an alternative approach for censored data is to substitute a value of one-half the LOD for a value reported as <LOD, but this substitution would not have an appreciable effect on the reported results.

37-mm open- and close-faced filter cassette

Twenty six half-shift or full-shift samples of airborne particles were collected in 12 different work areas using 37-mm cassette samplers. Eighteen of the 26 cassette samples were worn in the personal breathing zone of employees during the course of their normal work activities. The remaining eight cassette samples were collected at stationary locations in work areas during specific process activities. All 37-mm cassette samples were collected on MCE substrate. The 37-mm cassette samples were collected using either close- or open-faced cassette configuration. Note that close-faced sampling is standard practice for cobalt; however, open-faced cassette samples were collected to ensure even distribution of particles on the substrate, regardless of size, during sampling. One personal cassette sample was voided because the cassette fell on the ground for an unknown period of time during sampling.

All substrates were analyzed for cobalt, chromium, and nickel content in accordance with NIOSH Method 7300 by a laboratory accredited for metals analysis by the AIHA IHLAP. The LOD and LOQ for cobalt were 0.02 and 0.07 μg/filter, respectively; the LOD and LOQ for chromium were 0.06 and 0.2 μg/filter, respectively; and, the LOD and LOQ for nickel were 0.04 and 0.1 μg/filter, respectively.

Real-time particle size and number concentration

Fourteen samples of airborne particle size distribution and number concentration were determined in seven different work areas using real-time optical particle counters (Model 1.108, GRIMM Technologies Inc., Douglasville, GA). The particle counting instruments are capable of determining airborne particle size and particle number concentration but are unable to determine the chemical composition of the particles. Optical particle count samples were collected at stationary locations in work areas during specific process activities. The particle counting instruments spanned the physical size range 0.3 μm to >20 μm in 15 channels: >0.3 μm, >0.4 μm, >0.5 μm, >0.65 μm, >0.8 μm, >1.0 μm, >1.6 μm, >2.0 μm, >3 μm, >4 μm, >5 μm, >7.5 μm, >10 μm, >15 μm, and >20 μm. To provide a detailed temporal record of airborne particle concentration, two particle counting instruments were operated in parallel at each work area in the fast-sampling-time mode (collection of data every second). One unit covered channels 1 through 8: >0.3 μm, >0.4 μm, >0.5 μm, >0.65 μm, >0.8 μm, >1.0 μm, >1.6 μm, and >2.0 μm and the second unit covered channels 8 through 15: >2.0 μm, >3 μm, >4 μm, >5 μm, >7.5 μm, >10 μm, >15 μm, and >20 μm. Note that channel eight was overlapped by both sampling units. Note also that the particle diameter measured by the GRIMM instrument is optical or approximate physical diameter, which is generally smaller than the aerodynamic diameter measured by the cascade impactor. As a rule of thumb, the aerodynamic diameter of a particle is approximately equal to its physical diameter times the square root of its density. For example, a cobalt particle with physical diameter of 10 μm and density 8.9 g/cm^3 will have an aerodynamic diameter of approximately 29.8 μm.

Results

Bulk powders

As shown in Table I, the relationship between the measured and handbook density values depended on whether the powder samples consisted of a single material or a mixture of materials. For example, the density of WC feed stock material, 15.79 g/cm³, was similar to the reported handbook value (15.63 g/cm³), while densities of reclaimed WC powder (*i.e.*, 14.58 g/cm³ and 14.30 g/cm³) were lower than the density of pure WC but higher than the density of expected component materials such as cobalt (handbook density 8.9 g/cm³), nickel (handbook density 8.9 g/cm³), or molybdenum (handbook density 10.2 g/cm³). The lowest measured densities were 1.59 g/cm³ for the ammonium paratungstate (APT)/cobalt residue filter cake and 1.88 g/cm³ for carbon powder.

Micro-orifice uniform deposit impactor (MOUDI)

Total particle and total cobalt concentrations determined using MOUDI samplers are summarized in Table II. Total airborne particle mass concentration ranged from 55.0 μg/m³ (Grinding) to 3783.3 μg/m³ (Charging), whereas total cobalt in air ranged from 3.5 μg/m³ (Pressing) to 191.0 μg/m³ (Reclaim A). Nickel concentrations were generally low; the analytical LOD for nickel was exceeded in just two of the 17 samples (9.7 μg/m³ in Charging and 2.1 μg/m³ in Screening). Chromium levels were similar to background levels in substrate for all samples. Levels of total airborne particle mass were positively correlated with levels of total airborne cobalt mass collected on MOUDI samples (Figure 1).

The mass median aerodynamic diameter (MMAD) and geometric standard deviation (GSD) of particles determined using MOUDI samplers are summarized in Table II. Aerodynamic diameter is the diameter of a spherical particle with density 1 g/cm³ that has the equivalent settling velocity as the particle under study. The MMAD is the aerodynamic diameter above which 50% of the particles have greater mass and below which 50% of the particles have less mass. In a log-normal distribution, 68% of the particles fall within the size range MMAD/GSD to MMAD×GSD and 95% of particles fall within the size range MMAD/GSD² to MMAD×GSD². The MMAD of airborne dust ranged from 0.8 μm (Grinding) to 31.0 μm (Reclaim B- ball mill). Cobalt MMADs were generally greater than 10 μm (Table II), with the exception of samples in Grinding, and for a sample in Spray Drying and in Charging. Because most values of airborne nickel were below analytical detection limits, the MMAD could only be calculated for a sample collected in Charging (4.9 μm) and Screening (23.6 μm).

Of the 15 MOUDI samples collected using PVC substrate (Table II), a clear relationship was observed between the fraction of cobalt in airborne dust and aerodynamic particle diameter in four samples (see Figure 2). In general, the fraction of cobalt in airborne dust increased as aerodynamic particle diameter increased in Charging (3 samples) and in Screening (1 sample). , Variations in the fraction of cobalt in airborne dust among the three samples collected in charging may be due to differences in the proximity of samplers relative to a work activity and temporal variations in work activities. No clear relationship between the fraction of cobalt in airborne dust and aerodynamic particle diameter was observed for any of the remaining 11 MOUDI samples collected using PVC substrate.

Marple cascade impactor

Personal Breathing Zone Samples

Total cobalt, chromium, and nickel concentrations measured in the personal breathing zone of employees using

Marple impactor samplers are summarized in Table III. The levels of cobalt in air ranged from 16.4 (Shaping) to 319.8 µg/m³ (Milling at Gurley). Airborne chromium levels were very low: two samples were below the analytical limit of detection (Screening, Shaping), two samples were semi-quantitative, *i.e.*, between the LOD and LOQ (Charging and Tray Prep), and the sample in Milling was 8.1 µg/m³. Airborne nickel levels ranged from <LOD (Screening, Shaping, Tray Prep) to 105.5 µg/m³ (Charging).

The MMAD and GSD of cobalt and nickel particles are included in Table III. For all work areas sampled, calculated MMAD were greater than 10 µm. Variability between element concentrations and values of the MMAD estimated from MOUDI sample results and Marple impactor sample results may be attributable to the type of sample (personal versus area), placement of the sampler in the work area, and temporal variations (amount of material processed, open or closed doors and windows, etc.) Estimates of the MMAD and GSD were not calculated for chromium because most of the data was either below analytical method detection limits or semi-quantitative.

General Area Samples

Total cobalt concentrations measured at stationary locations in different work areas using Marple impactor samplers are summarized in Table IV. The level of cobalt in air ranged from <LOD (Sandblasting) to 142.8 µg/m³ (Spokane crusher in Reclaim B). Nickel and chromium levels in all samples were <LOD.

The MMAD and GSD of cobalt particles measured in area samples are also summarized in Table IV. The MMAD were greater than 10 µm for all work areas in which cobalt was measured, with the exception of Tray Prep.

37-mm open- and close-faced filter cassette

Personal Breathing Zone Samples

Total cobalt, chromium, and nickel concentrations measured in the personal breathing zones of employees using close- and open-faced 37-mm cassette samplers are summarized in Table V. In general, exposure levels were highest in Charging, Milling, and Spray Drying. Levels of cobalt ranged from 1.6 (Shipping at Grant) to 815.4 µg/m³ (Charging). Airborne cobalt levels were lowest in Shipping (at Grant) and Grinding, and generally exceeded 20 µg/m³ in most other work areas sampled. Chromium levels were generally low in all work areas sampled, with a maximum level of 2.9 µg/m³ in Milling at Gurley. Airborne nickel levels were generally low in all work areas sampled, except for Charging (maximum 804.7 µg/m³) and Milling (66.6 µg/m³).

General Area Samples

Total cobalt, chromium, and nickel concentrations measured at stationary locations in different work areas using close- and open-faced 37-mm cassette samplers are summarized in Table VI. The levels of airborne cobalt were lowest in Shaping, Sandblasting, and Tray Prep but exceeded 20 µg/m³ in the other work areas sampled. Chromium levels in air were generally below 6 µg/m³ in all work areas sampled and airborne nickel levels were below 3.5 µg/m³.

Real-time particle size and number concentration

Airborne particle size and number concentration samples were collected at stationary locations in Charging (4 samples), Screening (2 samples), Blending (2 samples), Grinding (1 samples), Shaping (1 sample), Tray Prep (1 sample), Reclaim A (1 sample), and Reclaim B (1 sample at Ball mill #7 and one sample at Blender). For each sample, the ratio of the count data from the overlapped channel 8 (>2 µm) from the two instruments was calculated. A ratio of 1.0 would indicate perfect agreement of data between the two instruments. In most cases, the ratio of the count data ranged from 0.8 to 1.2 allowing the use of an average of the channel 8 count data for plotting.

As expected, real-time particle count data indicated that specific work activities were associated with increased numbers of particles in air (Figures 3 to 5). For example, particle number concentration increased when charging was initiated, subsided during a work break, and increased when charging was resumed (Figure 3). When sintering trays were sprayed in the Tray Prep work area, particle number concentration increased (Figure 4). In Reclaim A, particle number concentration increased when furnace containers were loaded and unloaded (Figure 5). Particle number concentration also increased (data not shown) when a blender was unloaded (at Gurley), Ball Mill #7 was started (Gurley), powder was Screened (Gurley), material was Shaped, and parts were Chamfer ground.

Discussion

Particle size distribution

Analysis of particle mass distribution data (Tables I to III) indicate that airborne dust was generally respirable in size (*i.e.*, less than 10 μm in aerodynamic diameter). Cobalt and nickel aerosol particles generated during work activities surveyed were generally non-respirable (*i.e.*, greater than 10 μm in aerodynamic diameter), with the notable exception of cobalt aerosol generated during grinding activities. Respirable particles are more likely to deposit in the gas exchange region of the lung whereas non-respirable particles are more likely to deposit in the upper airways of the respiratory tract. In general, the MMAD will decrease as the energy imparted on the material during processing is increased. The observed small particle mass distributions were consistent with a higher-energy activity such as Grinding. The large particle size distributions were consistent with low-energy powder handling activities such as those performed during reclamation (*e.g.*, crushing), Blending, Milling, Screening, Pressing, and Shaping.

A strong positive relationship was observed between the fraction of cobalt in airborne dust and aerodynamic particle diameter for MOUDI samples collected in Charging and in Screening (Figure 2). This observation suggests that housekeeping and control measures that reduce ambient airborne dust could help to lower airborne cobalt levels.

Cobalt

As shown in Tables I to V, airborne cobalt levels exceeded the U.S. Occupational Safety and Health Administration (OSHA) permissible exposure limit (PEL) of 100 μg/m^3 in Reclaim A, Reclaim B, Charging, Milling, and Spray Drying. The NIOSH recommended exposure limit (REL) for cobalt (50 μg/m^3) was exceeded in the same areas as the PEL, and in Screening. The American Conference of Governmental Industrial Hygienists (ACGIH) threshold limit value (TLV) for cobalt (20 μg/m^3) was exceeded in the same areas as in which the PEL and REL were exceeded, and also in Tray Prep, Extrusion, Pressing, and Shaping. Values of the PEL, REL, and TLV for cobalt, chromium, and nickel were obtained from the *Guide to Occupational Exposure Values* published by the American Conference of Governmental Industrial Hygienists (Cincinnati, OH, 2002.)

Several MOUDI area samples were collected in Reclaim A and Reclaim B during the time in which specific activities were performed (Table II). From these data, specific activities may contribute disproportionately to measured exposure levels. For example, in Reclaim A, loading furnace containers generated higher levels of cobalt dust relative to operation of the cake crusher. In Reclaim B, operation of the ball mill, big Spokane crusher, and blender generated higher levels of cobalt dust relative to operation of the little Spokane crusher.

Chromium

Airborne chromium levels were well below the PEL, REL, and TLV in all work areas surveyed.

Nickel

Levels of airborne nickel were below the PEL, REL, and TLV in all work areas surveyed, except Charging and Milling, where the NIOSH REL for nickel (15 μg/m³) was exceeded.

Particle number concentration

Real-time particle count data indicated that specific work activities were associated with increased particle number concentration (Figures 3 – 5). Although the real-time particle counting instruments were not capable of discerning the chemical form of the particles counted, the data are potentially useful for identifying specific work activities with potential to generate airborne particles. Specific work activities that disproportionately generate aerosol could then be targeted for chemical-specific sampling to determine if cobalt is being generated in appreciable amounts. Information from sampling using a method specific for cobalt could be used to guide implementation of needed controls to reduce or eliminate release of cobalt aerosol from these work activities.

Note that when interpreting results from the GRIMM optical particle counter, it is conservative (*i.e.*, results in a higher estimate of respirable particle airborne mass) to assume that all particles are unit density. Use of the actual measured particle densities (Table I) to convert optical particle diameter to aerodynamic particle diameter will result in lower estimated concentrations of airborne mass in the respirable size range. Note that the cascade impactor results measure the aerodynamic size distributions directly.

NIOSH recommendations following the July 2003 and May 2004 surveys

Building on our recommendations from Interim Letter 1 (dated February 20, 2004) and Interim Letter II (dated March 2, 2005) previously sent to you, the following recommendations are made concerning exposure to MWF and metals at all three plants:

MWF

- Employee training
  - o As part of your existing employee training program, train employees on the potential adverse health effects associated with exposure to MWF, how to detect potential hazardous situations (*e.g.*, appearance of bacteria overgrowth and degradation of MWF), and appropriate work practices (*e.g.*, minimizing skin contact with MWF)
- Engineering
  - o Minimize the generation of MWF mists through appropriate operation and control of the MWF delivery system (see for example, *Mist Control Considerations for the Design, Installation, and Use of Machine Tools Using Metalworking Fluids*, American National Standards Institute Technical Report B11 TR 2-1997)
    - ▪ For control of exposure, utilize the industrial hygiene hierarchy of controls (ranked in order of most preferred to least preferred control method): elimination> substitution> engineering>work practices> personal protective equipment
- Work practices
  - o Augment your current MWF inspection protocol as appropriate to include a written MWF management plan that specifies procedures for maintenance of fluid chemistry (*e.g.*, pH, temperature, viscosity, storage, mixing and diluting MWF concentrate, preparing additives such as biocides and a cobalt agglomerator, and monitoring tramp oil contamination) and maintenance

of the fluid filtration and delivery systems (*e.g.*, fluid level in sump tank)

- Protective clothing and equipment
  - o Appropriate protective clothing should be worn when working with MWF (note that nitrile is thought to afford the most chemical resistance to MWF)
- Personal Hygiene
  - o Employees should periodically wash MWF-contaminated skin with mild soap and water and dry with clean towels
  - o Employees should be reminded to avoid placing their bare skin into MWF

Metals

- Continue to monitor inhalation exposure levels of cobalt and nickel in work areas where recognized professional and federal occupational exposure values are exceeded
  - o Inhalation exposure should be sampled in the personal breathing zone
- Reduce cobalt exposure levels to below recognized professional and federal occupational exposure values using the industrial hygiene hierarchy of controls (ranked in order of most preferred to least preferred control method): engineering>work practices> personal protective equipment
- Engineering
  - o In work areas with elevated cobalt exposures, use ventilation or other feasible engineering technologies to control exposure levels
  - o To aid in identification of specific work activities that may contribute disproportionately to metal exposure in a work area:
    - Dissect each job in a work area of elevated exposure into step-by-step activities (utilize employee input)
    - Use a portable real-time particle counter to identify the activities of a job that generate more aerosol than other activities
    - Implement a sampling strategy to characterize the chemical composition of the aerosol being generated by the activity
    - If cobalt is being generated in appreciable amounts, implement needed controls to reduce or eliminate aerosol
- Work practices
  - o Dedicate equipment (*e.g.*, hand tools) to specific work areas to prevent cobalt contamination migration from an area of higher cobalt to an area of lower cobalt contamination
  - o Provide a high-efficiency particulate air (HEPA) filtered vacuum in the pressing area for employees to clean their machines and work area. Use of a HEPA filtered vacuum will minimize transfer of cobalt from surfaces to air and unprotected areas of the skin when cleaning
  - o Employees in grinding should stand at a reasonable distance away from grinding machines during operation to minimize potential for exposure
  - o Ensure and routinely check the integrity of the sandblasting glove box air hoses and gloves
  - o Implement a skin protection program to minimize contamination of skin with metal powders
    - Use a non-latex material for gloves and other barriers.
- Personal protective clothing and equipment
  - o Use a non-latex glove material (*e.g.*, nitrile) with over gloves made of a resilient material when performing activities that require durable protection from substantial cobalt skin exposure
  - o Appropriate respiratory protection should be worn by properly trained personnel when job activities could result in metal aerosol exposure levels above recognized professional and federal occupational exposure values

- Respiratory protection may not perform as intended if it is not donned, used and maintained properly. As such, the use of personal protective equipment is not recommended as a primary means of reducing exposure levels on a long term basis
- Personal Hygiene
    - Employees should periodically wash metal-contaminated skin with mild soap and water and dry with clean towels
        - Especially before eating, smoking, or using the bathroom
    - Employees should be reminded to avoid placing their bare skin into metal powders
    - Shower soon after work
    - Improve cleanliness of non-production areas
        - Thoroughly clean and maintain lunch rooms and identify as "Clean Areas"
        - Minimize migration of cobalt from production to non-production areas

Table I. Density of bulk powder samples (May 2004)

Powder	Density (g/cm³) Measured	Density (g/cm³) Handbook	Density (g/cm³) Ratio (Measured/ Handbook)
Tungsten Carbide	15.79	15.63	1.01
Tungsten Carbide (reclaimed)	14.58	15.63	0.93
Tungsten Carbide (reclaimed)	14.30	15.63	0.91
Cobalt (0.5 μm)	8.18	8.90	0.92
Cobalt (extrafine)	9.26	8.90	1.04
Cobalt (400 mesh)	9.19	8.90	1.03
Nickel (regular)	8.93	8.90	1.00
Tantalum carbide	14.44	13.90	1.04
Molybdenum	10.36	10.20	1.02
Carbon	1.88	1.8 – 2.1	1.05 – 0.90
Torit dust (Grant)	13.52	NA	NA
APT/cobalt residue filter cake	1.59	NA	NA
Dry grinder duct dust (Grant)	10.48	NA	NA
Extrusion raw material (lot #76369)	14.09	NA	NA

NA = Not applicable for production–stream products or byproducts

Table II. Total mass concentration and mass median aerodynamic diameter of area samples collected using MOUDI samplers (May 2004)

Plant	Work Area	Total concentration, $(\mu g/m^3)^*$ Particle	Total concentration, $(\mu g/m^3)^*$ Cobalt	MMAD, μm (GSD)** Particle	MMAD, μm (GSD)** Cobalt
Huntsville	Reclaim A (container loading)	2310.5	191.0	4.9 (2.6)	29.2 (6.2)
Huntsville	Reclaim A (cake crusher)	977.2	27.4	4.4 (4.7)	10.5 (6.1)
Huntsville	Reclaim B (big Spokane)	2166.7	77.4	6.3 (2.7)	27.0 (5.9)
Huntsville	Reclaim B (little Spokane)	549.2	21.4	4.7 (4.8)	24.1 (6.3)
Huntsville	Reclaim B (ball mill)	2815.2	132.2	31.0 (5.8)	41.7 (5.4)
Gurley	Charging (near mixer)	825.4	70.5	4.5 (1.9)	10.8 (3.9)
Gurley	Charging (near mixer)	1917.1	108.3	6.1 (2.7)	19.3 (3.9)
Gurley	Charging (near mixer)	3783.3	145.2	6.9 (3.7)	7.0 (2.8)
Gurley	Charging (near mixer)	NA	91.5	NA	12.7 (3.7)
Gurley	Spray drying (sprayer #1)	142.2	9.4	8.2 (6.0)	7.2 (2.8)
Gurley	Screening (next to screener)	1898.1	81.2	1.8 (4.0)	11.2 (4.2)
Gurley	Screening (on table)	NA	8.2	NA	12.3 (5.6)
Grant	Pressing (outside 75-ton press)	191.4	3.5	1.2 (2.7)	NC
Grant	Pressing (inside 75-ton press)	471.6	12.1	1.6 (2.3)	63.1 (21.3)
Grant	Grinding (grinding area)	228.7	1.0	2.8 (3.6)	5.9 (8.4)
Grant	Grinding (dry grinder)	126.2	0.8	1.9 (2.4)	5.5 (10.3)
Grant	Grinding (center of plant)	55.0	0.7	0.8 (3.3)	6.2 (6.9)

NA = Not applicable for samples collected on mixed cellulose ester (MCE) substrate
NC = Value not calculated because less than 85% of cobalt mass was below the analytical LOQ
* Total concentration = sum of element mass on each impactor stage substrate for a given sample divided by air volume sampled
** MMAD = mass median aerodynamic diameter; GSD = geometric standard deviation

Table III. Total element concentration and mass median aerodynamic diameter of personal breathing zone samples collected using Marple series 290 8-stage cascade impactors (May 2004)

Plant	Work Area	Total concentration, (μg/m³)* Cobalt	Total concentration, (μg/m³)* Nickel	MMAD, μm (GSD)** Cobalt	MMAD, μm (GSD)** Nickel
Gurley	Charging	145.2	105.5	14.1 (2.4)	13.8 (2.4)
Gurley	Milling	319.8	46.7	16.3 (2.5)	17.0 (2.8)
Gurley	Screening	52.9	ND	19.1 (3.3)	NA
Grant	Shaping	16.4	ND	18.3 (4.7)	NA
Grant	Tray Prep	47.4	ND	13.5 (3.1)	NA

ND = Below the analytical method limit of detection (LOD)
NA = Not applicable because sample results were less than the analytical method limit of detection
* Total concentration = sum of element mass on each impactor stage substrate for a given sample divided by air volume sampled
** MMAD = mass median aerodynamic diameter; GSD = geometric standard deviation

Table IV. Total cobalt concentration and mass median aerodynamic diameter for area samples collected using Marple series 290 8-stage cascade impactors (May 2004)

Plant	Work Area	Total Cobalt (μg/m³)*	MMAD, μm (GSD)**
Huntsville	Reclaim B (Spokane)	142.8	13.8 (2.7)
Huntsville	Reclaim B (Ball mill)	133.6	17.7 (2.9)
Huntsville	Reclaim B (Blender)	113.7	12.1 (2.5)
Grant	Tray Prep	9.9	8.7 (3.5)
Grant	Sandblasting	ND	NA
Grant	Shaping	2.1***	NA

ND = Below the analytical method limit of detection (LOD)
NA = Not applicable because sample results were less than the analytical method limit of detection or semi-quantitative
* Total concentration = sum of element mass on each impactor stage substrate for a given sample divided by air volume sampled
** MMAD = mass median aerodynamic diameter; GSD = geometric standard deviation
*** Semi-quantitative (between the LOD and LOQ)

Table V. Total element concentration for samples collected in the personal breathing zone using close- and open-faced 37-mm filter cassettes (May 2004)

Plant	Work Area	Cassette	Total Concentration ($\mu g/m^3$) Cobalt	Total Concentration ($\mu g/m^3$) Chromium	Total Concentration ($\mu g/m^3$) Nickel
Huntsville	Reclaim B	Close-faced	43.2	ND	0.4
Huntsville	Reclaim B	Close-faced	57.2	0.7	0.4
Huntsville	Reclaim B	Close-faced	82.8	0.8	0.3
Huntsville	Reclaim B	Close-faced	107.8	1.1	1.0
Gurley	Charging	Close-faced	89.0	0.2	107.2
Gurley	Charging	Close-faced	815.4	0.8	804.7
Gurley	Milling	Close-faced	318.7	2.9	66.6
Gurley	Spray Drying	Open-faced	110.4	0.7	2.6
Grant	Extrusion	Close-faced	34.6	0.8	0.2
Grant	Pressing	Close-faced	37.5	1.0	0.7
Grant	Pressing	Close-faced	17.1	1.0	0.3
Grant	Shaping	Close-faced	9.5	0.0	0.3
Grant	Shaping	Close-faced	33.1	0.4	0.6
Grant	Grinding	Open-faced	1.8	0.5	0.7
Grant	Grinding	Open-faced	2.3	0.5	0.3
Grant	Shipping	Open-faced	1.6	0.5	0.3
Grant	Tray Prep	Close-faced	39.3	1.6	1.7
		OSHA PEL	100	1000	1000
		NIOSH REL	50	500	15
		ACGIH TLV	20	500	1500

ND = Below the analytical method limit of detection (LOD)

Table VI. Total element concentration for samples collected at stationary locations in work areas using close- and open-faced 37-mm filter cassettes (May 2004)

Plant	Work Area	Cassette	Total Concentration (µg/m³) Cobalt	Total Concentration (µg/m³) Chromium	Total Concentration (µg/m³) Nickel
Huntsville	Reclaim A	Close-faced	556.2	6.3	3.5
Huntsville	Reclaim B	Open-faced	65.4	0.6	0.3
Huntsville	Reclaim B	Close-faced	54.2	0.1	0.2
Huntsville	Reclaim B	Close-faced	183.8	1.0	0.3
Huntsville	Reclaim B	Close-faced	61.1	1.0	0.3
Grant	Shaping	Open-faced	4.3	0.7	0.2
Grant	Sandblasting	Open-faced	0.7	0.5	ND
Grant	Tray Prep	Open-faced	6.9	0.2	0.2
		OSHA PEL	100	1000	1000
		NIOSH REL	50	500	15
		ACGIH TLV	20	500	1500

ND = Below the analytical method limit of detection (LOD)

Figure 1. Relationship between total particle dust mass concentration and total cobalt concentration for area samples collected using MOUDI air samplers. Levels of total cobalt mass were positively related to levels of total particle mass in the work area as indicated by the positive R^2 values given in the plot. An R^2 value is an estimate of the relationship between two variables and can range from -1 (exact negative linear relationship) to 1 (exact positive linear relationship).

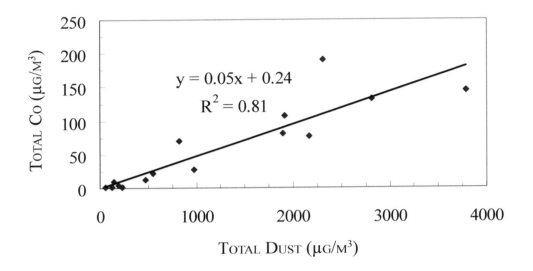

$$y = 0.05x + 0.24$$
$$R^2 = 0.81$$

Figure 2. Relationship between the fraction of cobalt in airborne dust and aerodynamic particle diameter for area samples collected using MOUDI air samplers using PVC substrate. The fraction of cobalt in airborne dust increased as aerodynamic particle diameter increased for (a) three samples collected in Charging and for (b) one sample collected in Screening. No clear relationship between the fraction of cobalt in airborne dust and aerodynamic particle diameter was observed for any other MOUDI samples.

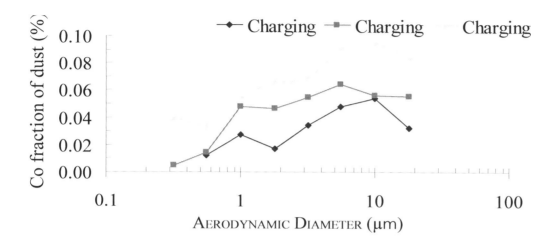

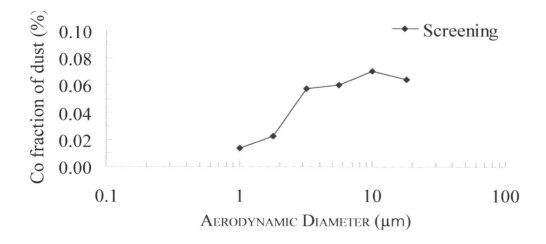

Figure 3. Example of fluctuations in particle number concentration during charging (May 20, 2004).

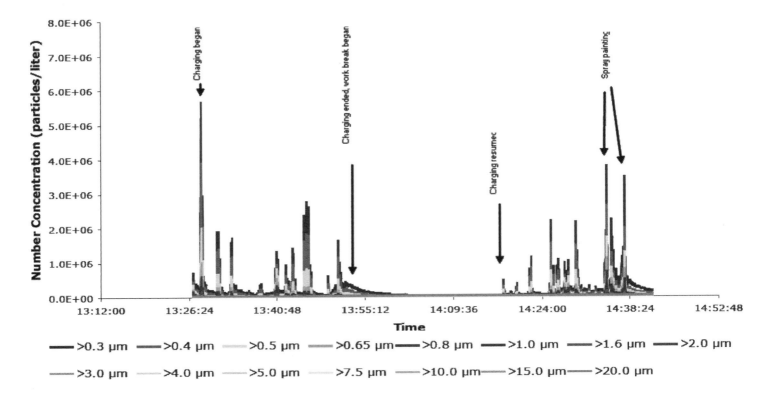

Figure 4. Example of fluctuations in particle number concentration during preparation of sintering trays in tray prep work area (May 24, 2004).

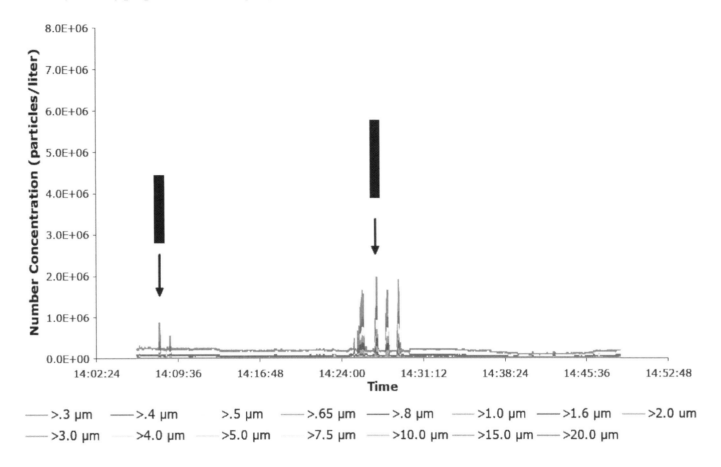

Figure 5. Example of fluctuations in particle number concentration during loading and unloading of furnace containers in Reclaim A work area (May 26, 2004).

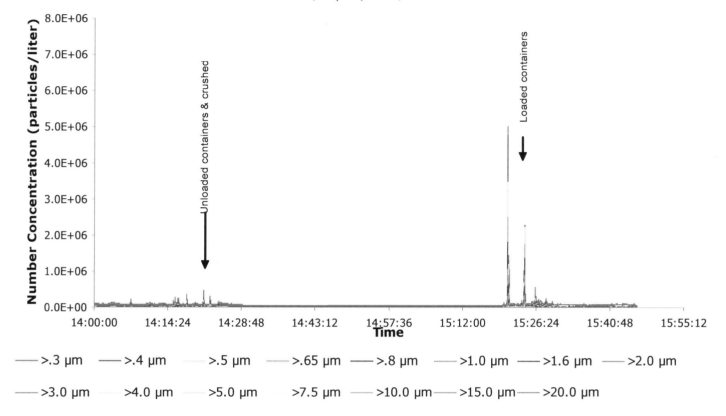

DEPARTMENT OF HEALTH & HUMAN SERVICES   **Public Health Service**

Phone: (304) 285-5751
  Fax: (304) 285-5820

Centers for Disease Control
  and Prevention (CDC)
National Institute for Occupational
Safety and Health (NIOSH)
1095 Willowdale Road
Morgantown, WV 26505-2888

September 1, 2005
HETA 2003-0257
Interim Letter VI

Mr. Steve Robuck, P.E.
Director of Safety and Environment
Metalworking Products
1 Teledyne Place
LaVergne, Tennessee 37086

Dear Mr. Robuck:

The National Institute for Occupational Safety and Health (NIOSH) conducted industrial hygiene surveys at the Alldyne Powder Technologies plants located in Huntsville and Gurley, Alabama and the Firth Sterling plant located in Grant, Alabama in July 2003, May 2004, October 2004, and November 2004. These surveys were in response to a confidential employee request concerning respiratory health effects and exposure to cobalt, nickel, chromium, tungsten carbide, and metalworking fluids.

This interim report includes the preliminary results for airborne tungsten fiber samples which were collected from October 26 to November 4, 2005. In accordance with the Code of Federal Regulations, Title 42, Part 85, copies of this letter must be posted by management in a prominent place accessible to employees for a period of 30 calendar days.

Sincerely,

Nancy Sahakian, M.D., M.P.H.
Lieutenant Commander, USPHS
Respiratory Disease Hazard Evaluation and
    Technical Assistance Program
Field Studies Branch
Division of Respiratory Disease Studies

Enclosure
cc:
Daryl Baker
Larry Hollingsworth
Junior Pugh
Confidential Employee Requestors
HETAB file (HETA 2003-0257)

Presence of Tungsten Oxide Fibers in Hard-Metal Processes

John McKernan, MSPH, CIH
National Institute for Occupational Safety and Health
Division of Surveillance, Hazard Evaluations and Field Studies
Industry-wide Studies Branch
Phone: 513-841-4212
Email: JMcKernan@cdc.gov

August 15, 2005

Purpose

To date, the existence of tungsten oxide fibers in the hard-metal industry (or any other tungsten-using industry) has not been evaluated in the United States. The purpose of this research project was to 1) perform a walk-through survey at the Alldyne Powder Technologies plants located in Huntsville and Gurley, Alabama and the Firth Sterling plant located in Grant, Alabama to understand the production processes and collect preliminary information; 2) conduct general area and personal breathing-zone (PBZ) air sampling to collect filter samples of airborne particles at various steps in the hard metal production processes; and 3) analyze the filter samples to determine the shape (morphology) and chemical composition of airborne particles collected in the three plants to determine if tungsten oxide fibers exist in the workplace atmosphere.

Background

To make tungsten metal (W), tungsten-containing material (*e.g.*, ore, reclaimed material in the form of ammonia paratungstate) is oxidized to form tungsten trioxide (WO_3). WO_3 is heated under an inert atmosphere and reduced to W. During calcination to form WO_3 and during reduction of WO_3, a series of lower tungsten oxide (referred to as WO_x in this report) compounds can be formed as byproducts of incomplete chemical reactions. Studies within the Swedish hard metal industry have shown that calcination of ammonium paratungstate and reduction of tungsten-containing compounds can generate WO_x compounds in the form of airborne fibers (Sahle, 1992; Sahle et al., 1994; Leanderson and Sahle, 1995; Sahle et al., 1996).

It is unknown if there are any potential adverse health effects related to human exposure to airborne WO_x fibers; however, one laboratory study conducted *in vitro* observed greater damage to human lung cells that were exposed to tungsten oxide fibers compared to human lung cells that were exposed to crocidolite asbestos fibers (Leanderson and Sahle 1995).

Methods

A specific validated method for collection and analysis of airborne WO_x fibers is lacking. As a result, all air samples were collected in accordance with National Institute for Occupational Safety and Health (NIOSH) Methods 7400 and 7402: Asbestos and other Fibers by Phase Contrast and Transmission Electron Microscopy (NIOSH 2003), which are standard methods for sampling and analysis of airborne asbestos-containing fibers.

Sampling Strategy

From the preliminary walk-through investigations of the facilities and available published data from the Swedish hard metal industry, 12 production processes with the potential to produce a broad range of fiber exposures were identified for air sampling (see Table I). Both general area samples and personal breathing zone (PBZ) samples for airborne WO_x fibers were collected. Sixty two area samples were collected at stationary locations in work areas to capture potential WO_x fiber generation during specific process activities. Seven PBZ samples were collected to capture potential WO_x fiber exposures during the course of normal employee work activities.

Sample Collection

Area and PBZ air samples were collected on 25 millimeter diameter electrically-conductive cassettes preloaded with mixed cellulose ester (MCE) 0.45 micrometer (μm) pore-size membrane filters (SKC Inc., Eighty Four, PA). The purpose of the electrically-conductive cassette was to ensure uniform deposition of fibers on the filter substrate. Air was drawn through the cassettes with battery operated pumps calibrated at 2 liters per minute (LPM) using a standard flow calibration device (BIOS International Corp., Butler, NJ).

In general, samples were collected over a full shift (e.g., 7 to 8 hours). The type and number (area or PBZ) of samples collected in each of the 12 production areas are provided in Table I.

Sample Analysis

Twelve area samples (out of the 69 total air samples) were selected for the preliminary analysis. Those selected represented processes that were determined by industrial hygienists to be the most likely to produce positive results (i.e., greatest potential to generate fibers).

Each MCE filter was removed from its sample cassette and prepared for analysis using the direct transfer method outlined in NIOSH Method 7402. After preparation, each sample was individually loaded into a transmission electron microscope (TEM) (Philips, Model 420, Eindhoven, Netherlands) for analysis.

Fibers were defined as particles having an aspect ratio of at least 3:1; that is, the fiber length was at least three times greater than the diameter. A modified version of the NIOSH counting rule "A" was used to count fibers on the sample. The "A" rule prescribes counting all particles that lie entirely in the field of view and have length >5 μm, diameter >0.25 μm, and aspect ratio (length to width) ≥3:1 (NIOSH, 2003). The modification to the "A" counting rule included counting fibers with lengths >0.5, >5, and >15 μm. These size cuts were based on fiber size distribution data previously reported by Sahle et al., and take into account the size of fibers that can be effectively cleared from the lung by lung macrophage cells. For counting purposes, the size cuts are cumulative sizes, e.g., a 7 μm fiber was counted as >0.5 and >5 μm. The recommended limit of detection (LOD) of NIOSH Method 7402 is 0.01 fibers per cubic centimeter of air (f/cm^3) for atmospheres free of interferences. The recommended quantitative working range of the method is 0.01 to 0.5 f/cm^3 per 1,000 L air sample (NIOSH 2003).

The elemental composition of fibers and particles were determined using an energy dispersive x-ray (EDX) spectrometer (PGT-EDAX, Model Avalon, Rocky Hill, NJ) connected to the TEM. This EDX detector can identify elements having atomic numbers greater than 11 (sodium).

Preliminary Results

Fibers composed of WO_x (see elemental composition data below) were present in quantifiable levels on 6 of 12 air samples that were analyzed (Table II). The concentration of airborne fibers ranged from <LOD (Carburizing, Spray drying, Screening, and Sintering) to 0.268 (Calcining of "blue" tungsten oxide at Huntsville) f/cm^3.

Overall, preliminary results indicate that average airborne fiber diameters are < 0.25 μm, and fiber lengths are < 5 μm. Figure 1 is a micrograph from an area sample collected near the 'blue' calcining process at the Huntsville facility. Although the fibers pictured are atypically long, their diameters are < 0.25 μm. The micrograph provides a very good illustration of the way most fibers were found on the samples. In general, the fibers were not in bundles, and were not agglomerated with other non-fibrous particles.

Using EDX analysis, it was determined that all fibers counted were composed of tungsten and oxygen. For the samples collected at processes where hard-metal binders were present (i.e., Charging, Screening, Spray drying, and Sintering), the number of cobalt-containing particles that were attached to WO_x fibers was similar to the number of cobalt-containing particles that were not attached to WO_x fibers. This result indicated that cobalt-containing particles were not attached preferentially to WO_x fibers. Cobalt was not detected on filter samples collected in work areas where tungsten oxides were reduced to W (i.e., calcining and reduction) or in work areas where tungsten carbide was formulated (i.e., carburizing plant).

Summary

The preliminary results indicate that WO_x fibers exist in the workplace air at concentrations up to 0.268 f/cm^3. Currently, the potential adverse health effects related to human exposure to WO_x fibers is unknown. Among the samples analyzed, those collected from high-temperature processes involved in the oxidation of ammonium paratungstate to tungsten oxide and the reduction of tungsten oxide to tungsten metal contained the highest number concentration of WO_X fibers. In general, WO_X fibers were < 5 µm in length by < 0.25 µm in diameter. Cobalt was detected in air samples collected from processes subsequent to and including Charging (*i.e.*, Spray drying, Screening, and Sintering). WO_X fibers were not preferentially agglomerated to cobalt particles.

Recommendations

Formation of WO_X fibers may be the result of incomplete oxidation of ammonia paratungstate or aerosolization of these fibers during reduction of WO_3 to tungsten metal. To be prudent, NIOSH recommends that engineering studies be undertaken to better understand the production process conditions (time, temperature, and oxygen content) under which WO_X fibers are formed. Adjustment of any or all of these operating conditions may eliminate the formation of WO_X fibers. In the interim, high efficiency particulate (HEPA) respirator use is prudent for workers exposed to fibers, since health effects of tungsten oxide fibers are unknown.

References

Leanderson, P. and W. Sahle (1995). "Formation of Hydroxyl Radicals and Toxicity of Tungsten Oxide Fibers." Toxic. in Vitro 9(2): 175-183.

NIOSH (2003). NIOSH Manual of Analytical Methods (NMAM). Cincinnati, OH, National Institute for Occupational Safety and Health.

Sahle, W. (1992). "Possible Role of Tungsten Oxide Whiskers in Hard-Metal Pneumoconiosis." Chest 102: 1310.

Sahle, W., et al. (1994). "Airborne Tungsten Oxide Whiskers in a Hard-Metal Industry. Preliminary Findings." Ann. Occup. Hyg. 38(1): 37-44.

Sahle, W., et al. (1996). "Preliminary Data on Hard Metal Workers Exposure to Tungsten Oxide Fibers." Sci. Total Environ. 191: 153-167.

Table I: Type and Number of Air Samples for Tungsten Oxide Fibers, by Plant and Production Process

Plant	Process	Type* (Sample)	N (Sample)
Huntsville	Ammonium paratungstate production	A	1
		P	0
Huntsville	Calcining (blue and yellow)	A	7
		P	0
Huntsville	Reduction	A	10
		P	1
Huntsville	Carburizing	A	5
		P	1
Gurley	Ball mill	A	2
		P	1
Gurley	Charging	A	3
		P	1
Gurley	Crushing	A	2
		P	0
Gurley	Reprocessing	A	1
		P	1
Gurley	Spray drying	A	5
		P	1
Gurley	Screening	A	11
		P	1
Grant	Pressing/Molding	A	7
		P	0
Grant	Sintering	A	8
		P	0

* A = Area air sample collected at stationary locations in work areas to capture potential WO_x fiber generation during specific process activities
P = Personal breathing zone air sample collected to capture potential WO_x fiber exposures during the course of normal employee work activities

Table II: Preliminary Results for Airborne Tungsten Oxide Fiber Concentrations

Process	Fiber Count Total	Fiber Count >0.5 μm	Fiber Count >5 μm	Fiber Count >15 μm	Concentration Filter (f/mm²)	Concentration Total Airborne (f/cm³)[A]	Cobalt?
Calcining (blue)	93	93	16	1	395	0.268	No
Calcining (yellow)	34	34	9	ND	72	0.048	No
Reduction	19	19	1	ND	35	0.025	No
Reduction	12	12	ND	ND	20	0.015	No
Carburizing	17	17	5	2	29	0.015	No
Carburizing	6	6	1	ND	10	<LOD	No
Charging	17	17	1	ND	30	0.012	Yes
Screening	6	6	ND	ND	10	<LOD	Yes
Screening	ND*	ND	ND	ND	<0.01	<LOD	Yes
Sintering	5	5	1	ND	8	<LOD	Yes
Spray drying	5	5	ND	ND	7	<LOD	Yes
Total	214	214	34	3			

[A] The quantitative working range of this technique is 0.01 to 0.5 f/cm³ as calculated using the number of fibers with length >0.5 μm and with a preferable fiber concentration range of 100 to 1200 f/mm²
ND = Not detected
* = Airborne fiber concentration calculated using the limit of detection (0.01 f/cm³) divided by $\sqrt{2}$ (NIOSH, 2003)
Note: 12 filter samples were submitted for analysis but 1 sample could not be analyzed because the filter was overloaded with material (area sample collected near APT dryer)

Figure 1: Airborne Tungsten Oxide Fibers from 'Blue' Calcination Process

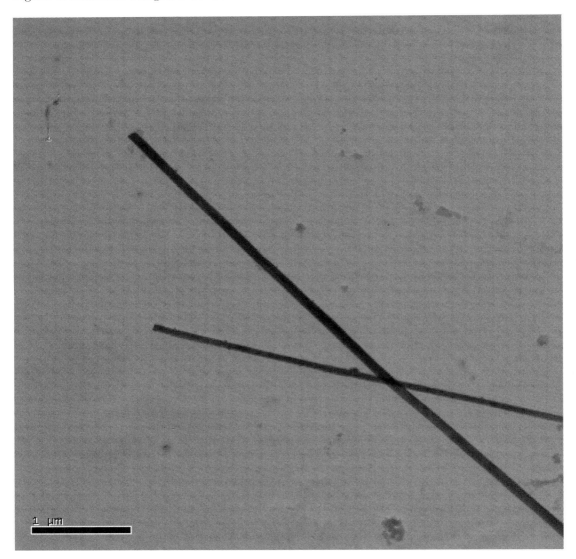

DEPARTMENT OF HEALTH & HUMAN SERVICES

Phone: (304) 285-5751
Fax: (304) 285-5820

Public Health Service

Centers for Disease Control
and Prevention (CDC)
National Institute for Occupational
Safety and Health (NIOSH)
1095 Willowdale Road
Morgantown, WV 26505-2888

November 8, 2005
HETA 2003-0257
Interim Letter VII

Mr. Steve Robuck
Director of Safety and Environment
Metalworking Products
1 Teledyne Place
La Vergne, Tennessee 37086

Dear Mr. Robuck:

The purpose of this letter is to report the progress of a National Institute for Occupational Safety and Health (NIOSH) industrial hygiene survey at the Alldyne Powder Technologies plants located in Huntsville and Gurley, Alabama and the Firth Sterling plant located in Grant, Alabama. NIOSH surveyed these plants from October 25 to November 2, 2004 in response to a confidential employee request concerning respiratory health effects and exposure to metalworking fluids, cobalt, nickel, chromium, and tungsten carbide.

Sincerely,

Nancy M. Sahakian, M.D., M.P.H.

Aleksandr Stefaniak, Ph.D., C.I.H.
Respiratory Disease Hazard Evaluation and
  Technical Assistance Program
Field Studies Branch
Division of Respiratory Disease Studies

cc:
Confidential Requesters

Survey goal:

Estimate personal breathing zone full-shift exposure to metal working fluid (MWF), cobalt, chromium, nickel, and tungsten using total dust and particle size-selective samplers in 21 pre-identified work areas throughout the Alldyne Powder Technologies plants located in Huntsville and Gurley, Alabama and the Firth Sterling plant located in Grant, Alabama.

Note that for purposes of this letter, the Gurley plant reprocessing and charging jobs were combined into a single category called "Powder Mixing", maintenance and janitor jobs were combined into a single category called "Maintenance", and the Building #2 Leadman job was grouped with Spray drying. The Grant plant round cell and shaping jobs were combined into a single category called "Shaping" and the receiving clerk and powder crib clerk jobs were combined into a single category called "Production Control."

Samples collected:

37-mm closed-face filter cassette for total dust and metal working fluids (MWF)

Sixteen (16) samples of airborne particles were collected in the grinding area at the Grant, AL plant using closed-face 37-mm cassette samplers. All samples were collected using pre-weighed polytetrafluoroethylene (PTFE) substrate at a flow rate of 2.0 liters per minute (Lpm). Eight (8) of the 16 closed-face cassette samples were positioned in the personal breathing zones of employees during the course of their normal work activities. The remaining eight cassette samples were general area samples collected at different stationary locations in the grinding work area.

All PTFE substrates were submitted for determination of total dust and MWF in accordance with NIOSH Analytical Method 5524. The analytical limit of detection (LOD) for total dust was 0.01 mg and the limit of quantification (LOQ) was 0.04 mg. The LOD for MWF was 0.01 mg and the LOQ was 0.03 mg.

The U.S. Occupational Safety and Health Administration (OSHA) has not promulgated a Permissible Exposure Limit (PEL) for MWF. The NIOSH Recommended Exposure Limit (REL) for MWF is 0.5 mg MWF/m^3 total particulate mass as a 10-hour TWA during a 40-hour workweek. The American Conference of Governmental Industrial Hygienists (ACGIH) has not recommended a Threshold Limit Value (TLV) for MWF.

37-mm closed-face filter cassette for total dust and elements

Two hundred fifty two (252) samples of airborne particles were collected from employees in 21 different work areas using closed-face 37-mm cassette samplers and analyzed for total dust and elements (cobalt, chromium, nickel, and tungsten). All samples were collected on pre-weighed polyvinyl chloride (PVC) substrate at a flow rate of 2.0 Lpm. Each 37-mm cassette sampler was positioned in the personal breathing zone of employees during the course of their normal work activities. In general, two 37-mm cassette samples were collected per employee, *i.e.*, one sample per day for two consecutive days. Of the 252 samples, one sample was discarded because the air sampling pump faulted during collection, yielding a net of 251 samples. Of the 251 samples, 71 (28%) were collected at Huntsville, 65 (26%) at Gurley, and 115 (46%) were collected at Grant.

All PVC substrates were submitted for determination of the following analytes: total dust in accordance with NIOSH Analytical Method 0500; cobalt, chromium, and nickel content in accordance with NIOSH Analytical Method 7300; and, tungsten content in accordance with NIOSH Analytical Method 7074. A laboratory accredited for metals analysis by the American Industrial Hygiene Association (AIHA) Industrial Hygiene Laboratory

Accreditation Program (IHLAP) was used for all metals analyses. The LOD for total dust was 0.02 mg (LOQ not available). For quantification of metals, the 251 PVC substrates were analyzed in multiple batches. A new instrument calibration curve was established prior to analyzing each batch of samples. Because the LOD and LOQ are unique to a given calibration curve, ranges are provided for these reporting limits: cobalt, LOD = 0.2 to 0.9 µg/filter, LOQ = 0.6 to 3 µg/filter; chromium, LOD = 0.3 to 0.6 µg/filter, LOQ = 1 to 2 µg/filter; nickel, LOD = 0.2 to 0.5 µg/filter, LOQ = 0.8 to 2 µg/filter; and tungsten LOD = 4 to 8 µg/filter, LOQ = 10 to 30 µg/filter.

The OSHA PEL, NIOSH REL, and ACGIH TLV, expressed as 8-hour time-weighted averages, for cobalt, chromium, nickel, and tungsten are:

Limit	8-hour time-weighted average concentration (mg/m^3)			
	Cobalt	Chromium	Nickel	Tungsten
PEL	0.1	1.0	1.0	--[A]
REL	0.05	0.5	0.5	5.0
TLV	0.02	0.5	0.5	5.0

[A] No PEL exists for this material

NIOSH defines cemented tungsten carbide or "hard metal" as a mixture of tungsten carbide, cobalt, and sometimes metal oxides or carbides and other metals (including nickel). Note that the NIOSH REL for cemented tungsten carbide containing >2% cobalt is 0.05 mg cobalt/m^3 (expressed as a 10-hour time-weighted average). NIOSH considers cemented tungsten carbide containing nickel to be a potential occupational carcinogen and recommends a REL of 0.015 mg nickel/m^3 (expressed as a 10-hour time-weighted average).

Marple cascade impactor

One hundred eight (108) samples of airborne particles were collected from employees in 21 different work areas using Marple series 290 8-stage cascade impactor samplers positioned in the personal breathing zones of employees during the course of their normal work activities. Only one impactor sample was collected per employee. The aerodynamic diameter cut points for the cascade impactor sampler at a flow rate of 2.0 Lpm were >21.3 µm (stage 1), 14.8 µm (stage 2), 9.8 µm (stage 3), 6.0 µm (stage 4), 3.5 µm (stage 5), 1.55 µm (stage 6), 0.93 µm (stage 7), 0.52 µm (stage 8), and <0.52 (final filter). All impactor samples were collected on pre-weighed PVC substrate that was sprayed with silicone prior to weighing to prevent particle bounce during sampling.

All filters and quality control samples (blank filters) were post-weighed at NIOSH using a microbalance in a temperature and humidity controlled chamber to estimate total dust mass. All impactor filters were submitted to a laboratory accredited for metals analysis by the AIHA IHLAP for quantification of cobalt, chromium, and nickel content in accordance with NIOSH Analytical Method 7300, and tungsten content in accordance with NIOSH Analytical Method 7074.

Results

37-mm closed-face filter cassette for total dust and metal working fluids (MWF)

Airborne total dust levels, MWF levels, and the fraction of dust concentration accounted by MWF are summarized in Table I for the personal breathing zone and area cassette samples collected in the Grinding work area. With one exception, total dust levels (average 0.43 ± 0.82 mg/m^3, range 0.09 to 3.47 mg/m^3) did not exceed 0.5 mg/m^3 in any of the samples. The one exception (3.47 mg/m^3 total dust) was a sample from an employee who spray painted during the early part of their shift. Note that excluding this employees' sample result yields an overall average total dust exposure of 0.23 ± 0.13 mg/m^3, range 0.09 to 0.49 mg/m^3. The MWF exposure concentration for the employee who spray painted was similar to levels measured for other employees and on the area samples, indicating that the elevated total dust exposure was probably due to paint overspray. MWF concentrations (average 0.15 ± 0.12 mg/m^3, range 0.04 to 0.42 mg/m^3) were generally below 0.4 mg/m^3. The mass fraction of total dust that was accounted for by MWF ranged from 0.09 to 0.88.

Figure 1 illustrates the relationship between MWF concentration and total dust concentration for personal breathing zone samples and for area samples collected in the Grinding work area. The plot of personal breathing zone sampling results does not include the sample from the employee who spray painted during his/her shift. In general, levels of MWF were positively related to levels of dustiness in the grinding work area as indicated by the positive R^2 values given in the plots (personal samples $R^2 = 0.89$; area samples $R^2 = 0.98$). An R^2 value is an estimate of the relationship between two variables and can range from -1 (exact negative linear relationship) to 1 (exact positive linear relationship).

37-mm closed-face filter cassette for total dust and elements

To calculate concentration levels for samples with analyte level below the LOD, a value of one-half the appropriate LOD was assigned to the sample.

Total dust

Total dust levels for the cassette samples are summarized by work area in Table II. Among all 251 samples, the average dust concentration was 0.91 ± 1.41 mg/m^3 (median = 0.33 mg/m^3), with range 0.01 mg/m^3 (Milling) to 10.86 mg/m^3 (Powder Mixing).

At Huntsville, the average concentration for 71 samples of airborne dust was 1.55 ± 1.78 mg/m^3, with range 0.01 mg/m^3 (Powder Laboratory) to 8.68 mg/m^3 (Metal Separation). At the Gurley plant, the average concentration of airborne dust for 65 samples was 1.21 ± 1.67 mg/m^3, with range 0.01 mg/m^3 (Milling) to 10.86 mg/m^3 (Powder Mixing). At Grant, the average concentration of airborne dust for 115 samples was 0.35 ± 0.47 mg/m^3, with range 0.07 mg/m^3 (Product Testing) to 3.26 mg/m^3 (Shaping). The dustiest work areas tended to be the areas where bulk material handling and comminution processes were performed (*e.g.*, Reclamation, Powder Mixing, and Screening). The least dusty areas tended to be areas where solid final product was handled and where engineering controls currently exist (*e.g.*, Sandblasting, Product Testing, and Shipping at Grant).

Cobalt

Airborne cobalt concentration levels for the cassette samples are summarized by work area in Table III. Levels of cobalt were quantifiable on 96% (242/251) of all samples collected at the three plants. Among all 251 samples, the average personal cobalt concentration was 0.049 ± 0.14 mg/m^3 (median = 0.014 mg/m^3), with range 0.00007 mg/m^3 (Powder Laboratory) to 1.62 mg/m^3 (Powder Mixing).

At Huntsville, the average concentration for 71 samples of airborne cobalt was 0.04 ± 0.05 mg/m^3, with range 0.00007 mg/m^3 (Powder Laboratory) to 0.28 mg/m^3 (Metal Separation). At the Gurley plant, the average concentration for 65 samples of airborne cobalt was 0.12 ± 0.25 mg/m^3, with range 0.0001 mg/m^3 (Milling) to 1.62 mg/m^3 (Powder Mixing). At Grant, the average concentration for 115 samples of airborne cobalt was 0.014 ± 0.027 mg/m^3, with range 0.0001 mg/m^3 (Sandblasting, Shipping) to 0.23 mg/m^3 (Production Control).

The percentages of airborne cobalt samples that exceeded the TLV for airborne cobalt in the work areas (numbers in parentheses) were: Metal Separation (43%), Reclamation A (60%), Reclamation B (89%), Reclamation A and B (67%), Powder Mixing (55%), Milling (90%), Spray Drying (83%), Screening (100%), Maintenance at Gurley (50%), Production Control (20%), Pressing (62%), Extrusion (40%), Shaping (26%), Breakdown (100%), Grinding (13%), Shipping at Grant (6%), and Maintenance (10%). The least dusty areas were areas where solid final product was handled and where engineering controls currently exist (*e.g.*, Grinding, Sandblasting, Product Testing, and Shipping at Grant).

Chromium

Airborne chromium concentration levels for the cassette samples are summarized by work area in Table IV. Levels of chromium were quantifiable on 70% (176/251) of all samples collected at the three plants. Among all 251 samples, the average personal chromium concentration was 0.002 ± 0.005 mg/m^3 (median = 0.0003 mg/m^3), with range 0.00004 mg/m^3 (Powder Laboratory) to 0.050 mg/m^3 (Metal Separation).

At Huntsville, the average concentration for 71 samples of airborne chromium was 0.041 ± 0.009 mg/m^3, with range 0.00004 mg/m^3 (Powder Laboratory) to 0.050 mg/m^3 (Metal Separation). At the Gurley plant, the average concentration for 65 samples of airborne chromium was 0.0009 ± 0.001 mg/m^3, with range 0.0001 mg/m^3 (Inventory Control, Powder Mixing, Spray Drying, Maintenance) to 0.005 (Spray Drying). At Grant, the average concentration for 115 samples of airborne chromium was 0.0004 ± 0.0007 mg/m^3, with range 0.00005 mg/m^3 (Shaping, Product Testing, Shipping) to 0.005 mg/m^3 (Shaping).

In general, levels of airborne chromium were at least an order of magnitude below the REL and TLV in all facilities (Table IV).

Nickel

Airborne nickel concentration levels for the cassette samples are summarized by work area in Table V. Levels of nickel were quantifiable on 68% (170/251) of all samples collected at the three plants. Among all 251 samples, average personal nickel concentration was 0.010 ± 0.047 mg/m^3 (median = 0.0005 mg/m^3), with range 0.00005 mg/m^3 (Reclamation A & B, Shaping, Grinding) to 0.45 mg/m^3 (Powder Mixing).

At Huntsville, the average concentration for 71 samples of airborne nickel was 0.008 ± 0.017 mg/m^3, with range 0.00005 mg/m^3 (Reclamation A and B) to 0.083 mg/m^3 (Metal Separation). At the Gurley plant, the average concentration for 65 samples of airborne nickel was 0.030 ± 0.088 mg/m^3, with range 0.00006 mg/m^3 (Inventory Control, Spray Drying) to 0.45 mg/m^3 (Powder Mixing). At Grant, the average concentration for 115 samples of airborne nickel was 0.0008 ± 0.001 mg/m^3, with range 0.00005 mg/m^3 (Shaping, Grinding) to 0.009 mg/m^3 (Shaping).

In general, levels of airborne nickel were low in all facilities. Only one sample (collected in Powder Mixing) approached the REL and TLV for nickel.

Tungsten

Airborne tungsten concentration levels for the cassette samples are summarized by work area in Table VI. Because of an administrative error by the analytical laboratory, tungsten was only quantified on 126 of the 251 samples collected at the three plants. Among these 126 samples, 64 (51%) were collected at Gurley and 62 (49%) were collected at Grant; the average personal tungsten concentration was 0.20 ± 0.26 mg/m^3 (median = 0.11 mg/m^3), with range 0.003 mg/m^3 (Product Testing) to 1.61 mg/m^3 (Screening).

At the Gurley plant, the average concentration for 64 samples of airborne tungsten was 0.28 ± 0.32 mg/m^3, with range 0.006 mg/m^3 (Milling) to 1.61 mg/m^3 (Screening). At Grant, the average concentration for 62 samples of airborne tungsten was 0.11 ± 0.12 mg/m^3, with range 0.003 mg/m^3 (Product Testing) to 0.47 mg/m^3 (Shaping).

In general, levels of airborne tungsten were at least a factor of three lower than the REL and TLV in all facilities.

Dust-metal relationships

For all 251 samples, levels of airborne cobalt, chromium, nickel, or tungsten were poorly correlated with levels of airborne dust. Additionally, for the 132 samples analyzed for tungsten, levels of airborne cobalt, chromium, or nickel were poorly correlated with levels of airborne tungsten.

Among all 251 samples, airborne dust mass was on average 0.2% (range: 0.01 to 3%) chromium, 0.6% (range: 0.002 to 16%) nickel, 4.5% (range: 0.03 to 34%) cobalt, and 36% (0.4 to 77%) tungsten.

Huntsville

Among all samples collected in Huntsville, levels of airborne cobalt and dust ($R^2 = 0.57$) and levels of airborne chromium and dust ($R^2 = 0.56$) were moderately correlated, but no correlation was observed between levels of airborne nickel and dust.

At the Huntsville plant, airborne dust mass was on average 0.3% (range: 0.01 to 3%) chromium, 0.6% (range: 0.002 to 5.5%) nickel, and 2.7% (range: 0.03 to 8%) cobalt. As summarized in Table VII, within individual work areas airborne chromium and nickel accounted for less than 1% of the mass of airborne dust. The fraction of cobalt in airborne dust varied by a factor of three among work areas, but accounted for less than 5% of airborne dust.

Gurley

Among all samples collected at Gurley, levels of airborne cobalt and dust ($R^2 = 0.87$) were strongly correlated, levels of airborne chromium and dust ($R^2 = 0.56$) and levels of airborne nickel and dust ($R^2 = 0.48$) were moderately correlated, and no correlation was observed between levels of airborne tungsten and dust. Levels of airborne nickel ($R^2 = 0.48$), but not cobalt or chromium, were positively correlated with levels of airborne tungsten.

Airborne dust mass was on average 0.1% (range: 0.01 to 1.5%) chromium, 1.2% (range: 0.03 to 15%) nickel, 8.6% (range: 1.2 to 34%) cobalt, and 39% (range: 0.4 to 77%) tungsten. Within individual work areas, airborne chromium and nickel accounted for less than 1% of the mass of airborne dust. The fraction of cobalt in airborne dust was higher in all work areas at Gurley compared to Huntsville (Table VII). The fraction of cobalt in airborne dust was highest in work areas where powders were handled (i.e., Powder Mixing and Milling). The fraction of tungsten in airborne dust varied by a factor of three among work areas in Gurley and accounted for approximately half the mass of airborne dust in Milling and Spray Drying.

With the exception of Powder Mixing, the ratios of cobalt to tungsten, chromium to tungsten, and nickel to tungsten were all generally less than 0.6. In Powder Mixing, the ratio of airborne cobalt to tungsten was 4.5 and the ratio of airborne nickel to tungsten was 1.4, consistent with an operation where powdered cobalt or nickel is poured into a drum containing tungsten powder.

Grant

Levels of airborne cobalt and dust ($R^2 = 0.60$) and levels of airborne chromium and dust ($R^2 = 0.60$) were moderately correlated; however, levels of airborne nickel or tungsten were poorly correlated with levels of airborne dust. Additionally, levels of airborne cobalt ($R^2 = 0.66$), but not chromium or nickel, were positively correlated with levels of airborne tungsten. Airborne dust mass was on average 0.2% (range: 0.01 to 0.6%) chromium, 0.3% (range: 0.005 to 3.5%) nickel, 3.4% (range: 0.08 to 13%) cobalt, and 32% (range: 1.4 to 72%) tungsten.

Within individual work areas, airborne chromium and nickel accounted for less than 1% of the mass of airborne dust (Table VII). The fraction of cobalt in airborne dust was highest in work areas where powders were handled (*i.e.*, Pressing, Shaping, and Extrusion) and lowest in work areas where solid final product were handled (*i.e.*, Grinding, Sandblasting, Product Testing, and Shipping). Similarly, the fraction of tungsten in airborne dust was highest in work areas where powders were handled (*i.e.*, Pressing, Shaping, and Extrusion) and lowest in work areas where solid final product were handled (*i.e.*, Sandblasting, Product Testing, and Shipping). In Grinding, the fraction of tungsten in airborne dust (25.3%) was intermediate between work areas that handle powders and work areas that handle solid finished product.

With the exception of Breakdown, the ratios of cobalt to tungsten, chromium to tungsten, and nickel to tungsten were all generally less than 0.6. In Breakdown, the ratio of airborne cobalt to tungsten was 1.3.

Marple cascade impactor

At the time of writing this letter, all impactor filter samples are being analyzed for cobalt, chromium, nickel, and tungsten content.

Discussion

Metal Working Fluids (MWF)

All personal breathing zone and area sample measurements collected in the October 2004 survey were below 0.4 mg MWF/m³ of air. NIOSH recommends that exposure to MWF be limited to 0.5 mg MWF/m³ total particulate mass as a 10-hour TWA during a 40-hour workweek (NIOSH Criteria for a Recommended Standard: Occupational Exposure to Metalworking Fluids, January 1998). Note that endotoxin and culturable fungi and bacterial levels were not assessed for samples collected during our October 2004 survey.

As demonstrated in Figure 1, levels of airborne MWF were positively associated with airborne total dust. This finding suggests that engineering, good housekeeping, and good work practice efforts in the grinding area to control dust levels should concurrently decrease MWF exposure levels.

Metals

Levels of airborne chromium, nickel, and tungsten were generally well below the PEL, REL, and TLV (Tables IV to VI). In contrast, as presented in Table III, levels of airborne cobalt levels exceeded the TLV (20 µg/m³) on at least one sample in 16 of 21 work areas sampled. The only areas where no samples exceeded the TLV for airborne cobalt were Powder Laboratory, Inventory Control, Product Testing, and Sandblasting.

Within each plant, levels of airborne cobalt were positively associated with levels of airborne total dust. This association between airborne cobalt and airborne dust suggests that engineering, good housekeeping, and good work practice efforts to control dust levels should concurrently decrease cobalt exposure levels.

The contribution of chromium and nickel to airborne dust mass was generally low (<1%) and constant among plants, whereas the cobalt and tungsten content of airborne dust was variable. In general, the fraction of cobalt in airborne dust was highest in work areas where employees engaged in powder handling. Note that employee personal breathing zone exposures to cobalt often exceeded the TLV in work areas where powder is handled. Thus, efforts to minimize aerosolization of powders and implementation of controls to prevent dispersion of cobalt-containing dust and to remove airborne cobalt-containing dust should help to reduce airborne personal exposure levels.

Recommendations

As described in detail in the document "Criteria for a Recommended Standard: Occupational Exposure to Metalworking Fluids" (NIOSH, 1998), the following recommendations are made regarding exposures to MWF:

- Routine monitoring of inhalation and skin MWF exposures of affected employees
    o At least annually and whenever any major process change takes place
        ▪ Inhalation exposure should be sampled in the personal breathing zone
        ▪ Skin exposure should be qualitatively evaluated
- Employee training
    o As part of your existing employee training program, train employees on the potential adverse health effects associated with exposure to MWF, how to detect potential hazardous situations (*e.g.*, appearance of bacteria overgrowth and degradation of MWF), and appropriate work practices (*e.g.*, minimizing skin contact with MWF)
- Engineering
    o Minimize the generation of MWF mists through appropriate operation and control of the MWF delivery system (see for example, *Mist Control Considerations for the Design, Installation, and Use of Machine Tools Using Metalworking Fluids*, American National Standards Institute Technical Report B11 TR 2-1997)
        ▪ For control of exposure, utilize the industrial hygiene hierarchy of controls (ranked in order of most preferred to least preferred control method): elimination> substitution> engineering>work practices> personal protective equipment
- Work practices
    o Augment your current MWF inspection protocol as appropriate to include a written MWF management plan that specifies procedures for maintenance of fluid chemistry (*e.g.*, pH, temperature, viscosity, storage, mixing and diluting MWF concentrate, preparing additives such as biocides and a cobalt agglomerator, and monitoring tramp oil contamination) and maintenance of the fluid filtration and delivery systems (*e.g.*, fluid level in sump tank)
    o Employees in grinding should stand at a reasonable distance away from grinding machines during operation. Distance between the operator and the machine should be optimized to permit employees to oversee machine processes while minimizing the amount of MWF in the breathing zone
- Protective clothing and equipment
    o Appropriate protective clothing should be worn when working with MWF (note that nitrile is thought to afford the most chemical resistance to MWF)
    o If MWF exposure exceeds $0.5 - 5.0$ mg MWF/m^3 use an air-purifying, half-mask respirator

equipped with any P-or R-series particulate filter (P95, P99, P100, R95, R99, and R100)
- o If MWF exposure exceeds 5.0 – 12.5 mg MWF/m³ use a powered air-purifying respirator equipped with a hood or helmet and a high efficiency particulate air (HEPA) filter
- Personal Hygiene
  - o Employees should periodically wash MWF-contaminated skin with mild soap and water and dry with clean towels
  - o Employees should be reminded to refrain from placing their bare skin repeatedly into MWF
  - o The use of a barrier cream to protect skin from MWF is not recommended. Barrier creams do not universally protect the skin from MWF.

Building on our recommendations from previous interim letters sent to you, the following recommendations are made concerning inhalation exposure to cobalt at all three plants:

- Routinely monitor inhalation exposure to metals
  - o At least annually and whenever any major process change takes place
    - ▪ Inhalation exposure should be sampled in the personal breathing zone
- Engineering
  - o In work areas with elevated cobalt exposures, reduce cobalt exposure levels to below the current OSHA PEL (or to a lower professionally recognized level)
    - ▪ Utilize the industrial hygiene hierarchy of controls (ranked in order of most preferred to least preferred control method): elimination> substitution> engineering>work practices> personal protective equipment
  - o To aid in identification of specific work activities that may contribute disproportionately to cobalt exposure in a work area:
    - ▪ Dissect each job in a work area of elevated exposure into step-by-step activities (utilize employee input)
    - ▪ Use a portable real-time particle counter to identify the activities of a job that generate more aerosol than other activities
- Work practices
  - o Dedicate equipment (*e.g.*, hand tools) to specific work areas to prevent cobalt contamination migration from an area of higher cobalt to an area of lower cobalt contamination
  - o Provide a high-efficiency particulate air (HEPA) filtered vacuum in the pressing area for employees to clean their machines and work area. Use of a HEPA filtered vacuum will minimize transfer of cobalt from surfaces to air and unprotected areas of the skin when cleaning
  - o Employees in grinding should stand at a reasonable distance away from grinding machines during operation. Distance between the operator and the machine will permit employees to oversee machine processes while minimizing the amount of cobalt in the breathing zone
  - o Ensure and routinely check the integrity of the sandblasting glove box door seals, exhaust air hoses and gloves
- Personal protective clothing and equipment
  - o Appropriate respiratory protection should be worn by properly trained personnel when job activities could result in cobalt aerosol exposure levels above the pertinent OSHA PEL (or a lower feasible professionally recognized level) that could not be controlled to an acceptable level by engineering and work practice controls
  - o NIOSH in the document "Pocket Guide to Chemical Hazards" (NIOSH, 2004) recommends the following levels of respiratory protection for exposure to cemented tungsten carbides containing >2% cobalt by mass:

- Up to 0.25 mg Co/m^3: Any dust or mist respirator with an assigned protection factor (APF) of 5
- From 0.25 to 0.5 mg Co/m^3: Any dust and mist respirator (except single use and quarter-mask respirators) with an APF of 10; any dust, mist, and fume respirator with an APF of 10; or any supplied-air respirator with an APF of 10
- From 0.5 to 1.25 mg Co/m^3: Any supplied-air respirator operated in continuous-flow mode with an APF of 25; any powered, air-purifying respirator with a dust and mist filter with an APF of 25; or any powered, air-purifying respirator with a dust, mist, and fume filter with an APF of 25
- From 1.25 to 2.5 mg Co/m^3: Any air-purifying, full-facepiece respirator with a high-efficiency particulate air (HEPA) filter with APF of 50; any self-contained breathing apparatus with a full facepiece with APF of 50; or, any supplied-air respirator with a full facepiece with APF of 50
- Respiratory protection may not perform as intended if it is not donned, used and maintained properly. As such, the use of personal protective equipment is not recommended as a primary means of reducing exposure levels on a long term basis

- Personal Hygiene
  - Shower soon after work
  - Improve cleanliness of non-production areas
    - Thoroughly clean and maintain lunch rooms and identify as "Clean Areas"
    - Minimize migration of cobalt from production to non-production areas

Table I. Total dust level, metal working fluid (MWF) level, and the fraction of dust mass accounted for by MWF ($f_{MWF/Dust}$) for the personal breathing zone and area polytetrafluoroethylene (PTFE) cassette samples collected in the Grinding work area at the Grant plant (October 2004)

Sample	Total dust (mg/m³)	MWF (mg/m³)	$f_{MWF/Dust}$
Personal	0.20	0.08	0.39
Personal	0.41	0.29	0.69
Personal	0.15	0.04	0.25
Personal	0.19	0.08	0.45
Personal	0.32	0.12	0.38
Personal	0.35	0.24	0.69
Personal[1]	3.47	0.30	0.09
Personal	0.16	0.08	0.47
Area	0.11	0.09	0.77
Area	0.14	0.07	0.55
Area	0.13	0.11	0.85
Area	0.39	0.35	0.88
Area	0.09	0.07	0.78
Area	0.49	0.42	0.85
Area	0.15	0.07	0.46
Area	0.11	0.07	0.69

[1] Employee spray painted during first half of shift

Table II. Total dust levels summarized by work area for samples collected in the personal breathing zone using closed-face 37-mm filter cassettes (October 2004)

Plant	Work Area[1]	Samples	Dust (mg/m³) Avg ± St Dev	Dust (mg/m³) Minimum	Dust (mg/m³) Maximum
Huntsville	Metal Separation	30	2.48 ± 2.20	0.34	8.68
Huntsville	Reclamation A	5	1.54 ± 0.96	0.18	2.49
Huntsville	Reclamation B	9	1.38 ± 0.82	0.04	2.51
Huntsville	Reclamation A and B	9	1.55 ± 1.01	0.18	2.92
Huntsville	Powder Laboratory	18	0.11 ± 0.12	0.01	0.43
Gurley	Inventory Control	2	0.10 ± 0.02	0.08	0.12
Gurley	Powder Mixing	20	2.03 ± 2.60	0.17	10.86
Gurley	Milling	10	0.56 ± 0.44	0.01	1.54
Gurley	Spray Drying	18	0.85 ± 0.63	0.18	2.47
Gurley	Screening	7	1.87 ± 1.27	0.74	4.28
Gurley	Shipping	2	0.24 ± 0.01	0.23	0.25
Gurley	Maintenance	6	0.55 ± 0.50	0.03	1.19
Grant	Production Control	5	0.15 ± 0.10	0.07	0.33
Grant	Pressing	13	0.44 ± 0.19	0.22	0.78
Grant	Extrusion	5	0.45 ± 0.53	0.09	1.36
Grant	Shaping	27	0.44 ± 0.71	0.09	3.26
Grant	Breakdown	1	0.98		
Grant	Grinding	15	0.54 ± 0.71	0.11	2.82
Grant	Sandblasting	8	0.26 ± 0.20	0.10	0.70
Grant	Product Testing	15	0.15 ± 0.05	0.07	0.22
Grant	Shipping	16	0.23 ± 0.18	0.07	0.80
Grant	Maintenance	10	0.31 ± 0.24	0.11	0.89

[1] Location that employee reported working on the day sample was collected

Table III. Total cobalt levels summarized by work area for samples collected in the personal breathing zone using closed-face 37-mm filter cassettes (October 2004)

Plant	Work Area[1]	Samples	Cobalt (mg/m³) Avg ± St Dev	Cobalt (mg/m³) Minimum	Cobalt (mg/m³) Maximum
Huntsville	Metal Separation	30	0.040 ± 0.059	0.002	0.28
Huntsville	Reclamation A	5	0.053 ± 0.053	0.005	0.12
Huntsville	Reclamation B	9	0.074 ± 0.050	0.001	0.16
Huntsville	Reclamation A and B	9	0.050 ± 0.040	0.003	0.13
Huntsville	Powder Laboratory	18	0.004 ± 0.005	0.00007	0.02
Gurley	Inventory Control	2	0.006 ± 0.0004	0.006	0.01
Gurley	Powder Mixing	20	0.29 ± 0.40	0.01	1.62
Gurley	Milling	10	0.051 ± 0.040	0.0001	0.13
Gurley	Spray Drying	18	0.058 ± 0.045	0.02	0.16
Gurley	Screening	7	0.094 ± 0.045	0.05	0.16
Gurley	Shipping	2	0.018 ± 0.003	0.02	0.02
Gurley	Maintenance	6	0.023 ± 0.020	0.003	0.06
Grant	Production Control	5	0.008 ± 0.008	0.003	0.23
Grant	Pressing	13	0.026 ± 0.012	0.01	0.06
Grant	Extrusion	5	0.030 ± 0.044	0.003	0.11
Grant	Shaping	27	0.028 ± 0.046	0.001	0.20
Grant	Breakdown	1	0.029		
Grant	Grinding	15	0.007 ± 0.008	0.002	0.05
Grant	Sandblasting	8	0.002 ± 0.001	0.0001	0.003
Grant	Product Testing	15	0.003 ± 0.002	0.005	0.01
Grant	Shipping	16	0.003 ± 0.008	0.0001	0.03
Grant	Maintenance	10	0.007 ± 0.014	0.002	0.05

[1] Location that employee reported working on the day sample was collected

Table IV. Total chromium levels summarized by work area for samples collected in the personal breathing zone using closed-face 37-mm filter cassettes (October 2004)

Plant	Work Area[1]	Samples	Chromium (mg/m^3) Avg ± St Dev	Chromium (mg/m^3) Minimum	Chromium (mg/m^3) Maximum
Huntsville	Metal Separation	30	0.008 ± 0.012	0.0004	0.050
Huntsville	Reclamation A	5	0.001 ± 0.001	0.0003	0.003
Huntsville	Reclamation B	9	0.002 ± 0.001	0.0003	0.004
Huntsville	Reclamation A and B	9	0.003 ± 0.003	0.0004	0.008
Huntsville	Powder Laboratory	18	0.0002 ± 0.0002	0.00004	0.0007
Gurley	Inventory Control	2	0.0002 ± 0.00002	0.0001	0.0002
Gurley	Powder Mixing	20	0.0009 ± 0.0009	0.0001	0.003
Gurley	Milling	10	0.0008 ± 0.001	0.0002	0.003
Gurley	Spray Drying	18	0.0001 ± 0.002	0.0001	0.005
Gurley	Screening	7	0.002 ± 0.001	0.0005	0.003
Gurley	Shipping	2	0.0002 ± 0.000004	0.0002	0.0002
Gurley	Maintenance	6	0.0003 ± 0.0002	0.0001	0.0008
Grant	Production Control	5	0.0003 ± 0.0002	0.0002	0.0007
Grant	Pressing	13	0.0004 ± 0.0003	0.00008	0.0009
Grant	Extrusion	5	0.0007 ± 0.001	0.0002	0.003
Grant	Shaping	27	0.0006 ± 0.001	0.00005	0.005
Grant	Breakdown	1	0.0002		
Grant	Grinding	15	0.0004 ± 0.0003	0.0002	0.001
Grant	Sandblasting	8	0.0002 ± 0.0002	0.0002	0.0007
Grant	Product Testing	15	0.0003 ± 0.0003	0.00005	0.0009
Grant	Shipping	16	0.0002 ± 0.0001	0.00005	0.0006
Grant	Maintenance	10	0.0004 ± 0.0004	0.0002	0.002

[1] Location that employee reported working on the day sample was collected

Table V. Total nickel levels summarized by work area for samples collected in the personal breathing zone using closed-face 37-mm filter cassettes (October 2004)

Plant	Work Area[1]	Samples	Nickel (mg/m³) Average ± St Dev	Nickel (mg/m³) Minimum	Nickel (mg/m³) Maximum
Huntsville	Metal Separation	30	0.017 ± 0.023	0.0008	0.083
Huntsville	Reclamation A	5	0.001 ± 0.002	0.0002	0.004
Huntsville	Reclamation B	9	0.0006 ± 0.0004	0.00006	0.001
Huntsville	Reclamation A and B	9	0.0008 ± 0.0009	0.00005	0.003
Huntsville	Powder Laboratory	18	0.0005 ± 0.0004	0.00006	0.001
Gurley	Inventory Control	2	0.0002 ± 0.0002	0.00006	0.0003
Gurley	Powder Mixing	20	0.089 ± 0.14	0.00007	0.45
Gurley	Milling	10	0.007 ± 0.008	0.0003	0.025
Gurley	Spray Drying	18	0.002 ± 0.003	0.00006	0.015
Gurley	Screening	7	0.004 ± 0.003	0.0003	0.010
Gurley	Shipping	2	0.0009 ± 0.0007	0.0004	0.001
Gurley	Maintenance	6	0.002 ± 0.001	0.0004	0.004
Grant	Production Control	5	0.0004 ± 0.0002	0.0002	0.0005
Grant	Pressing	13	0.001 ± 0.002	0.00006	0.005
Grant	Extrusion	5	0.0005 ± 0.0002	0.0002	0.0007
Grant	Shaping	27	0.001 ± 0.002	0.00005	0.009
Grant	Breakdown	1	0.00006		
Grant	Grinding	15	0.0009 ± 0.0009	0.00005	0.003
Grant	Sandblasting	8	0.0004 ± 0.0002	0.0002	0.0006
Grant	Product Testing	15	0.0004 ± 0.0002	0.00006	0.0008
Grant	Shipping	16	0.0005 ± 0.0002	0.00006	0.0007
Grant	Maintenance	10	0.0004 ± 0.0002	0.00006	0.0006

[1] Location that employee reported working on the day sample was collected

Table VI. Total tungsten levels summarized by work area for samples collected in the personal breathing zone using closed-face 37-mm filter cassettes (October 2004)

Plant	Work Area[1]	Samples	Tungsten (mg/m^3) Average ± St Dev	Tungsten (mg/m^3) Minimum	Tungsten (mg/m^3) Maximum
Huntsville	Metal Separation	--[2]	--	--	--
Huntsville	Reclamation A	--	--	--	--
Huntsville	Reclamation B	--	--	--	--
Huntsville	Reclamation A and B	--	--	--	--
Huntsville	Powder Laboratory	--	--	--	--
Gurley	Inventory Control	2	0.016 ± 0.010	0.010	0.023
Gurley	Powder Mixing	20	0.25 ± 0.38	0.035	1.34
Gurley	Milling	10	0.24 ± 0.19	0.006	0.66
Gurley	Spray Drying	18	0.29 ± 0.21	0.030	0.79
Gurley	Screening	7	0.61 ± 0.50	0.062	1.61
Gurley	Shipping	2	0.092 ± 0.005	0.088	0.095
Gurley	Maintenance	6	0.19 ± 0.18	0.049	0.50
Grant	Production Control	3	0.094 ± 0.090	0.035	0.20
Grant	Pressing	9	0.22 ± 0.11	0.11	0.46
Grant	Extrusion	3	0.097 ± 0.076	0.031	0.18
Grant	Shaping	17	0.15 ± 0.13	0.033	0.47
Grant	Breakdown	1	0.022		
Grant	Grinding	9	0.070 ± 0.077	0.014	0.26
Grant	Sandblasting	3	0.013 ± 0.010	0.007	0.025
Grant	Product Testing	5	0.017 ± 0.014	0.003	0.039
Grant	Shipping	6	0.052 ± 0.11	0.006	0.27
Grant	Maintenance	6	0.094 ± 0.16	0.013	0.42

[1] Location that employee reported working on the day sample was collected
[2] Not analyzed

Table VII. Contribution of cobalt (Co), chromium (Cr), nickel (Ni), and tungsten (W) to total dust levels summarized by work area for samples collected in the personal breathing zone using closed-face 37-mm filter cassettes (October 2004)

Plant	Work Area[1]	Co/dust (%)	Cr/dust (%)	Ni/dust (%)	W/dust (%)
Huntsville	Metal Separation	1.8	0.4	0.7	--[2]
Huntsville	Reclamation A	2.9	0.1	0.1	--
Huntsville	Reclamation B	5.2	0.2	0.1	--
Huntsville	Reclamation A and B	3.3	0.2	0.1	--
Huntsville	Powder Laboratory	2.6	0.4	1.0	--
Gurley	Inventory Control	6.0	0.2	0.3	16.0
Gurley	Powder Mixing	12.2	0.1	2.8	28.9
Gurley	Milling	8.7	0.3	1.6	54.4
Gurley	Spray Drying	6.9	0.1	0.2	45.0
Gurley	Screening	5.6	0.1	0.2	41.6
Gurley	Shipping	7.8	0.1	0.4	38.7
Gurley	Maintenance	6.3	0.1	0.6	36.6
Grant	Production Control	4.6	0.3	0.3	45.2
Grant	Pressing	6.3	0.1	0.3	52.4
Grant	Extrusion	4.8	0.1	0.2	33.6
Grant	Shaping	6.0	0.2	0.5	47.7
Grant	Breakdown	3.0	0.02	0.01	2.2
Grant	Grinding	2.1	0.1	0.4	25.3
Grant	Sandblasting	0.8	0.2	0.2	6.6
Grant	Product Testing	2.0	0.2	0.3	11.5
Grant	Shipping	0.7	0.1	0.3	10.8
Grant	Maintenance	1.6	0.2	0.2	18.4

[1] Location that employee reported working on the day sample was collected
[2] Not analyzed

Figure 1. Relationship between levels of MWF and levels of total dust for personal breathing zone sample and area samples collected in the Grinding area at the Grant plant (October 2004). Levels of MWF were positively related to levels of dustiness in the grinding work area as indicated by the positive R^2 values given in the plots. An R^2 value is an estimate of the relationship between two variables and can range from -1 (exact negative linear relationship) to 1 (exact positive linear relationship).

Personal Breathing Zone Samples

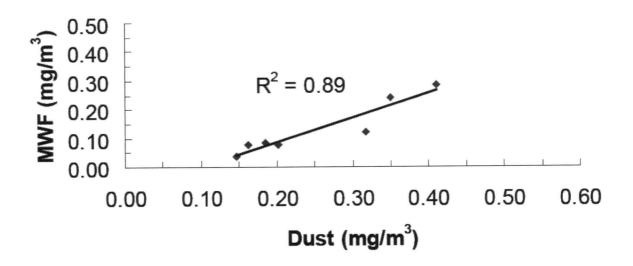

Area Samples

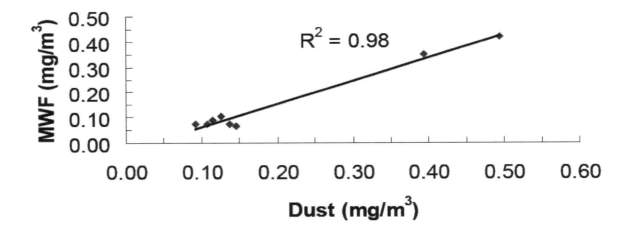

DEPARTMENT OF HEALTH & HUMAN SERVICES

Phone: (304) 285-5751
Fax: (304) 285-5820

Public Health Service

Centers for Disease Control
and Prevention (CDC)
National Institute for Occupational
Safety and Health (NIOSH)
1095 Willowdale Road
Morgantown, WV 26505-2888

May 8, 2006
HETA 2003-0257
Interim Letter VIII

Mr. Jim Doherty
Interim Director of Health, Safety and Environment
Alldyne Powder Technologies
7300 Highway 20
Huntsville, Alabama 35806

Dear Mr. Doherty:

The purpose of this letter is to report the results of a National Institute for Occupational Safety and Health
(NIOSH) industrial hygiene survey to assess potential skin exposures at the Alldyne Powder Technologies
facilities located in Huntsville and Gurley, Alabama and the Firth Sterling facility located in Grant, Alabama.
NIOSH surveyed these three facilities from November 6-12, 2004, in response to a confidential employee request
concerning respiratory health effects and exposure to metalworking fluids, cobalt, nickel, chromium, and tungsten
carbide.

Sincerely,

Nancy M. Sahakian, M.D., M.P.H.

Gregory A. Day, Ph.D.
Respiratory Disease Hazard Evaluation and
  Technical Assistance Program
Laboratory Research Branch
Division of Respiratory Disease Studies

Enclosure

cc:
Confidential Requesters

Rationale and survey goal:

It is known that cobalt can get onto the skin and enter the body, possibly influencing the development of adverse health effects among hard metal workers. However, there are no standards regarding levels of cobalt or tungsten on work surfaces or skin. Our goal was to measure levels of cobalt and tungsten on work surfaces and on workers' skin in the Alldyne Powder Technologies facilities located in Huntsville and Gurley, Alabama, and the Firth Sterling facility located in Grant, Alabama. We selected participants from pre-identified work areas or job categories throughout the three facilities and collected wipe samples from routinely-handled work surfaces and from participants' hands and necks. All samples were submitted for analysis of cobalt and tungsten to a laboratory accredited by the American Industrial Hygiene Association Industrial Hygiene Laboratory Accreditation Program for determination of cobalt and tungsten.

Samples collected:

Surface wipes for cobalt and tungsten

Each facility was surveyed for two days as follows: November 7-8 at Gurley, November 9-10 at Grant, and November 11-12 at Huntsville. A total of 156 wipe samples were collected in 26 separate work areas or job categories across facilities for analysis of cobalt and tungsten. Thirty-six (36) of the 156 samples were collected at Huntsville, 48 at Gurley, and 72 at Grant. All surface wipe samples were collected following procedures consistent with NIOSH Method 9100. Briefly, after putting on a pair of clean nitrile gloves, each sample was collected by wiping a surface with a Wash 'n Dri® moist disposable towelette (First Brands Corporation, Danbury, CT) and when possible with a 10-cm x 10-cm disposable template. Each towelette was then placed into an individually-labeled and sealed plastic bag and held for sample analysis.

The analytical limit of detection (LOD) for cobalt was 0.6 µg/wipe and the limit of quantification (LOQ), the lowest value that the laboratory could confidently report, was 2 µg/wipe by NIOSH Analytical Method 7300. Because the wipe samples are often analyzed in multiple batches, each batch may be associated with a unique instrument calibration curve and a range of values of the LOD and LOQ occurs. Such a range of values was the case for tungsten: LOD = 4 to 7 µg/wipe, LOQ = 10 to 20 µg/wipe. Surface wipe result masses (in µg cobalt and tungsten) were normalized to concentrations per 100 square centimeters ($\mu g/100\ cm^2$), the area of the template.

Hand and neck wipes for cobalt and tungsten

On the same days that surface wipe samples were collected at each facility, we also collected skin wipe samples from the hands and necks of employees for cobalt and tungsten analysis. Forty-one (41) first-shift employees participated in the study: ten at the Huntsville facility, 15 at Gurley, and 16 at Grant. Some employees at Huntsville and Grant provided more than one sample by participating on both days. All skin wipe samples were collected using Wash 'n Dri moist disposable towelettes identical to those used to collect work surface wipe samples. All participants provided a hand and neck wipe sample before starting to work (baseline samples) and a hand and neck wipe sample before lunchtime (follow-up samples), for a total of four samples per person per day. Each person wiped both of their hands (palm and back) from the top of the wrist to the tip of the fingers for no more than one minute and placed the sample into an individually-labeled and sealed plastic bag. Each person then put on a clean pair of nitrile gloves and wiped his or her neck from ear to ear and under the chin down to the top of the Adam's apple for no more than one minute and placed that sample into a separate plastic bag. Follow-up samples were collected, typically just before going to lunch, using the same procedure. Additionally, each participant provided an estimate of the number of pairs of nitrile gloves worn since the beginning of the shift. Note that the outside of nitrile gloves was not wiped, only the skin of the hands after gloves were removed. From these samples, we determined the amount of cobalt and tungsten that accumulated on the participants' skin (the amount at follow-up minus the amount at baseline).

All baseline and follow-up skin wipe samples (114 hand; 114 neck) were submitted for determination of cobalt and tungsten in accordance with NIOSH Analytical Method 7300. For hand wipes, the LOD for cobalt ranged from 0.08 to 1 µg/wipe and the LOQ from 0.3 to 4 µg/wipe; the LOD for tungsten from 1 to 10 µg/wipe and the LOQ from 4 to 40 µg/wipe. For neck wipes, the LOD for cobalt was 0.7 µg/wipe and the LOQ was 2 µg/wipe; the LOD for tungsten was 8 µg/wipe and the LOQ was 30 µg/wipe.

Results:

All results in this report are presented as figures. More detailed data are provided in tabular form in Appendix A.

Surface wipes

Cobalt

Amounts of cobalt were measured above the LOQ on all (156/156) sampled work surfaces. We used the median, defined as the 50th percentile of a set of measurements, as the summary measure for each work area or job category by facility. When a set of measurements is ranked from smallest to largest, then half of the values are greater than or equal to the median and the other half are less than or equal to it. Figure 1 illustrates median cobalt concentrations arranged by facility and work area or job category. (The corresponding data are summarized in Table I - Appendix A). Overall, levels of cobalt on surfaces were higher at the Gurley facility compared to either Huntsville or Grant. Huntsville: the median cobalt concentration among 36 surface wipe samples was 137 µg/100 cm², and ranged from 4 µg/100 cm² (Administration) to 1,359 µg/100 cm² (Reclamation B). Gurley: the median cobalt concentration among 48 surface wipe samples was 670 µg/100 cm², and ranged from 74 µg/100 cm² (Receiving) to 4,400 µg/100 cm² (Screening). Grant: the median cobalt concentration among 72 surface wipe samples was 246 µg/100 cm², and ranged from 11 µg/100 cm² (Administration) to 1,582 µg/100 cm² (Shaping).

Tungsten

Amounts of tungsten were above the LOQ on nearly all (155/156) sampled work surfaces. The only sample below the LOQ was collected from a desktop in Administration at the Grant facility. Figure 2 illustrates median tungsten concentrations, arranged by facility and work area or job category. (Corresponding data are summarized in Table II - Appendix A). Median levels of tungsten were similar across the three facilities. Huntsville: the median tungsten concentration among 36 surface wipes was 1,288 µg/100 cm², and ranged from 97 µg/100 cm² (Administration) to 3,269 µg/100 cm² (Reclamation B). Gurley: the median tungsten concentration among 48 surface wipes was 1,400 µg/100 cm², and ranged from 585 µg/100 cm² (Receiving) to 3,150 µg/100 cm² (Reprocessing). Grant: the median tungsten concentration among 72 surface wipes was 1,165 µg/100 cm², and ranged from 75 µg/100 cm² (Administration) to 3,826 µg/100 cm² (Extrusion).

Hand wipes

Cobalt

Amounts of cobalt were equal to or greater than the LOQ on nearly all (55/57) baseline and all (57/57) follow-up hand wipe samples. Figure 3 illustrates median levels of cobalt accumulated on participants' hands, arranged by facility and work area or job category. (Corresponding data are summarized in Table III - Appendix A). Overall, levels of cobalt on hands were higher at the Gurley facility compared to either Huntsville or Grant. Huntsville: the median cobalt mass that accumulated on participants' hands was 154 µg, and ranged from 4 µg

(Administration) to 1,280 µg (Metal Separation). During an approximate five-hour sampling period, participants reported wearing a median one pair of nitrile gloves (range was zero to three pairs of gloves).

Gurley: the median cobalt mass that accumulated on participants' hands was 489 µg, and ranged from 68 µg (Reprocessing) to 22,334 µg (Charging). During an approximate five-hour sampling period, participants reported wearing three pairs of nitrile gloves (range was zero to ten pairs of gloves).

Grant: the median cobalt mass that accumulated on participants' hands was 94 µg, and ranged from 12 µg (Shaping) to 4,579 µg (Powder Inventory). During an approximate four-hour sampling period, participants reported wearing three pairs of nitrile gloves (range was zero to nine pairs of gloves).

Tungsten

Tungsten levels were above the LOQ on nearly all (55/57) baseline and nearly all (56/57) follow-up hand wipe samples. Figure 4 illustrates median amounts of tungsten accumulated on participants' hands, arranged by facility and work area or job category. (Corresponding data are summarized in Table III - Appendix A). Overall, levels of tungsten on hands were higher at the Huntsville facility compared to either Gurley or Grant.

Huntsville: the median tungsten mass that accumulated on the participants' hands was 2,555 µg, and ranged from 192 µg (Administration) to 6,010 µg (Maintenance).

Gurley: the median tungsten mass that accumulated on participants' hands was 890 µg, and ranged from 301 µg (Reprocessing) to 2,765 µg (Screening).

Grant: the median tungsten mass that accumulated on participants' hands was 961 µg, and ranged from 33 µg (Tray Preparation) to 5,575 µg (Powder Inventory).

Neck wipes

Cobalt

We measured cobalt on most, but not all participants' neck wipe samples. In the three facilities combined, 70% (40/57) of the baseline measurements were above the LOD and 49% (28/57) were equal to or greater than the LOQ. In contrast, 95% (54/57) of the follow-up measurements were above the LOD and 89% (51/57) were equal to or greater than the LOQ, suggesting the accumulation of cobalt on skin while at work. Figure 5 illustrates median amounts of cobalt accumulated on participants' necks, arranged by facility and work area or job category. (Corresponding data are summarized in Table IV - Appendix A). Overall, levels of cobalt on necks were higher at the Gurley facility compared to either Huntsville or Grant.

Huntsville: the median cobalt mass that accumulated on participants' necks was 25 µg, and ranged from 4 µg (Carbide Plant) to 939 µg (Metal Separation).

Gurley: the median cobalt mass that accumulated on participants' necks was 90 µg, and ranged from 9 µg (Receiving) to 601 µg (Charging).

Grant: the median cobalt mass that accumulated on participants' necks was 5 µg, and ranged from 2 µg (CNC Pressing and Extrusion) to 14 µg (Breakdown).

Tungsten

Tungsten was measured on most, but not all participants' neck wipe samples. In the three facilities combined, 67% (38/57) of the baseline measurements were above the LOD and 40% (23/57) were equal to or greater than the LOQ. At follow-up, 92% (52/57) of the measurements were above the LOD and 77% (44/57) were equal to or greater than the LOQ. Figure 6 illustrates median accumulated masses of tungsten on participants' necks, arranged by facility and work area or job category. (Corresponding data are summarized in Table IV - Appendix A).

Huntsville: all samples provided by the participant in Administration were below the LOQ. The median tungsten mass that accumulated on participants' necks was 1305 µg, and ranged from 128 µg (Reclamation B) to 1229 µg

(Reclamation A).

Gurley: the median tungsten mass that accumulated on participants' necks was 526 μg, and ranged from 59 μg (Receiving) to 1430 μg (Charging).

Grant: Four participants in different work areas (Administration, CNC Pressing, Sandblasting, and Tray Preparation) provided all baseline and follow-up neck wipe measurements below the LOQ. The median tungsten mass that accumulated on participants' necks was 42 μg, and ranged from 22 μg (Extrusion) to 261 μg (Maintenance).

Relationships between contamination on work surfaces and on skin

Figure 7 illustrates relationships between (a) median levels of cobalt on work surfaces and accumulated masses of cobalt on participants' hands by work area or job category, (b) median levels of cobalt on work surfaces and accumulated masses of cobalt on necks, and (c) median levels of cobalt accumulated on hands and necks at the three facilities combined. In each plot, the r-value provides an estimate of the relationship between two variables that can range from -1 (exact negative linear relationship) to +1 (exact positive linear relationship). An r-value equal to zero suggests that there is no relationship between the two variables, whereas r-values approaching +1 or -1 suggest that the two variables are closely associated with one another.

We observed a weak relationship between median levels of cobalt on work surfaces and participants' hands (r = 0.22) and a moderate relationship between levels of cobalt on work surfaces and participants' necks (r = 0.66). Levels of cobalt on hands and necks were also moderately related (r = 0.51).

Recommendations:

Although there are no standards or professional guidelines regarding safe levels of surface contamination for cobalt, good housekeeping practices are necessary in operational areas where cobalt is used or handled to prevent the accumulation of cobalt-containing dust on surfaces throughout the workplace. Such accumulations, if not controlled, may lead to the spread of contamination on surfaces and the re-suspension of cobalt-containing particles into the air, both in the area where the dusts were originally generated and in other work areas.

Similarly, there are no standards or professional guidelines regarding skin exposure to cobalt or tungsten. Because cobalt can be absorbed across skin, contaminated skin could potentially contribute to total-body exposure. As a consequence, skin contamination could influence biological exposure monitoring results.

Building on our recommendations from previous interim letters sent to you, the following recommendations are made concerning cobalt exposures at all three facilities:
- Minimize cobalt levels in air and on work surfaces
    o Utilize the industrial hygiene hierarchy of controls (ranked in order of most preferred to least preferred control method): elimination> substitution> engineering>work practices> personal protective equipment.
- Augment the current management-supported skin protection program with the following elements:
    o Ensure that supervisors are trained on all elements of the skin protection program.
    o Reinforce and update initial employee training with periodic re-training in regard to the protective actions that workers must take to reduce their potential for exposure.
- Work practices
    o Dedicate equipment (for example, hand tools) to specific work areas to prevent the migration of cobalt contamination from areas of higher contamination to areas of lower contamination.
    o Replace contaminated shop packets with clean packets before bringing paperwork into administrative areas for processing.
    o Improve general cleanliness of production areas through good housekeeping measures (for example, all employees routinely clean their work areas on a daily basis).

- o Utilize a high-efficiency particulate air (HEPA) filtered vacuum for employees to clean their machines and work areas. HEPA-filtered vacuuming will minimize transfer of cobalt from surfaces to air and unprotected areas of the skin when cleaning.
- Personal protective clothing and equipment
  - o Wear long-sleeved shirts while passing through or working in production areas.
  - o Wear nitrile gloves before handling contaminated clothing (for example, while putting on or taking off work boots and clothes) and while working in production areas.
  - o Do not reuse disposable protective gloves.
  - o Replace nitrile gloves with new gloves when they become damaged or torn.
  - o Avoid placing contaminated hands into clean gloves.
- Personal Hygiene
  - o Routinely wash hands at work.
  - o Avoid contacting other areas of exposed skin with hands while working.
  - o Shower soon after work.

Figure 1. Median cobalt levels on all surface wipe samples by facility and work area or job category (November 2004).

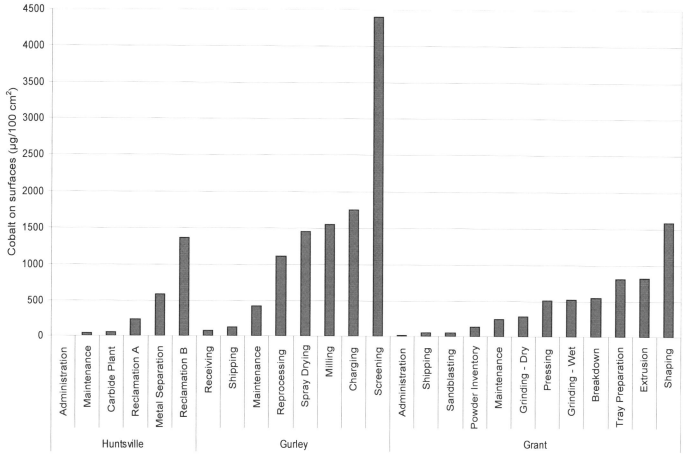

Figure 2. Median tungsten levels on all surface wipe samples by facility and work area or job category (November 2004).

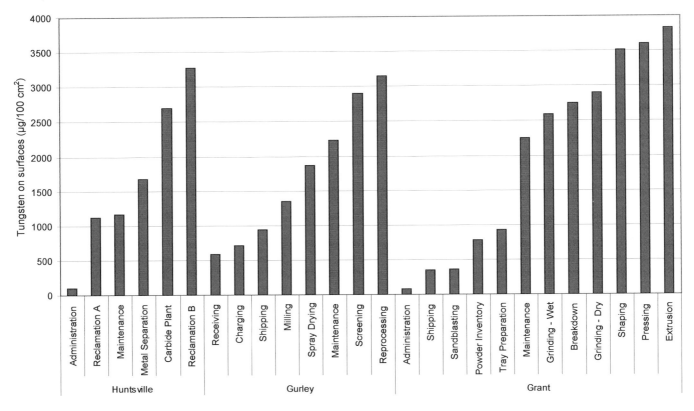

Figure 3. Median amounts of cobalt accumulated on hands by facility and work area or job category (November 2004).

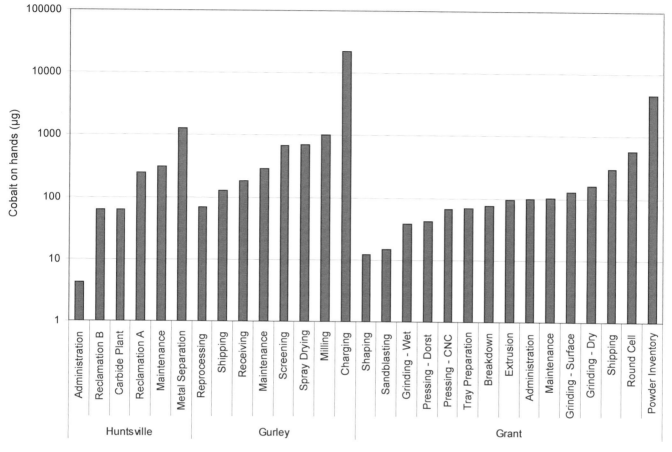

Figure 4. Median amounts of tungsten accumulated on hands by facility and work area or job category (November 2004).

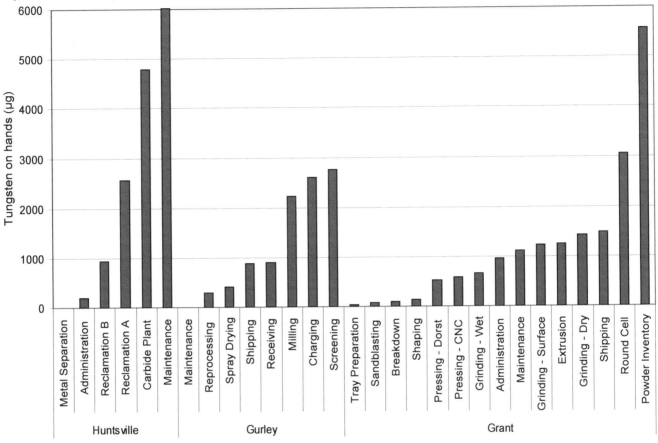

* Follow-up measurements lower than baseline.

Figure 5. Median amounts of cobalt accumulated on necks by facility and work area or job category (November 2004).

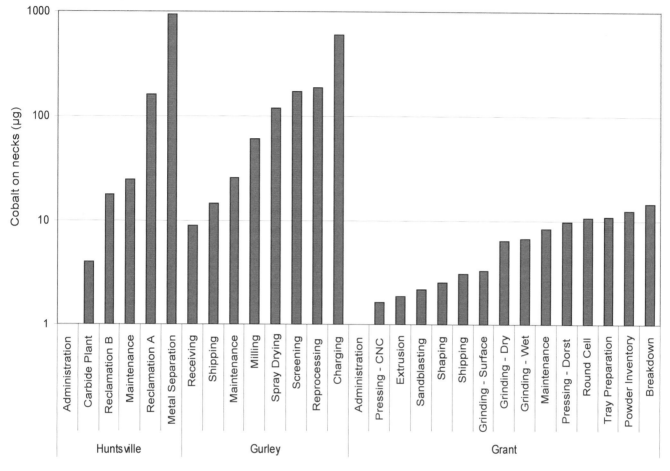

Figure 6. Median amounts of tungsten accumulated on necks by facility and work area or job category (November 2004).

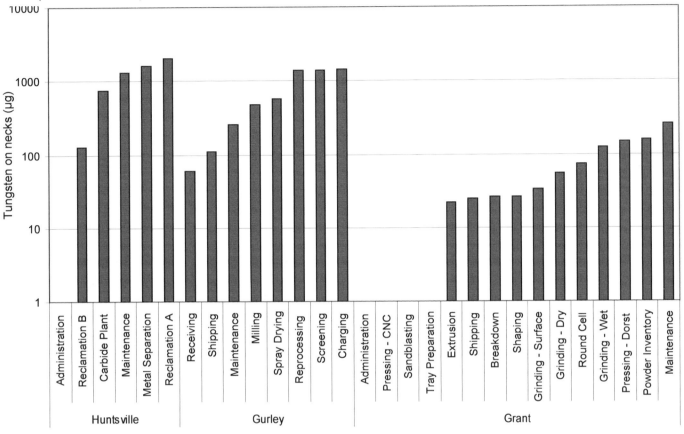

* All measurements < LOQ.

Figure 7. Relationships between median cobalt levels (a) accumulated on hands and levels on surfaces, (b) accumulated on necks and levels on surfaces, and (c) accumulated on necks and hands. All samples collected at the Huntsville, Gurley, and Grant facilities (November 2004).

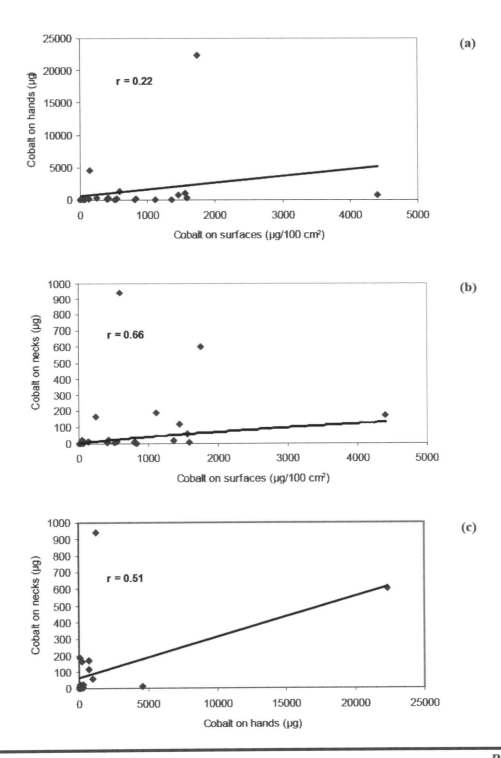

Appendix A

Table I. Levels of cobalt by facility and work area or job category for samples collected from work surfaces (November 2004)

Facility	Work Area or Job Category	Median	Cobalt (µg/100 cm²) Median	Cobalt (µg/100 cm²) Minimum	Cobalt (µg/100 cm²) Maximum
Huntsville	Administration	6	4	2	8
Huntsville	Metal Separation	6	586	93	17000
Huntsville	Carbide Plant	6	56	10	580
Huntsville	Maintenance	6	39	9	400
Huntsville	Reclamation A	6	242	32	7000
Huntsville	Reclamation B	6	1359	220	3004
Gurley	Charging	6	1744	466	22000
Gurley	Maintenance	6	420	120	1300
Gurley	Milling	6	1550	550	3200
Gurley	Receiving	6	74	16	275
Gurley	Reprocessing	6	1105	340	9900
Gurley	Screening	6	4400	670	14000
Gurley	Shipping	6	130	46	330
Gurley	Spray Drying	6	1446	75	4900
Grant	Administration	6	11	3	59
Grant	Breakdown	6	545	130	630
Grant	Extrusion	6	821	430	5455
Grant	Grinding – Dry	6	290	160	3600
Grant	Grinding – Wet	6	520	206	1574
Grant	Maintenance	6	245	71	470
Grant	Powder Inventory	6	137	17	400
Grant	Pressing	6	510	140	2900
Grant	Sandblasting	6	51	6	500
Grant	Shaping	6	1582	100	2800
Grant	Shipping	6	49	10	97
Grant	Tray Preparation	6	805	219	1656

Table II. Levels of tungsten by facility and work area or job category for samples collected from work surfaces (November 2004)

Facility	Work Area or Job Category	Samples	Tungsten (μg/100 cm^2) Median	Tungsten (μg/100 cm^2) Minimum	Tungsten (μg/100 cm^2) Maximum
Huntsville	Administration	6	97	26	150
Huntsville	Metal Separation	6	1675	670	5600
Huntsville	Carbide Plant	6	2696	980	12248
Huntsville	Maintenance	6	1165	198	7600
Huntsville	Reclamation A	6	1032	330	2200
Huntsville	Reclamation B	6	3269	1092	9300
Gurley	Charging	6	719	301	1402
Gurley	Maintenance	6	2227	1163	5300
Gurley	Milling	6	1350	310	7300
Gurley	Receiving	6	585	89	2000
Gurley	Reprocessing	6	3150	732	5400
Gurley	Screening	6	2900	2000	4700
Gurley	Shipping	6	935	310	1500
Gurley	Spray Drying	6	1865	447	7800
Grant	Administration	6	75	< LOQ	410
Grant	Breakdown	6	2750	470	4000
Grant	Extrusion	6	3826	961	8700
Grant	Grinding – Dry	6	2900	130	7500
Grant	Grinding – Wet	6	2600	254	5600
Grant	Maintenance	6	2250	710	3500
Grant	Powder Inventory	6	778	100	3000
Grant	Pressing	6	3600	960	8000
Grant	Sandblasting	6	365	31	4400
Grant	Shaping	6	3514	770	12000
Grant	Shipping	6	356	100	600
Grant	Tray Preparation	6	926	439	5400

Table III. Levels of cobalt and tungsten on wipe samples collected from participants' hands at baseline and follow-up by facility and work area or job category (November 2004)

Facility	Work Area or Category	Worker	No. Samples	Cobalt Mass (μg)* Baseline	Cobalt Mass (μg)* Follow-up	Tungsten Mass (μg)* Baseline	Tungsten Mass (μg)* Follow-up
Huntsville	Administration	A	2	1	5	48	240
Huntsville	Metal Separation	A	1**	120	1400	920	840
Huntsville	Metal Separation	B	1**	210	140	1800	1000
Huntsville	Carbide Plant	A	1	4	29	530	7500
Huntsville	Carbide Plant	B	1	10	110	1500	4100
Huntsville	Maintenance	A	2**	113	425	2445	3505
Huntsville	Reclamation A	A	1	7	48	100	710
Huntsville	Reclamation A	B	1	90	540	1000	5500
Huntsville	Reclamation B	A	1	5	26	76	370
Huntsville	Reclamation B	B	1	67	170	700	2300
Gurley	Charging	A	1	41	44000	150	3100
Gurley	Charging	B	1	31	740	160	2400
Gurley	Maintenance	A	1	410	700	2300	2300
Gurley	Maintenance	B	1**	140	34	1100	370
Gurley	Milling	A	1	31	1900	240	2700
Gurley	Milling	B	1	20	190	190	2200
Gurley	Receiving	A	1	77	260	610	1500
Gurley	Receiving	B	1**	210	93	1600	770
Gurley	Reprocessing	A	1	4	72	69	370
Gurley	Screening	A	1	26	150	200	1600
Gurley	Screening	B	1	49	1300	470	4600
Gurley	Shipping	A	1	15	180	240	1400
Gurley	Shipping	B	1	70	160	690	1300
Gurley	Spray Drying	A	1	100	800	880	1300
Gurley	Spray Drying	B	1**	320	310	2800	2200
Grant	Administration	A	2	9	109	85	1045
Grant	Breakdown	A	2	49	125	155	260
Grant	Extrusion	A	2	76	170	495	1750
Grant	Grinding – Dry	A	2	26	185	315	1750
Grant	Grinding – Wet	A	2	21	60	255	915
Grant	Grinding – Grant Surface	A	2	64	191	420	1650
Grant	Maintenance	A	2	16	118	166	1285
Grant	Powder Inventory	A	2	172	4750	1175	6750
Grant	Pressing – CNC	A	2	16	83	169	760
Grant	Pressing – Dorst	A	2	21	63	225	750
Grant	Round Cell	A	2**	56	318	565	1750
Grant	Sandblasting	A	2	8	23	64	145
Grant	Shaping	A	1**	86	43	930	420
Grant	Shaping	B	1	38	50	440	580
Grant	Shipping	A	2	56	360	415	1900
Grant	Tray Preparation	A	2**	37	105	299	160

* Reported masses are medians when participants submitted more than one sample.
** Samples contained higher baseline than follow-up measurements for cobalt and/or tungsten.

Table IV. Levels of cobalt and tungsten on wipe samples collected from participants' necks at baseline and follow-up by facility and work area or job category (November 2004)

Facility	Work Area or Job Category	Worker	No. Samples	Cobalt Mass (µg)* Baseline	Cobalt Mass (µg)* Follow-up	Tungsten Mass (µg)* Baseline	Tungsten Mass (µg)* Follow-up
Huntsville	Administration	A	2	< LOD	< LOQ	< LOD	< LOQ
Huntsville	Metal Separation	A	1	7	300	71	1700
Huntsville	Metal Separation	B	1**	15	1600	130	37
Huntsville	Carbide Plant	A	1	< LOD	5	90	970
Huntsville	Carbide Plant	B	1	< LOD	3	1500	4100
Huntsville	Maintenance	A	2	14	39	410	1715
Huntsville	Reclamation A	A	1	3	47	53	810
Huntsville	Reclamation A	B	1	7	290	200	3500
Huntsville	Reclamation B	A	1	3	13	42	170
Huntsville	Reclamation B	B	1**	9	34	110	75
Gurley	Charging	A	1	< LOQ	210	< LOQ	1500
Gurley	Charging	B	1	7	1000	< LOQ	1400
Gurley	Maintenance	A	1	13	60	130	610
Gurley	Maintenance	B	1	< LOQ	6	< LOQ	68
Gurley	Milling	A	1	3	67	34	590
Gurley	Milling	B	1	3	61	50	460
Gurley	Receiving	A	1**	5	5	60	39
Gurley	Receiving	B	1	4	13	41	100
Gurley	Reprocessing	A	1	< LOQ	190	69	370
Gurley	Screening	A	1	4	20	52	200
Gurley	Screening	B	1	2	330	34	2700
Gurley	Shipping	A	1	8	14	96	140
Gurley	Shipping	B	1	2	25	< LOQ	200
Gurley	Spray Drying	A	1**	130	310	860	800
Gurley	Spray Drying	B	1	2	59	41	610
Grant	Administration	A	2	< LOD	< LOQ	< LOD	< LOD
Grant	Breakdown	A	2**	2	17	< LOD	39
Grant	Extrusion	A	2**	< LOQ	4	< LOQ	31
Grant	Grinding – Dry	A	2**	< LOQ	5	< LOQ	42
Grant	Grinding – Wet	A	2**	< LOQ	8	< LOD	80
Grant	Grinding – Surface	A	2	< LOQ	5	< LOQ	51
Grant	Maintenance	A	2**	< LOQ	9	< LOQ	145
Grant	Powder Inventory	A	2**	7	19	1175	6750
Grant	Pressing – CNC	A	2**	< LOQ	< LOQ	< LOD	< LOD
Grant	Pressing – Dorst	A	2**	< LOQ	11	< LOQ	105
Grant	Round Cell	A	2	< LOQ	12	< LOQ	93
Grant	Sandblasting	A	2	< LOD	3	< LOD	< LOQ
Grant	Shaping	A	1**	< LOD	3	150	< LOQ
Grant	Shaping	B	1	< LOQ	4	< LOD	30
Grant	Shipping	A	2	< LOQ	4	< LOQ	32
Grant	Tray Preparation	A	2	< LOQ	12	< LOD	< LOQ

*Reported masses are medians when participants submitted more than one sample.
** Samples contained higher baseline than follow-up measurements for cobalt and/or tungsten.

DEPARTMENT OF HEALTH & HUMAN SERVICES

Phone: (304) 285-5751
Fax: (304) 285-5820

Public Health Service

Centers for Disease Control
and Prevention (CDC)
National Institute for Occupational
Safety and Health (NIOSH)
1095 Willowdale Road
Morgantown, WV 26505-2888

May 9, 2006
HETA 2003-0257
Interim Letter IX

Mr. James Doherty
Interim Director of Health, Safety and Environment
Alldyne Powder Technologies
7300 Highway 20
Huntsville, Alabama 35806

Dear Mr. Doherty:

From January 23 to February 2, 2005, researchers from the National Institute for Occupational Safety and Health (NIOSH) performed a medical survey of Metalworking Products employees of the Grant, Gurley, and Huntsville, Alabama plants. This survey (referred to subsequently as the January 2005 survey) included: a questionnaire; a spirometry test (breathing test); a methacholine challenge test (a breathing test sometimes used in the diagnosis of asthma); tests for metal in urine, blood, exhaled breath, and wrist wipes; lung inflammation tests of exhaled breath condensate; blood antibody tests; and genetic tests. From April 11 to May 6, 2005, eleven employees completed a three-week serial spirometry test. We have notified employees of their individual spirometry, methacholine challenge, serial spirometry, and cobalt urine and blood results.

Enclosure A provides summary information concerning methods and test results from the January 2005 medical survey and the subsequent serial spirometry tests. In addition to results from the questionnaire and the spirometry and methacholine tests, available results include: 1) urine cobalt and tungsten levels; 2) blood and exhaled breath cobalt, tungsten, and nickel levels; 3) blood chromium levels; 4) total immunoglobulin E levels (antibody levels which are frequently elevated in individuals who have allergic conditions, including asthma); and 5) inflammation biomarker levels (leukotriene β-4 (LTB-4), interleukin-8 (IL-8), malondialdehyde (MDA)) in exhaled breath. Results for metal tests from skin wipe samples obtained during the medical survey, metal antibody tests, and genetic tests are not yet available.

In a previous interim letter dated March 25, 2005, we identified possible higher-risk work areas for the development of occupational asthma, based on our September 2003 survey. With the addition of results from the January 2005 survey, we have now updated and slightly revised our analysis as follows: 1) we included an additional 22 employees who first participated in our study in the January 2005 survey; 2) we included employees who completed questionnaires but did not complete spirometry tests; 3) we excluded all former employees (two had been included in the previous analysis); and 4) we excluded all employees with non-current post-hire asthma (one had been included in the previous analysis). Based on this analysis, we identified five possible higher-risk work areas for the development of occupational asthma:

maintenance (Gurley), product testing, milling/spray drying, pressing, and sintering (Table 3 in Enclosure A).

Thus, some work processes do seem riskier than others. Compared to data representing the national population, we have demonstrated a greater than 2-fold excess in ever-diagnosed asthma and about a 3-fold excess in new-onset asthma among workers employed at these three plants. But our attempts to find exposure or dose correlates of risk have not been successful. Our investigation of novel biomarkers of inflammation, atopy (allergic asthma or hayfever to common allergens), and physiological response have also contributed little to date. Possible explanations are that we have not classified occupational asthma correctly and that occupational asthma may have diverse exposure etiologies (including metalworking fluid). As we continue to analyze our environmental and biological exposure results, we hope to better understand what specific exposures in sintering, grinding, and product testing are associated with apparent risk of occupational lung disease among workers. Despite the uncertainties, the observed excess of disease among employees warrants attempts to lower workplace exposures to cobalt.

Based on what we have learned to date, the following summarizes our current recommendations. More detail regarding these recommendations are included in the recommendations listed in Enclosure A:

- Reduce airborne cobalt exposure levels in all work areas to below recognized professional and federal occupational exposure limits and monitor levels on a regular basis

- Reduce potential air and skin exposures in identified higher-risk work areas to as low as technically feasible

- Prevent the migration of cobalt contamination from areas of higher contamination to areas of lower contamination

- Improve general cleanliness of both production and non-production areas through good housekeeping measures

- Use a high-efficiency particulate air (HEPA) filtered vacuum to clean machines and work areas and curtail use of sweeping/brushing

- Ensure that appropriate respiratory protection is worn by properly trained personnel when job activities could result in exposure levels above recognized professional and federal occupational exposure limits for cobalt in air and such exposures can not be controlled to an acceptable level by engineering and work practice controls

- Augment the current skin protection program with the following elements:
    - Train supervisors on elements and implementation of the skin protection program
    - Have workers wear long-sleeved shirts when working in production areas
    - Have workers use nitrile gloves before handling contaminated clothing (for example, while putting on or taking off work boots and clothes) and while working in production areas
    - Have workers discard (not reuse) used protective gloves
    - Encourage workers to shower soon after work

- After changes in engineering controls, work practices, general housekeeping, and personal protective clothing and equipment have been instituted, repeat employee urine or whole blood cobalt tests in work areas in which we found a high proportion of employees with urine or whole blood cobalt levels in excess of the American Conference of Governmental Industrial Hygienists (ACGIH) biological exposure indices (BEIs).

- In our reports of individual cobalt test results to participating employees, we suggested that those with urine and/or blood cobalt levels greater than or equal to the relevant ACGIH BEI(s) seek repeat testing from their personal physician. We further suggested that workers whose repeat results remain greater than or equal to the relevant BEI wear a respirator at work. If they had already been wearing a respirator at work, we recommended that they make sure that they had been fit-tested within the last year and that they always use their respirator at work. We also recommended that, while at work, they wash their hands frequently and use nitrile gloves.

- In our reports of individual spirometry or methacholine challenge test results to participating employees, we suggested that those with abnormal or work-related test results share the results with their personal physicians. We also suggested that they seek evaluation by a lung doctor (pulmonologist) if they had a work-related pattern on their serial spirometry test or if they had airways hyper-responsiveness and their asthma symptoms began or worsened after beginning to work in the hard metal industry.

- Any current or future workers with respiratory symptoms that the worker believes are work-related should be medically evaluated by a physician. The company's director of safety and environment should establish a mechanism to monitor respiratory symptoms and disease reported by workers.

NIOSH recommends that copies of this letter and enclosures, including the interim letter summary sheet for workers (Enclosure B) be posted by management in a prominent place accessible to the employees for a period of at least 30 calendar days. NIOSH does not actively disseminate letter reports such as this beyond this initial mailing. However, this letter would be releasable if requested under the Freedom of Information Act.

My colleagues and I thank Metalworking Products for helping us during our January-February and April-May 2005 medical surveys. We are continuing to analyze data from all of our surveys of your three facilities and will report further findings in additional interim letters or a final report. Please feel free to contact me at (304) 285-6383 with any questions or concerns you may have.

Sincerely,

Nancy Sahakian, M.D., M.P.H.
Lieutenant Commander
U.S. Public Health Service
Field Studies Branch
Division of Respiratory Disease Studies

Enclosures

cc:
Daryl Baker
Larry Hollingsworth
Junior Pugh
Confidential Employee Requestors
HETAB file (HETA 2003-0257)

ENCLOSURE A
HETA 2003-0257

METHODS (JANUARY – MAY 2005 SURVEYS)

We invited Grant and Gurley plant employees in production, maintenance, product testing, powder laboratory, shipping, and supervisory jobs and Huntsville employees in reclamation, metal separation, maintenance, powder laboratory, and supervisory jobs to participate in all or any individual survey components. A small group of employees from the above work areas were chosen (based on a range of reported symptoms) to complete the methacholine challenge and 3-week serial spirometry tests. A signed informed consent was obtained from all participants. The study protocol was approved by the NIOSH Human Subjects Research Board.

Employees who had participated in the September 2003 medical survey completed a short paper questionnaire. The questionnaire asked about physician-diagnosed asthma, current asthma symptoms, and work history after September 2003. Employees who had not participated in the September 2003 medical survey completed a longer computerized questionnaire and a spirometry test. The computerized questionnaire included the same questions as the September 2003 questionnaire with regard to worker symptoms, medical diagnoses, smoking history, and work history.

Spirometry Test

Spirometry tests were done according to the 1995 recommendations of the American Thoracic Society.[1] Quality was assessed based on reproducibility of curves, absence of cough and hesitation, and expiration of at least 6 seconds. We chose the largest forced vital capacity (FVC) and forced expiratory volume in one second (FEV1) from a minimum of three acceptable trials. We calculated predicted and lower limit of normal values using reference values derived from asymptomatic never-smokers in the 3rd National Health and Nutrition Examination Survey (NHANES III).[2, 3] Test results were compared to the lower limit of normal values to identify employees with abnormal spirometry patterns.[4] We defined airways obstruction as both an FEV1 and an FEV1/FVC ratio below the respective lower limits of normal; borderline obstruction as a normal FEV1 with an FEV1/FVC ratio below the lower limit of normal; and restriction as a normal FEV1/FVC ratio and an FVC below the lower limit of normal. A mixed obstructive and restrictive pattern was defined as both an FEV1/FVC ratio and an FVC below the respective lower limits of normal.

Methacholine Challenge Test

The methacholine challenge test can determine the sensitivity (hyper-responsiveness) of the airways in the lungs. A spirometry test is done before and after each administered dose of the drug methacholine. Increasingly higher concentrations of methacholine are breathed in until the FEV1 is decreased by 20%, the individual experiences side effects, or a maximum concentration dose is administered.[5] We defined airways hyper-responsiveness as a 20% or greater drop in FEV1 at a methacholine concentration less than or equal to 16.0 mg/ml.

Serial Spirometry Test

Serial spirometry was performed using a portable spirometer (EasyOne™, ndd Medical Technologies,

Chelmsford, MA). Individuals were instructed to blow forcefully into the portable spirometer a minimum of three times per test session, with five test sessions daily for a 3-week period. The five test times were on arising, on arrival at work, before lunch, at the end of work, and before going to bed (and at comparable times on non-work days). On-site coaching was provided by NIOSH technicians. Serial spirometry records were reviewed to determine whether peak expiratory flow rate (PEF) or FEV1 decreased or whether the daily variation in PEF or FEV1 increased during times at work. Two NIOSH physicians and one NIOSH researcher independently reviewed the serial spirometry records. We defined a work-related pattern of spirometry results as agreement of at least two of the 3 reviewers that work-relatedness was present.

Case Definitions

We defined "healthy" workers as those: 1) whose most recent spirometry test was normal; 2) who did not have airways hyper-responsiveness; and 3) who reported that they had never been diagnosed with asthma, did not have current asthma symptoms, were not troubled by shortness of breath, did not have shortness of breath when hurrying on level ground, did not have a usual cough, had never been diagnosed with chronic bronchitis, and were not currently using breathing medication.

We defined "probable current asthma" cases as employees who at least 3 of 9 asthma symptoms, current use of medication for their breathing, or who had weak airways hyper-responsiveness on methacholine challenge testing (PC20 > 4 and $\leq$ 16mg/ml) and who did not have current physician-diagnosed asthma. We defined "current asthma" cases as employees who reported current physician-diagnosed asthma or who had very strong airways hyper-responsiveness (PC20 $\leq$ 4 mg/ml) on methacholine challenge testing.

We defined "suspected occupational asthma" for new participants as one or more of the following: a methacholine challenge test that demonstrated airways hyper-responsiveness, current physician-diagnosed asthma, 3 or more asthma symptoms,[6] or current use of asthma medication. (For employees who participated for the first time in September 2003, we defined "suspected occupational asthma" similarly; however, we used reversibility of airways obstruction or borderline obstruction instead of a positive methacholine challenge test.)

Updated Analysis of Incidence Rates of Suspected Occupational Asthma by Work Area

We revised inclusion and exclusion criteria used in our previous analysis of suspected occupational asthma incidence rates as follows: 1) we included an additional 22 employees who first participated in our study in the January 2005 survey; 2) we included employees who completed questionnaires but did not complete spirometry tests; 3) we excluded all former employees (two had been included in the previous analysis); and 4) we excluded all employees with non-current post-hire asthma (one had been included in the previous analysis). After excluding all employees with a pre-hire asthma diagnosis, pre-hire wheeze, pre-hire shortness of breath, or unknown dates of asthma diagnosis or symptom onset, we then combined the remaining new participants and employees who participated in the September 2003 survey, and used work tenure only up to September 2003 to calculate suspected occupational asthma incidence rates as described in our Revised Interim Letter I dated March 25, 2004.

Biological Sample Collection

We collected urine, blood, exhaled breath condensate, and wrist wipe samples during the last two hours of an employee's shift and on one of the last two days of their work week. For urine collection, employees were instructed to wash their hands, remove the collection container from a plastic bag, put on a pair of nitrile gloves (also in a plastic bag), and then collect their urine sample in a sterile container. Urine samples were refrigerated on-site, packed with cooler packs, and shipped to a NIOSH-contracted laboratory where they were analyzed for cobalt and tungsten content, specific gravity (a measure of how concentrated the urine sample was), and creatinine (a measure of the amount of body fluids that were cleared by the kidney to produce the urine sample).

Whole blood samples for metal and genetic (HLA-DPβ_1^{GLU69}) testing were drawn in disodium EDTA tubes and CPT tubes, respectively, refrigerated on-site, and packed in insulated containers with cooler packs. Blood samples for metal testing were shipped to a NIOSH-contracted laboratory and blood samples for genetic testing were shipped to NIOSH for analysis. Blood samples for metal antibody and total immunoglobulin E tests were drawn in serum tubes and centrifuged on-site to separate the serum from the blood cells. The serum was transferred to cryo vials which were packed in insulated containers with dry ice and shipped to NIOSH for analysis.

We collected exhaled breath condensate samples over a 20-minute period using a TURBO DECCS™ (Transportable Unit for Research on Biomarkers Obtained from Disposable Exhaled Condensate Collection Systems unit (Ital Chill, Parma, Italy)) with a chilling temperature of -5° Centigrade. Employees rinsed their mouth with water prior to collection and wore a pair of nitrile gloves during collection of the sample. Individual samples were transferred on-site to Eppendorf tubes, which were packed with dry ice and shipped to a collaborating research laboratory for analysis.

To obtain wrist wipe samples, a NIOSH employee technician put on a clean pair of nitrile gloves and wiped the underside of the employee's wrist for 30 seconds with a Wash 'n Dri™ moistened towelette (First Brands Corporation, Danbury, CT). Wipes were subsequently placed in individual zip-locked plastic bags that were shipped to a NIOSH-contracted laboratory for metal analysis.

Laboratory Analysis

All laboratory analyses were performed in research laboratories not regulated by the Clinical Laboratory Improvements Advisory Committee (CLIA), and as such are not held to the standards set for clinical laboratories. Because of this, individual reported results are not definitive. However, results are useful for comparing work area exposures. Limit of detection (LOD) values, limit of quantitation (LOQ) values, and working ranges (ranges within which results are accurate) for analytes are listed in Table 1.

In the analysis of chromium in whole blood, samples were initially tested using the Inductively Coupled Plasma – Mass Spectrometry (ICP-MS). However, due to technical problems with this technique, the remaining samples were analyzed using Inductively Coupled Plasma – Atomic Emission Spectrometry (ICP-AES). We only report whole blood chromium results for which ICP-AES was used.

Background Information

Biological Exposure Indices (BEIs®)

The American Conference of Governmental Industrial Hygienists (ACGIH) defines biological exposure indices (BEIs) for specific occupational exposures. These BEIs are urine and/or blood levels of occupational chemicals that should not be exceeded if the occupational exposures are kept below the ACGIH threshold limit value for cobalt (20 µg (micrograms) of cobalt per cubic meter of air). The

ACGIH BEIs for cobalt in urine and whole blood samples collected at the end of shift on the end of the work week are 15 µg cobalt per L (liter) of urine and 1 µg cobalt/L of whole blood. ACGIH defines "end of shift" as "as soon as possible after exposure ceases" and "end of work week" as "after four or five consecutive working days with exposure." There are no ACGIH BEIs for tungsten, nickel, or total chromium in urine or blood or for any metal levels in exhaled breath condensate.

The concentration of metal in urine can vary depending on the amount of liquid recently consumed. The creatinine content in urine, which reflects the amount of body fluid filtered by the kidneys to produce the urine sample, can vary depending on the urine concentration and health of the kidneys. ACGIH considers urine samples to be acceptable for measuring BEIs if the urine specific gravity is between 1.010 and 1.030 or the urine creatinine level is between 0.3 and 3.0 grams per liter of urine.

Reasons for Differences in Employee's Urine, Blood, and Exhaled Breath Condensate Metal Levels

Employees working in the same work area may have different urine, blood, and exhaled breath condensate metal levels for a variety of reasons. In addition to different work tasks, worker differences that might result in variable levels include differences in: 1) work habits; 2) use of respiratory protection; 3) speed at which the body is able to eliminate individual metals; 4) personal hygiene; 5) outside sources of cobalt (such as from multivitamins, vitamin B12, and artificial joints); and 6) contamination of the urine sample with metal from the skin or clothing.

Statistical Analysis

In our analyses of biological indices of metal exposures, we excluded: employees who reported working in more than one work area (n=13); employees who provided samples at the beginning of their workshift (n=2); and employees who worked in a different work area two days prior to the test (n=1) or who had returned to work after an extended absence (n=1). We reported results for work areas for which we received at least 3 samples.

We included all blood nickel and tungsten levels in our analysis. Otherwise we restricted our analyses of blood and urine metal levels to: 1) urine cobalt values from urine samples with specific gravities between 1.010 and 1.030 and creatinine levels between 0.3 and 3.0 g/L which came from employees who reported not taking multivitamins or vitamin B12 and not having an artificial joint; 2) urine nickel and tungsten values from urine samples with specific gravities between 1.010 and 1.030 and creatinine levels between 0.3 and 3.0 g/L; and 3) blood cobalt levels from blood samples from employees who reported not taking multivitamins or vitamin B12 and not having an artificial joint.

We calculated the percent of urine and blood cobalt samples with levels at or above the ACGIH BEIs for cobalt. We also calculated geometric means (averages) for urine, blood, and exhaled breath condensate metals for all participants and by work areas, using the SAS QLIM function to calculate geometric means for work areas with values below the limit of detection. This statistical function allowed us to statistically estimate these low values.

For some biological exposure measurements that do not have BEIs (urine cobalt per gram creatinine, blood nickel, and exhaled breath condensate levels of cobalt, nickel, and tungsten), we calculated the percent of samples with levels at or above the workforce geometric mean. The one exception was that, because of a large number of urine tungsten values below the limits of detection and quantitation, we calculated the percent of samples with tungsten at or above these limits.

For cobalt in urine and whole blood, and cobalt and tungsten in exhaled breath condensate, we also calculated and compared the geometric mean value for workers in higher-risk work areas with the geometric mean value for workers in other work areas for which risk could be assessed (reclamation, shaping, powder mixing, shipping (Grant), maintenance (Grant), and metal separation).

We constructed scatterplots and tested the log-transformed data for correlations between: 1) urine and blood cobalt; 2) urine cobalt per gram creatinine and blood cobalt; 3) urine and exhaled breath condensate cobalt; and 4) urine cobalt per gram creatinine and exhaled breath condensate cobalt. We considered Pearson Correlation Coefficient (r) values between 0.80 and 1.00 to represent very strong correlations, between 0.60 and 0.79 to represent strong correlations, between 0.40 and 0.59 to represent moderate correlations, and between 0.20-0.39 to represent weak correlations. We also constructed scatter plots of average work area data for personal breathing zone total airborne cobalt levels from closed-face cassette samples collected in October 2004 (see Interim Letter VII dated March 20, 2006) versus work area averages of urine cobalt per gram creatinine, blood cobalt, and exhaled breath condensate cobalt from samples collected in the January 2005 survey. For all these scatter plots, we excluded data for employees who reported current use of respiratory protection. For scatter plots of urine and blood cobalt, we additionally excluded employees who reported use of vitamins or the presence of an artificial joint.

We used 100 kilo units (kU) or more of total immunoglobulin E per liter of serum to suggest allergic asthma, hayfever, or eczema. We calculated geometric mean total immunoglobulin E levels for: 1) suspected occupational asthma cases; 2) pre-hire asthma cases; and 3) the remainder of the workforce. We then tested whether there was any statistically significant difference among these three mean values.

We used Student's t test and the Wilcoxon Rank Sum test to compare inflammation biomarker levels in exhaled breath condensate from "healthy" workers and probable current asthma and current asthma cases combined; and from "healthy" workers and current asthma cases (as defined above in "Case Definitions"). For MDA, we used all values (all values were greater than the limit of quantitation). For LTB-4 and IL-8, we used 1) values greater than the limit of quantitation; or 2) all measurements (substituting a value of one-half the limit of detection for all measurements that were less than the limit of detection).

RESULTS

Demographic Data and Participation Rates

Of the 267 employees eligible for the January 2005 medical survey, 150 (56%) participated. Demographics of these participants are included in Table 2. Of 243 employees eligible for the September 2003 medical survey, 197 (81%) participated in either our September 2003 or January 2005 surveys.

Questionnaire Responses for Employees Participating in the Medical Survey for the First Time in January 2005

During the January 2005 survey, 46 employees who did not participate in the September 2003 survey completed a long questionnaire for the first time. Ever physician-diagnosed asthma was present in 3 of 46 (7%), current physician-diagnosed asthma in 2 of 46 (4%), and physician-diagnosed asthma with post-hire onset in 0 of 46 (0%) participants. Three or more current asthma symptoms were reported by 7 of 46 (15%) participants.

All 3 employees with suspected occupational asthma had 3 or more current asthma symptoms. They reported that either wheezing or shortness of breath began while working in spray drying, milling, or pressing.

Incidence Rates of Suspected Occupational Asthma by Work Area

Of the 43 employees who completed a long questionnaire and who provided us a hire date, 26 (60%) had hire dates prior to September 2003 and reported having worked during September 2003 in one of the work areas included in our 2003 survey. Inclusion of these 26 employees increased the participation rate for our incidence rate analysis from 69% (results included in Revised Interim Letter I dated March 25, 2005) to 81% of those employed in September 2003. Based on our updated analysis, we identified five possible higher-risk work areas for the development of occupational asthma: maintenance (Gurley), product testing, milling/spray drying, pressing, and sintering (Table 3).

Spirometry Results for Employees Participating in the Medical Survey for the First Time in January 2005

During the January 2005 survey, 41 employees who did not participate in the September 2003 survey completed a spirometry test. Spirometry results for the 41 tested employees were as follows: restriction was present in 6 (15%); obstruction or borderline obstruction was present in 7 (17%); and a mixed obstructive and restrictive pattern was present in 1 (2%).

Methacholine Challenge Test

Five of 15 (33%) employees who completed a methacholine challenge test and who had suspected occupational asthma had airways hyper-responsiveness. Two of 45 (4%) of employees without suspected occupational asthma had airways hyper-responsiveness (one of these employees reported having wheeze prior to being hired).

Serial Spirometry

Agreement among reviewers as to the presence of a work-related pattern was reached for 9 of the 11 employee tests. The 2 tests for which there was not complete agreement were rated based on agreement of two out of the three reviewers. Of 8 suspected occupational asthma cases who completed serial spirometry of sufficient quality to interpret, 2 (25%) had a work-related pattern. Both of these employees were identified as having the onset of their suspected occupational asthma while working in pressing. The use of an asthma inhaler may obscure work-related changes in FEV1 and PEF. Of the 6 suspected occupational asthma cases who did not have a work-related pattern on serial spirometry, 3 used an asthma inhaler multiple times (range: 13-26) during the 3 weeks of serial spirometry testing.

Urine Cobalt and Tungsten Levels

After excluding 61 (of 122) urine samples with specific gravity measurements or creatinine levels that were out of the acceptable ranges and urine samples from employees who indicated that they were taking vitamins or had an artificial joint, 4 work areas had more than 75% of their employee urine samples with cobalt levels at or above the ACGIH BEI (Table 4). These work areas were milling, spray drying, pressing, and reclamation. Of the 6 higher-risk work areas (pressing, sintering, grinding for hard metal disease; and maintenance (Gurley), product testing, milling/spray drying, pressing, and sintering for suspected occupational asthma), we had acceptable urine results for 5. None of the employee urine samples in 3 (sintering, grinding, and product testing) of the 5 represented higher-risk work areas exceeded the ACGIH BEI. The geometric mean urine cobalt value for employees in higher-risk work areas was 17.1 µg/L; for employees in other-risk work areas it was 14.9 µg/L. There was no statistically significant difference between these two means.

After excluding 37 (of 122) urine samples from employees who indicated that they were taking vitamins or had an artificial joint, 5 work areas had more than 75% of their employee urine cobalt per gram creatinine measurements in excess of the workforce geometric mean of 9.6 µg cobalt/gram creatinine (Table 5). These work areas were milling, spray drying, pressing, shaping, and reclamation. Of the 6 higher-risk work areas, we had acceptable urine results for 5. None of the employee urine samples in 3 (sintering, grinding, and product testing) of these 5 higher-risk work areas exceeded the workforce geometric mean value. The geometric mean urine cobalt per gram creatinine value for employees in higher-risk work areas was 11.5 µg/L, and for employees in other-risk work areas it was 9.9 µg/L. There was no statistically significant difference between these two geometric means.

After excluding 31 (of 122) urine samples with specific gravity or creatinine levels that were out of the acceptable ranges, urine tungsten levels exceeded the limit of quantitation in some employees in milling, spray drying, pressing, shaping, grinding, reclamation, metal separation, and the "other" work areas (Table 6). All of the samples from employees in metal separation and most of the samples from employees in spray drying had urine tungsten levels that exceeded the limit of quantitation. The highest recorded urine tungsten level was for an employee in the metal separation work area. Of the 6 higher-risk work areas, we had acceptable urine results for 5. All of the employee urine samples in 2 (sintering and product testing) of these 5 higher-risk work areas were below the limit of quantitation.

Whole Blood Cobalt, Tungsten, Nickel, and Chromium Levels

After excluding 40 (of 125) whole blood samples from employees who indicated that they were taking vitamins or had an artificial joint, 8 work areas had more than 75% of their employee blood samples at or above the ACGIH BEI for cobalt. These work areas were powder mixing, milling, spray drying, pressing, shaping, maintenance (Grant), reclamation, and metal separation (Table 7). Of the 6 higher-risk work areas, we had acceptable blood cobalt results for 5. Three (sintering, grinding, and product testing) of these 5 higher-risk work areas had less than 50% of their employee blood cobalt levels above the ACGIH BEI. The geometric mean whole blood cobalt level for employees in higher-risk work areas was 2.1 µg/L, and for employees in other-risk work areas it was 2.3 µg/L. There was no statistically significant difference between these two geometric means.

All whole blood tungsten levels were below the limit of detection. Results for nickel levels are provided in Table 8. Of 96 whole blood samples analyzed for chromium using the ICP-AES technique, 8 were from employees who did not work 100% of the time in one work area and 2 were from employees who did not provide a work history. All 86 remaining blood chromium levels were below the limit of quantitation; 26 were greater or equal to the limit of detection. All whole blood tungsten levels were below the limit of detection.

Exhaled Breath Condensate Cobalt, Tungsten, and Nickel Levels

Work areas with more than 75% of their exhaled breath condensate samples with metal levels at or above the workforce geometric mean values were: powder mixing, milling, and spray drying (for cobalt) (Table 9); milling, spray drying, reclamation, and metal separation (for tungsten) (Table 10); and milling, spray drying, reclamation, and metal separation (for nickel)(Table 11). Three higher-risk work areas (sintering, grinding, and product testing) had one-third or less of their employees with exhaled breath condensate cobalt levels at or above the workforce geometric mean; and one higher-risk work area (product testing) had 17% of their employees with exhaled breath condensate tungsten levels at or above the workforce geometric mean.

The geometric mean exhaled breath condensate cobalt value for employees in higher-risk work areas was 6.2 µg/L, and for employees in other-risk work areas it was 5.5 µg/L; these two geometric means were not statistically different. The geometric mean exhaled breath condensate tungsten value for employees in higher-risk work areas was 2.3 µg/L, and for employees in other-risk work areas it was 10.2 µg/L; these two geometric mean values were statistically different.

Urine, Blood, Exhaled Breath Condensate, and Air Level Comparisons

There were very strong correlations between urine cobalt and blood cobalt (Figure 1) and between urine cobalt per gram creatinine and blood cobalt (Figure 2). There was a weak correlation between urine cobalt and exhaled breath condensate cobalt (Figure 3) and between urine cobalt per gram creatinine and exhaled breath condensate cobalt (Figure 4). Sparse work area data (only 7 to 8 data points per scatter plot) were insufficient to assess correlations between work area airborne cobalt levels and urine cobalt per gram creatinine, blood cobalt, and exhaled breath condensate cobalt.

Total Immunoglobulin E Levels

Of 140 employees, total immunoglobulin E levels ranged from < 2 kU/L to 1,050 kU/L and 32 (23%) had levels of 100 kU or more per liter. Geometric means were 81.4 kU/L for participants with pre-hire physician-diagnosed asthma, 28.0 kU/L for participants with suspected occupational asthma cases, and 40.3 kU/L for other participants. There was no statistically significant difference among these geometric mean values.

Exhaled Breath Condensate Inflammation Biomarkers

Geometric mean values of LTB-4, IL-8, and MDA did not differ significantly between probable current asthma cases and current asthma cases combined and "healthy" workers; or between current asthma cases and "healthy" workers (Table 12).

DISCUSSION AND CONCLUSIONS

Serial Spirometry

Only one-fourth of serial spirometry tests completed in employees with suspected occupational asthma were interpreted as having a work-related pattern. Factors that may have interfered with our identification of a work-related pattern in individuals with occupational asthma include: variable exposures, use of asthma medication on workdays, short work weeks, short non-work periods, and short period of serial spirometry. In fact, of the 6 employees with suspected occupational asthma who did not have a work-related pattern, 3 reported using an asthma inhaler multiple times during the 3-week test period. Of course, it is possible some or all of the 6 employees with suspected occupational asthma who did not have a work-related spirometry pattern may not, in fact, have had occupational asthma.

Total Immunoglobulin E

Total immunoglobulin E measures all immunoglobulin E antibodies in the serum. Since these antibodies usually are specific to common allergens (e.g., pollens, molds, and dust mites), high total immunoglobulin E levels are often found in the serum of individuals who are atopic (i.e., have allergic asthma or hayfever specific to common allergens). Antibodies to less common allergens (e.g., cobalt,[7] nickel, and other occupational substances) also contribute to total immunoglobulin E levels. However, based on a study of 9 hard metal workers,[8] it is unlikely that an allergy to cobalt alone would result in an excessively high total immunoglobulin E level. That study of 9 hard metal workers with confirmed cobalt asthma showed that all 4 with elevated total immunoglobulin E levels were atopic. Among the 4 workers with immunoglobulin E antibodies specific to cobalt, the one worker who was not atopic did not have an elevated total immunoglobulin E level. An epidemiological study of hard metal workers demonstrated that atopic workers were more likely to have asthmatic symptoms.[9] Another study demonstrated similar total immunoglobulin E levels in cobalt-exposed workers compared to non-cobalt-exposed workers, however the study did not indicate which part of the industry was studied (i.e., cobalt ore production, hard metal production, etc.).[10]

Contrary to the results of the study[9] above that concluded that atopy predisposed workers to hard metal asthma, our not finding higher total immunoglobulin E levels in workers with suspected occupational asthma compared to other participants suggests that atopy does not place workers at increased risk for occupational asthma in the hard metal industry. It may be that occupational asthma in the hard metal industry may be due to a non-IgE-related mechanism. Also, our suspected occupational asthma definition may misclassify some individual participants with respect to their true status as either having or not having occupational asthma, which could contribute, at least in part, to our finding of a lack of association between total IgE and suspected occupational asthma.

Cobalt and Tungsten Exposures

Exposures to cobalt, nickel, and chromium metals can cause occupational asthma. The current understanding within the scientific community is that co-exposure to cobalt and tungsten causes hard metal disease.

Cobalt can be absorbed from the environment through breathing, swallowing, and touching. Urine and whole blood cobalt levels measure the amount of cobalt that has been absorbed by any of these exposure mechanisms. Within a few weeks, the body is able to eliminate (in the urine) a large proportion of previously absorbed cobalt. In other studies, cobalt air levels have been shown to be associated with urine and blood cobalt levels. Due to few data points, we did not have sufficient data to test associations between work area cobalt air levels and urine and blood cobalt levels. In addition, misclassification of exposures (the air levels were measured three months before the urine and blood samples were collected) could contribute to the observed scatter of data points.

Urine cobalt levels exceeded the ACGIH BEI in 46% of the workforce; and whole blood cobalt levels exceeded the ACGIH BEI in 74% of the workforce. These findings suggest that many workers may be exposed to levels of cobalt in the air greater than the ACGIH Threshold Limit Value of 20 µg/cubic meter of air or may have absorbed large amount of cobalt through the skin or from ingestion. Urine and blood cobalt levels of employees in higher-risk work areas and other-risk work areas were similar.

It is unknown what metal levels in exhaled breath condensate signify. An initial study[11] failed to demonstrate a correlation between cobalt levels in exhaled breath condensate and in air. Researchers have speculated that the lack of correlation may be due to cobalt quickly leaving the lung and entering the circulatory system (i.e., "fast kinetics"). These researchers have postulated that cobalt in exhaled breath condensate may reflect the amount of cobalt retained in the lung and able to damage the lung. In our study, exhaled breath condensate cobalt levels of employees in higher-risk work areas and other-risk work areas were similar. Exhaled breath condensate tungsten levels were lower for employees in higher-risk work areas compared to other-risk work areas.

Our observation of similar or lower urine, blood, or exhaled breath condensate levels of cobalt and tungsten for employees in higher-risk work areas, compared to employees in other-risk work areas, suggests that some unique characteristic of exposure (not an absolute level of cobalt absorbed by the lungs) may be responsible for occupational lung disease in exposed workers. Relevant exposure characteristics may include: exposure to cobalt and tungsten with different particle characteristics; exposure to other metals, such as nickel or chromium; exposure to other chemicals or substances (such as metalworking fluid); co-exposure of several metals; co-exposure to metals and chemicals; and co-exposures by inhalation and skin exposure.

Our data indicates that biological exposure levels for metal differ substantially among higher-risk work areas. Two higher-risk work areas (sintering and product testing) had no employee urine cobalt levels greater than or equal to the BEI; whereas one higher-risk work area (milling/spray drying) had all employee urine cobalt levels greater than or equal to the BEI. The work areas with the lowest and highest geometric mean exhaled breath condensate cobalt and tungsten levels were both higher-risk work areas. Likewise, Table 13 indicates that three higher-risk work areas (sintering, grinding, and product testing) did not have excessively high proportions of elevated employee urine, blood, and exhaled breath condensate metal levels, and the three other higher-risk work areas did.

As we continue to analyze our environmental and biological exposure results, we hope to better understand what specific exposures in sintering, grinding, and product testing are associated with apparent risk of occupational lung disease among workers.

SUMMARY

Based on all information available to date, some work processes at these three plants do seem riskier than others. Compared to data representing the national population, we have demonstrated a greater than 2-fold excess in ever-diagnosed asthma and about a 3-fold excess in new-onset asthma among workers employed at these three plants. But our attempts to find exposure or dose correlates of risk have not been successful. Our investigation of novel biomarkers of inflammation, atopy, and physiological response have also contributed little to date. Possible explanations are that we have not classified occupational asthma correctly or that occupational asthma may have diverse exposure etiologies (including metalworking fluid). Despite the uncertainties, the observed excess of disease among employees warrants attempts to lower workplace exposures to cobalt.

RECOMMENDATIONS

Based on what we have learned to date, the following summarizes our current recommendations:

- Reduce airborne cobalt exposure levels in all work areas to below recognized professional and federal occupational exposure limits and monitor levels on a regular basis

- Reduce potential air and skin exposures in identified higher-risk work areas to as low as technically feasible

- Prevent the migration of cobalt contamination from areas of higher contamination to areas of lower contamination. Possible routes of cross contamination include the transfer of cobalt from shoes, clothing, hands, equipment, and paperwork to less contaminated work areas.

- Improve general cleanliness of both production and non-production areas through good housekeeping measures

- Use a high-efficiency particulate air (HEPA) filtered vacuum to clean machines and work areas and curtail use of sweeping/brushing

- Ensure that appropriate respiratory protection is worn by properly trained personnel when job activities could result in exposure levels above recognized professional and federal occupational exposure limits for cobalt in air and such exposures can not be controlled to an acceptable level by engineering and work practice controls

- Augment the current skin protection program with the following elements:
    o Train supervisors on elements and implementation of the skin protection program
    o Have workers wear long-sleeved shirts when working in production areas
    o Have workers use nitrile gloves before handling contaminated clothing (for example, while putting on or taking off work boots and clothes) and while working in production areas
    o Have workers discard (not reuse) used protective gloves
    o Encourage workers to shower soon after work

- After changes in engineering controls, work practices, general housekeeping, and personal protective clothing and equipment have been instituted, repeat employee urine or whole blood cobalt tests in work areas with a high proportion of workers with cobalt levels in excess of the ACGIH BEIs. These work areas would be milling, spray drying, pressing, and reclamation for urine samples; and powder mixing, milling, spray drying, pressing, shaping, maintenance (Grant), reclamation, and metal separation for whole blood samples. Urine and whole blood samples need to be obtained at the end of the shift and the end of the work week. Note that if no preventive interventions are made, biological samples collected more stringently at the end of the shift and end of the work week (compared to our collection methods of within 2 hours of the end of the shift and within the last two days of the end of the work week) may yield slightly higher cobalt levels than we measured. However, if effective changes are instituted in the workplace, levels should be lower than those reported in Attachment A.
- In our reports of individual cobalt test results to participating employees, we suggested that those

with urine and/or blood cobalt levels greater than or equal to the relevant ACGIH BEI(s) seek repeat testing from their personal physician. We further suggested that workers whose repeat results remain greater than or equal to the relevant BEI wear a respirator at work. If they had already been wearing a respirator at work, we recommended that they make sure that they had been fit-tested within the last year and that they always use their respirator at work. We also recommended that, while at work, they wash their hands frequently and use nitrile gloves.

- In our reports of individual spirometry or methacholine challenge test results to participating employees, we suggested that those with abnormal or work-related test results share the results with their personal physicians. We also suggested that they seek evaluation by a lung doctor (pulmonologist) if they had a work-related pattern on their serial spirometry test or if they had airways hyper-responsiveness and their asthma symptoms began or worsened after beginning to work in the hard metal industry. This would provide an opportunity for their physician to determine whether they had a work-related illness and, if so, to possibly suggest a job reassignment.

- Any current or future workers with respiratory symptoms that the worker believes are work-related should be medically evaluated by a physician. The company's director of safety and environment should establish a mechanism to monitors respiratory symptoms and disease reported by workers.

REFERENCES

1. American Thoracic Society [1995]. Standardization of spirometry: 1994 update. Am J Resp Crit Care Med 152:1107-1136.

2. Hankinson JL, Odencrantz JR, Fedan KB [1999]. Spirometric reference values from a sample of the general U.S. population. Am J Resp Crit Care Med 159:179-187.

3. CDC [1996]. Third National Health and Nutrition Examination Survey, 1988-1994, NHANES III Examination Date File [CD-ROM]. Hyattsville, Maryland: U.S. Department of Health and Human Services, Public Health Service, Centers for Disease Control and Prevention. (Public use data file documentations No. 76300).

4. American Thoracic Society [1991]. Lung function testing: selection of reference values and interpretive strategies. Am Rev Resp Dis 144:1202-1218.

5. American Thoracic Society. [2000]. Guidelines for methacholine and exercise challenge testing – 1999. Am J Respir Crit Care Med 161:309-329.

6. Venables K, Farrer N, Sharp L. et al. [1993]. Respiratory symptoms questionnaire for asthma epidemiology: validity and reproducibility. Thorax 48:214-219.

7. Shirakawa T, Kusaka Y, Fujimura N et al. [1988]. The existence of specific antibodies to cobalt in hard metal asthma. Clin Allergy 18:451-460.

8. Kusaka Y, Nakano Y, Shirakawa T, et al. [1989]. Lymphocyte transformation with cobalt in hard metal asthma. Ind Health 27:155-163.

9. Kusaka Y, Iki M, Kumagai W, et al. [1996]. Epidemiological study of hard metal asthma. Occup Environ Med 53:188-193.

10. Benco V, Wagner V, Wagnerova M et al. [1986]. Human exposure to nickel and cobalt: biological monitoring and immunobiochemical response. Environ Res 40:399-410.

11. Goldoni M, Catalani S, De Palma G, et al. [2004]. Exhaled breath condensate as a suitable matrix to assess lung dose and effects in workers exposed to cobalt and tungsten. Environ Health Perspect 112:1293-1298.

Table 1. Limits of detection, limits of quantitation, and working ranges for analytes

Analyte	Urine LOD	Urine LOQ	Whole Blood LOD	Whole Blood LOQ	Serum LOD	Exhaled breath condensate LOD	Exhaled breath condensate LOQ	Exhaled breath condensate Working range
Cobalt	0.4 µg/L	2.0 µg/L	0.1 µg/L	0.4 µg/L	-	0.003 µg/L	0.009 µg/L	-
Tungsten	10 µg/L	40 µg/L	20 µg/L	50 µg/L	-	0.003 µg/L	0.009 µg/L	-
Nickel	-	-	0.7 µg/L	3.0 µg/L	-	0.003 µg/L	0.009 µg/L	-
Chromium	-	-	20 µg/L	60 µg/L	-	-	-	-
LTB-4	-	-	-	-	-	2.5 ng/L	-	2.5-800 ng/L
IL-8	-	-	-	-	-	0.05 ng/L	-	0.15-25 ng/L
MDA	-	-	-	-	-	1 nmol/L	3 nmol/L	-
Total IgE	-	-	-	-	2 kU/L	-	-	-

LOD, limit of detection; LOQ, limit of quantitation; working range, range in which results are accurate; LTB-4, leukotriene B-4; IL-8, interleukin-8; MDA, malondialdehyde; IgE, immunoglobulin E; µg/L, microgram per liter; ng/L, nanogram per liter; nmol/L, nanomoles per liter; kU/L, kilo units per liter.

Table 2. Demographics of participants, January 2005 (N=150)

Demographics	Participants
Age (years)	
- Median	44
- Range	21-66
Gender (number, percent)	
- Males	109 (72.7%)
- Females	41 (27.3%)
Smoking Status (number, percent)	
- Current smokers	50 (33.3%)
- Former smokers	33 (22.0%)
- Never smokers	67 (44.7%)
Pack-years (for ever-smokers)	
- Median	19
- Range	0.1-64
Tenure (years)*	
- Median	8.8
- Range	0.17-32.6
Race (number, percent)	
- White	110 (73.3%)
- Black	23 (15.3%)
- Native American, Native Hawaiian, or Asian	4 (2.7%)
- White and Native American †	13 (8.7%)
Ethnicity (number, percent)	
- Hispanic	4 (2.7%)
- Non-Hispanic	146 (97.3%)

* Three employees did not provide their work histories; † employees indicated that they were both White and Native American.

Table 3. Suspected occupational asthma incidence rates by work area, September 2003 and January 2005 surveys combined

Work Area	Number of Cases	Person-Years	Suspected Occupational Asthma Incidence Rate (cases per 1000 person-years)
Screening *	1	11	90.9
Maintenance (Gurley)	2	50	40.0
Product Testing	2	79	25.3
Milling/Spray Drying	3	131	22.9
Pressing	7	315	22.2
Sintering	2	91	22.0
Reclamation	3	177	16.9
Shaping	2	119	16.8
Powder Mixing	1	62	16.1
Other	4	295	13.6
Shipping (Grant)	1	82	12.2
Grinding	1	229	4.4
Powder Laboratory *	0	42	0
Shipping (Gurley) *	0	37	0
Sandblasting*	0	12	0
Maintenance (Grant)	0	96	0
Metal Separation (APT)	0	82	0
All Work Areas	29	1910	15.2

*Work area risk levels were not designated in these four areas due to small person-year denominators.
Suspected possible higher-risk work areas (shaded in dark gray) had the highest incidence rates of suspected occupational asthma for all work areas where case numbers were sufficient to provide stable estimates; work area shaded in light gray had a high suspected occupational asthma incidence rate but this rate was based on only one case. Calculations were based on information for 163 participants.
Five participants had incomplete work histories with a range of 3% to 25% of their work history unaccounted for; this resulted in 8 of a total of 1910 (0.4%) person-years unaccounted for among all the work-time used in these calculations.

Table 4. Urine cobalt levels in micrograms cobalt per liter (μg/L) of urine by work area for urine samples with acceptable specific gravity and creatinine levels from employees with no known background source of cobalt, January 2005

Work Area	N	N ≥ 15.0* μg/L	% ≥ 15.0* μg/L	Min (μg/L)	Max (μg/L)	N ≥ LOQ	%_ ≥ LOQ	GM	CI for GM
Powder Mixing (n=5)	4	3	75	5.1	120	4	100	26.6	3.4-207.5
Milling (n=5)	4	4	100	150	290	4	100	185.1	112.8-303.8
Spray Drying (n=3)	2	2	100	36	56	2	100	44.9	2.7-743.6
Pressing (n=16)	7	6	86	14.0	190	7	100	46.8	20.9-104.8
Shaping (n=8)	4	3	75	5.5	100	4	100	26.0	3.8-176.4
Sintering (n=6)	2	0	0	5.3	5.4	2	100	5.4	4.8-6.0
Grinding (n=16)	11	0	0	1.0	14.0	9	81.8	4.8	2.9-7.7
Product Testing (n=7)	1	0	0	2.1	2.1	1	100	2.1	-
Grant Shipping (n=3)	2	0	0	2.3	4.3	2	100	3.1	0.1-167.5
Grant Maintenance (n=4)	2	0	0	10.0	14.0	2	100	11.8	1.4-100.3
Reclamation (n=9)	6	5	83	6	210	6	100	30.5	9.6-101.8
Metal Separation (n=12)	5	1	20	4.2	29	5	100	8.3	3.1-22.7
Other (n=28)	11	4	36	2.0	140	10	90.9	9.7	4.3-21.9
Total (n=122)	61	28	46	1.0	290	58	95.1	15.2	10.7-21.7

Urine samples were from employees who denied use of multivitamins (or vitamin B12) and presence of artificial joints and which had specific gravity values between 1.010 and 1.030 and creatinine values between 0.3 and 3.0 grams per liter urine; 17 employees were excluded (13 employees who reported working in more than one work area, 2 employees who provided a urine sample at the beginning of their workshift, 1 employee who worked in a different work area two days prior to the test, and 1 employee who had returned to work after an extended absence); there were fewer than 3 urine samples for screening, Gurley shipping, and Huntsville maintenance, so results from these work areas were included in the other work area; we had no urine samples for powder laboratory and Gurley maintenance; 3 samples were received for sandblasting but all were not acceptable; n, number of samples received for analysis; N, number of samples included in tabled results; Min, minimum value; Max, maximum value; GM, geometric mean; CI, 95% confidence interval; LOQ, limit of quantitation (2.0 μg cobalt/ liter urine). *Biological exposure index which is comparable to an exposure of 20 μg cobalt per cubic meter of air.

Table 5. Urine cobalt/creatinine levels in micrograms cobalt per gram creatinine (µg Co/g creat) for urine samples from employees with no known background source of cobalt, January 2005

Work Area	N	N ≥ 9.6* µg Co/g creat	% ≥ 9.6* µg Co/g creat	Min (µg Co/g creat)	Max (µg Co/g creat)	GM	CI for GM
Powder Mixing (n=5)	5	3	60	2.8	137.9	14.5	2.5-84.9
Milling (n=5)	5	5	100	105.9	214.3	134.7	95.8-189.4
Spray Drying (n=3)	2	2	100	15.7	25.5	20	0.9-438.4
Pressing (n=16)	10	9	90	7.4	144.7	30.3	14.9-61.8
Shaping (n=8)	4	4	100	9.7	109.9	25.7	5.0-133.5
Sintering (n=6)	3	0	0	3.1	7.1	4.7	1.7-13.0
Grinding (n=16)	12	0	0	1.0	8.2	3.2	2.2-4.7
Product Testing (n=7)	4	0	0	1.5	7.8	3.1	1.1-9.3
Grant Shipping (n=3)	2	0	0	2.9	4.2	3.5	0.3-38.1
Grant Maintenance (n=4)	2	0	0	3.6	6.7	4.9	0.1-257.3
Reclamation (n=9)	7	6	85.7	4.3	123.5	25.2	8.7-73.2
Metal Separation (n=12)	8	1	12.5	1.0	12.1	4.2	2.3-7.8
Other (n=28)	20	6	30.0	1.4	87.9	6.1	3.5-10.0
Total (n=122)	84	36	42.9	1.0	214.3	9.6	7.1-12.8

Urine samples were from employees who denied use of multivitamins (or vitamin B12) and presence of artificial joints; 17 employees were excluded (13 employees who reported working in more than one work area, 2 employees who provided a urine sample at the beginning of their workshift, 1 employee who worked in a different work area two days prior to the test, and 1 employee who had returned to work after an extended absence); there were fewer than 3 urine samples for screening, Gurley shipping, and Huntsville maintenance so results for these work areas were included in the other work area; there were no urine samples for powder laboratory and Gurley maintenance; 3 samples were received for sandblasting but all were not acceptable; n, number of samples received for analysis; N, number of samples included in tabled results; Min, minimum value; Max, maximum value; GM, geometric mean; CI, 95% confidence interval; LOQ, limit of quantitation (2.0 µg cobalt/liter urine). *Workforce geometric mean.

Table 6. Urine tungsten levels by work area for urine samples with acceptable specific gravity and creatinine levels, January 2005

Work Area	N	N ≥ LOD	% ≥ LOD	N ≥ LOQ	% ≥ LOQ	Range (µg/L)
Powder Mixing (n=5)	4	2	50	0	0	< LOD-< LOQ
Milling (n=5)	4	4	100	2	50	< LOQ-110
Spray Drying (n=3)	3	3	100	2	67	< LOQ-220
Pressing (n=16)	11	11	100	4	36	< LOQ-160
Shaping (n=8)	7	5	71	2	29	< LOD-88
Sintering (n=6)	4	0	0	0	0	< LOD
Grinding (n=16)	14	12	86	3	21	< LOD-96
Sandblasting (n=3)	3	1	33	0	0	< LOD-<LOQ
Product Testing (n=7)	4	0	0	0	0	< LOD
Grant Shipping (n=3)	2	1	50	0	0	< LOD-< LOQ
Grant Maintenance (n=4)	4	3	75	0	0	< LOD-< LOQ
Reclamation (n=9)	7	7	100	2	29	< LOQ-250
Metal Separation (n=12)	8	8	100	8	100	66-1500
Other (n=25)	16	11	69	4	25	< LOD-110
Total (n=122)	91	68	75	27	30	< LOD-1500

Urine samples had specific gravity values between 1.010 and 1.030 and creatinine values between 0.3 and 3.0 grams per liter urine; 17 employees were excluded (13 employees who reported working in more than one work area, 2 employees who provided a urine sample at the beginning of their workshift, 1 employee who worked in a different work area two days prior to the test, and 1 employee who had returned to work after an extended absence); there were fewer than 3 urine samples for screening, Gurley shipping, and Huntsville maintenance so results for these work areas were included in the other work area; we had no urine samples for powder laboratory and Gurley maintenance; n, number of samples received for analysis; N, number of samples included in tabled results; LOD, limit of detection (10µg tungsten/liter urine; LOQ, limit of quantitation (40µg tungsten/liter urine).

Table 7. Blood cobalt levels in micrograms per liter (μg/L) whole blood for blood samples from employees with no known background source of cobalt, January 2005

Work Area	N	N ≥1.0* μg/L	% ≥ 1.0* μg/L	Min (μg/L)	Max (μg/L)	N ≥ LOQ	%_ ≥ LOQ	GM	CI for GM
Powder Mixing (n=5)	5	4	80	0.73	41	5	100	3.7	0.6-23.6
Milling (n=5)	5	5	100	11	21	5	100	15.6	11.2-21.7
Spray Drying (n=3)	2	2	100	3.1	3.4	2	100	3.2	1.8-5.8
Pressing (n=18)	11	11	100	1.4	7.0	11	100	3.7	2.6-5.2
Shaping (n=8)	4	4	100	2.3	4.1	4	100	3.3	2.2-5.1
Sintering (n=6)	3	1	33	0.44	1.7	3	100	0.9	0.2-4.7
Grinding (n=16)	12	5	42	0.2	2.6	11	91.7	0.9	0.6-1.5
Product Testing (n=7)	4	1	25	0.2	1.8	3	75	0.7	0.2-2.9
Grant Shipping (n=4)	2	1	50	0.6	2.5	2	100	1.23	< 0.1-9629.6
Grant Maintenance (n=4)	2	2	100	1.0	2.9	2	100	1.7	< 0.1-1475.2
Reclamation (n=8)	7	6	86	0.4	19	7	100	4.0	1.2-13.2
Metal Separation (n=11)	7	6	86	0.56	3.0	7	100	1.4	0.9-2.27
Other (n=30)	21	15	71	0.1	31	19	90.5	1.3	0.8-2.3
Total (n=125)	85	63	74	0.1	41	81	95.3	2.0	1.5-2.5

Whole blood samples were obtained from employees who denied use of multivitamins (or vitamin B12) and presence of artificial joints; 7 employees were excluded (13 employees who reported working in more than one work area, 2 employees who provided a blood sample at the beginning of their workshift, 1 employee who worked in a different work area two days prior to the test, and 1 employee who had returned to work after an extended absence); there were fewer than 3 whole blood samples for screening, Gurley shipping, Gurley maintenance, and Huntsville maintenance so results from these work areas were included in the other work area; we had no whole blood samples for the powder laboratory; 4 samples were received for sandblasting but all were not acceptable; n, number of samples received for analysis; N, number of samples included in tabled results; Min, minimum value; Max, maximum value; GM, geometric mean; CI, 95% confidence interval; LOD, limit of detection (0.1 μg cobalt/liter whole blood); LOQ, limit of quantitation (0.4 μg cobalt/liter whole blood). *Biological exposure index which is comparable to an exposure of 20 μg cobalt per cubic meter of air.

Table 8. Blood nickel levels in micrograms per liter (μg/L) whole blood, January 2005

Work Area	N	N ≥ 11.8* μg/L	% ≥ 11.8* μg/L	Min (μg/L)	Max (μg/L)	N ≥ LOQ	% ≥ LOQ	GM	CI for GM
Powder Mixing	5	3	60	9	13	5	100	11.3	9.2-13.9
Milling	5	3	60	9.7	28	5	100	14.1	8.3-24.1
Spray Drying	3	3	100	12	13	3	100	12.3	11.0-13.8
Pressing	18	11	61	5.6	17	18	100	11.6	10.1-13.3
Shaping	8	3	38	7	25	8	100	12.5	8.8-17.7
Sintering	6	4	67	3.0	14	6	100	9.4	5.0-17.8
Grinding	16	6	38	3.5	30	16	100	9.5	7.2-12.5
Sandblasting	4	4	100	13	19	4	100	14.8	11.1-19.7
Product Testing	7	4	57	5.9	20	7	100	10.9	7.5-15.8
Grant Shipping	4	4	100	13	15	4	100	14.0	12.7-15.3
Grant Maintenance	4	3	75	5.7	16	4	100	11.5	5.4-24.7
Reclamation	8	5	63	9.8	18	8	100	13.1	10.7-16.1
Metal Separation	11	10	91	11	17	11	100	13.2	12.1-14.3
Other	26	17	65	4.7	31	26	100	12.3	10.6-14.3
Total	125	80	64	3.0	31	125	100	11.8	11.1-12.6

17 employees were excluded (13 employees who reported working in more than one work area, 2 employees who provided a blood sample at the beginning of their workshift, 1 employee who worked in a different work area two days prior to the test, and 1 employee who had returned to work after an extended absence); there were fewer than 3 whole blood samples for screening, Gurley shipping, Gurley maintenance, and Huntsville maintenance so results from these work areas were included in the other work area; we had no whole blood samples for the powder laboratory; N, number; Min, minimum value; Max, maximum value; GM, geometric mean; CI, 95% confidence interval; LOD, limit of detection (0.7 μg nickel/liter whole blood); LOQ, limit of quantitation (3.0 μg nickel/liter whole blood). *Workforce geometric mean.

Table 9. Exhaled breath condensate cobalt levels in micrograms/liter (µg/L), January 2005

Work Area	N	N ≥ 5.9* µg/L	% ≥ 5.9* µg/L	Min (µg/L)	Max (µg/L)	GM	CI for GM
Powder Mixing	4	4	100	6.0	25	11.0	3.7-32.8
Milling	3	3	100	270	296	282.5	252-316.7
Spray Drying	3	3	100	38	60	50.4	27.3-92.8
Pressing	16	8	50	0.6	49	7.5	3.9-14.4
Shaping	5	2	40	1.4	16	3.9	1.2-13.2
Sintering	3	1	33	0.5	25	2.1	< 0.1-449.7
Grinding	15	5	33	0.2	41	2.8	1.3-6.2
Sandblasting	4	2	50	1.9	75	9.8	0.6-152.3
Product Testing	6	1	17	0.6	13.50	2.4	0.7-7.6
Grant Shipping	4	1	25	1.0	7.80	2.2	0.52-9.5
Grant Maintenance	3	2	67	3.0	36	10.0	0.5-220.2
Reclamation	5	3	60	1.2	118	15.9	1.6-163.6
Metal Separation	12	5	42	0.5	48	4.7	2.3-9.8
Other	19	7	37	0.7	126	4.6	2.6-8.1
Total	102	47	46	0.2	296	5.9	4.4-7.9

15 employees were excluded (13 employees who reported working in more than one work area and 2 employees who provided an exhaled breath condensate sample at the beginning of their workshift); there were fewer than 3 samples for screening, Gurley Shipping, and Huntsville maintenance; N, number; Min, minimum value; Max, maximum value; GM, geometric mean; CI, 95% confidence interval. *Workforce geometric mean.

Table 10. Exhaled breath condensate tungsten levels in micrograms/liter (µg/L), January 2005

Work Area	N	N ≥ 3.1* µg/L	% ≥ 3.1* µg/L	Min (µg/L)	Max (µg/L)	GM	CI for GM
Powder Mixing	4	0	0	< 0.1	2.6	0.4	< 0.1-21.0
Milling	3	3	100	18	31	25.6	12.0-54.5
Spray Drying	3	3	100	5.2	44	15.4	1.1-219.0
Pressing	16	9	56	0.4	40	3.1	1.4-7.3
Shaping	5	3	60	0.6	15	3.0	0.6-14.3
Sintering	3	2	67	0.1	3.8	1.1	< 0.1-185.8
Grinding	15	8	53	< 0.1	54	1.2	0.3-5.1
Sandblasting	4	3	75	0.1	7	2.0	0.1-60.5
Product Testing	6	1	17	0.1	6	0.8	0.1-4.1
Grant Shipping	4	0	0	1.1	2.4	1.7	1.0-2.8
Grant Maintenance	3	2	67	0.4	17	2.9	< 0.1-312.9
Reclamation	5	4	80	1.9	149	13.0	1.5-115.7
Metal Separation	12	11	92	< 0.1	473	38.1	6.2-232.6
Other	19	7	37	< 0.1	72	1.8	0.7-4.9
Total	102	58	55	< 0.1	473	3.1	2.0-4.9

15 employees were excluded (13 employees who reported working in more than one work area and 2 employees who provided an exhaled breath condensate sample at the beginning of their workshift); there were fewer than 3 samples for screening, Gurley Shipping, and Huntsville maintenance; N, number; Min, minimum value; Max, maximum value; GM, geometric mean; CI, 95% confidence interval. *Workforce geometric mean.

Table 11. Exhaled breath condensate nickel levels in micrograms/liter (µg/L), January 2005

Work Area	N	N ≥ 0.2* µg/L	% ≥ 0.2* µg/L	Min (µg/L)	Max (µg/L)	GM	CI for GM
Powder Mixing	4	3	75	0.08	0.30	0.2	0.1-0.4
Milling	3	3	100	0.30	1.80	0.6	0.1-6.6
Spray Drying	3	3	100	0.40	0.70	0.5	0.3-1.0
Pressing	16	12	75	0.06	4.30	0.4	0.2-0.6
Shaping	5	1	20	0.07	0.30	0.1	0.1-0.2
Sintering	3	2	67	0.04	0.60	0.2	< 0.1-5.0
Grinding	15	7	47	0.02	0.80	0.1	0.1-0.2
Sandblasting	4	3	75	0.10	1.50	0.3	< 0.1-1.8
Product Testing	6	3	50	0.10	0.60	0.2	0.1-0.4
Grant Shipping	4	3	75	0.05	0.50	0.2	< 0.1-0.8
Grant Maintenance	3	2	67	0.08	1.80	0.4	< 0.1-18.5
Reclamation	5	4	80	0.10	2.30	0.5	0.1-2.9
Metal Separation	12	10	83	0.06	1.80	0.3	0.2-0.5
Other	19	12	63	0.05	2.20	0.2	0.1-0.3
Total	102	68	67	0.02	4.30	0.2	0.2-0.3

15 employees were excluded (13 employees who reported working in more than one work area and 2 employees who provided an exhaled breath condensate sample at the beginning of their workshift); there were fewer than 3 samples for screening, Gurley Shipping, and Huntsville maintenance; N, number; Min, minimum value; Max, maximum value; GM, geometric mean; CI, 95% confidence interval. *Workforce geometric mean.

Table 12. Exhaled breath condensate inflammation biomarker levels in "healthy" workers and cases, January 2005

Biomarkers	"Healthy" workers* (N = 30) Geometric mean (SD)	"Healthy" workers* (N = 30) Median	Probable Current Asthma Cases† (N = 30) & Current Asthma Cases (N = 17) Total N = 47 Geometric mean (SD)	Probable Current Asthma Cases† (N = 30) & Current Asthma Cases (N = 17) Total N = 47 Median	Probable Current Asthma Cases† (N = 30) & Current Asthma Cases (N = 17) Total N = 47 t test (p-value)	Probable Current Asthma Cases† (N = 30) & Current Asthma Cases (N = 17) Total N = 47 Rank sum test (p-value)	Current Asthma Cases ‡ (N = 17) Geometric mean (SD)	Current Asthma Cases ‡ (N = 17) Median	Current Asthma Cases ‡ (N = 17) t test (p-value)	Current Asthma Cases ‡ (N = 17) Rank sum test (p-value)
LTB-4 §	5.40 ng/L (1.85)	7.00	6.67 ng/L (1.76)	8.00	0.24	0.24	6.87 ng/L (1.94)	8.00	0.20	0.27
LTB-4**	5.56 ng/L (1.78)	6.65	6.42 ng/L (1.84)	7.95	0.24	0.24	6.25 ng/L (2.11)	7.55	0.39	0.39
IL-8 §	0.42 ng/L (2.13)	0.36	0.37 ng/L (1.59)	0.37	0.31	0.81	0.34 ng/L (1.42)	0.37	0.32	0.64
IL-8**	0.13 ng/L (4.22)	0.20	0.14 ng/L (3.33)	0.20	0.23	0.42	0.14 ng/L (3.12)	0.20	0.15	0.47
MDA §	8.52 nmol/L (1.56)	7.95	8.64 nmol/L (1.53)	8.90	0.93	0.93	9.02 nmol/L (1.54)	8.90	0.71	0.69

ng/L, nanograms per liter; SD, standard deviation; LTB-4, leukotriene B4; IL-8, interleukin-8; MDA, malondialdehyde; p-values less than 0.05 indicate statistical significance.

* "Healthy" workers were defined as employees: 1) whose most recent spirometry test was normal; 2) who reported to never have been diagnosed with asthma or chronic bronchitis, to not have current asthma symptoms, shortness of breath, usual cough, or to currently be using breathing medications; and 3) who had a negative methacholine challenge test (PC20 >16), if this was performed.

† Probable Current Asthma cases were defined as employees with at least 3 of 9 asthma symptoms, current use of medication for their breathing, or a methacholine challenge test PC20 > 4 and ≤ 16 mg/ml and who did have current physician-diagnosed asthma.

‡ Current Asthma cases were defined as employees with current physician-diagnosed asthma or a methacholine challenge test PC20 of ≤ 4 mg/ml.

§ Measurements within working ranges (2.5-800 ng/liter for LTB-4; 0.15 to 25 ng/L for IL-8) or greater than the limit of quantitation (3 nmol/L for MDA) were used. All MDA values were above the limit of detection.

**All measurements were used; for measurements below the limit of detection, one half the limit of detection was used.

Table 13. Summary table for urine, whole blood, and exhaled breath condensate samples, January 2005

Work Area	> 75% urine cobalt levels ≥ BEI *	> 75% urine µg cobalt/ gram creatinine levels ≥ WGM †	> 50% urine tungsten levels ≥ LOQ §	> 75% whole blood cobalt levels ≥ BEI ‡	> 75% exhaled breath condensate cobalt levels ≥ WGM	> 75% exhaled breath condensate tungsten levels ≥ WGM
Powder Mixing				x	x	
Milling•	x	x		x	x	x
Spray Drying•	x	x	x	x	x	x
Pressing •	x	x		x		
Shaping		x		x		
Sintering •						
Grinding •						
Sandblasting	no acceptable samples	no acceptable samples		no acceptable samples		
Product Testing •						
Grant Shipping						
Grant Maintenance				x		
Reclamation	x	x		x		x
Metal Separation			x	x		x
Other						
Total			x			

BEI, Biological Exposure Index; WGM, workforce geometric mean; LOQ, limit of quantitation; * urine samples had acceptable specific gravity and creatinine levels and were from employees who denied use of multivitamins (or vitamin B12) and the presence of artificial joints; † urine samples were from employees who denied use of multivitamins (or vitamin B12) and the presence of artificial joints; § urine samples had acceptable specific gravity and creatinine levels; ‡ whole blood samples were from employees who denied use of multivitamins (or vitamin B12) and the presence of artificial joints; BEI for urine cobalt is 15 µg/L; BEI for whole blood cobalt is 1 µg/L. Designated higher-risk work areas for suspected occupational asthma and hard metal disease are shaded in gray/•.

Figure 1. Scatter plot showing the correlation between log values of urine cobalt and blood cobalt, January 2005

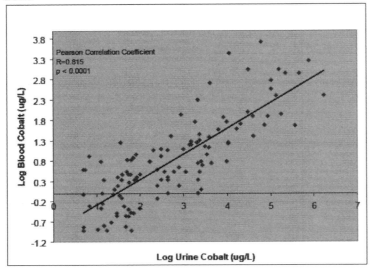

Data points with urine cobalt or blood cobalt values less than the respective limits of quantitation (urine cobalt, 2.0 µg/L; blood cobalt, 0.4 µg/L) were excluded.

Figure 2. Scatter plot showing the correlation between log values of urine cobalt per gram creatinine and blood cobalt, January 2005

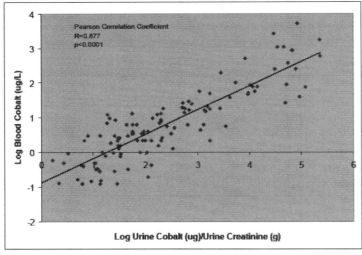

Data points with urine cobalt or blood cobalt values less than the respective limits of quantitation (urine cobalt, 2.0 µg/L; blood cobalt, 0.4 µg/L) were excluded.

Figure 3. Scatter plot showing the correlation between log values of urine cobalt and exhaled breath condensate cobalt, January 2005

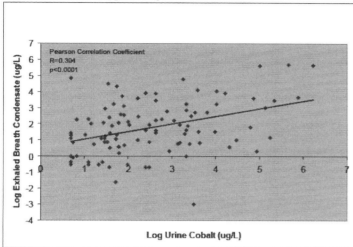

Data points with urine cobalt or exhaled breath condensate values less than the respective limits of quantitation (urine cobalt, 2.0 µg/L; exhaled breath condensate cobalt, 0.009 µg/L) were excluded.

Figure 4. Scatter plot showing the correlation between the log values of urine cobalt per gram creatinine and exhaled breath condensate cobalt, January 2005

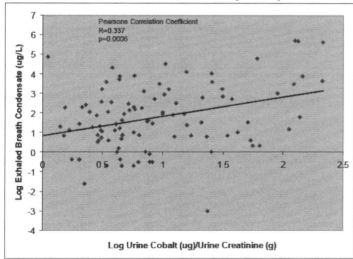

Data points with urine cobalt or exhaled breath condensate values less than the respective limits of quantitation (urine cobalt, 2.0 µg/L; exhaled breath condensate cobalt, 0.009 µg/L) were excluded.

ENCLOSURE B

Interim Letter IX Summary Sheet
HETA 2003-0257
May 9, 2006

In June 2003, the National Institute for Occupational Safety and Health (NIOSH) received a Health Hazard Evaluation request from employees at three Metalworking Products plants in Grant, Gurley, and Huntsville, Alabama who were concerned about respiratory health effects potentially associated with work exposures. NIOSH conducted two medical surveys of the three plants in September 2003 and January 2005. These are our preliminary findings. After all analyses are completed, a full report will be sent to Metalworking Products for posting at the workplace.

What NIOSH Did

- We administered health and work history questionnaires to workers.
- We performed breathing tests on workers.
- We collected urine, blood, and breath samples from employees and tested the samples for metals.

What NIOSH Found

- More than a 2-fold excess of ever-diagnosed asthma and about a 3-fold excess of new-onset asthma in employees, compared to national data.
- Five work areas were at higher-risk for the development of suspected occupational asthma. These work areas were Maintenance and Milling/Spray Drying in the Gurley plant, and Pressing, Sintering, and Product Testing in the Grant plant.
- Three work areas were at higher-risk for the development of hard metal disease, based on where workers with this suspected lung disease developed their symptoms or disease. These work areas were Pressing, Sintering, and Grinding in the Grant plant.
- 46% of all urine samples and 74% of all blood samples had cobalt levels that suggested exposure to more than 20 micrograms cobalt per cubic meter of air.
- Workers in higher-risk work areas did not have higher levels of cobalt in their urine or blood, compared to workers in lower-risk work areas.

- Workers in higher-risk work areas did not have higher levels of cobalt in their exhaled breath, compared to workers in lower-risk work areas. Findings suggest that low levels of cobalt may cause disease in some or all of the higher-risk work areas, and that in some work areas disease may be due to certain, as yet unknown, characteristics of exposure.

What Plant Managers Can Do

- Reduce cobalt air levels to below the occupational exposure limits in all work areas
- Reduce worker skin exposures to metals
  o Require gloves
  o Prevent dust contamination of work surfaces and non-production areas
- Reduce exposures in higher-risk work areas to as low as possible
- After changes have been made in engineering, work practices, housekeeping, and glove and respirator use, retest workers and collect air samples for work areas in which a high proportion of workers had high cobalt levels

What Employees Can Do

- Wear long-sleeved shirts
- Wear nitrile gloves at work; gloves should be put on over clean hands
- Shower as soon as possible after work
- Be evaluated by a lung doctor (pulmonologist) if breathing symptoms began or worsened after beginning to work in the hard metal industry

If you have any questions, please contact Dr. Nancy Sahakian at (304) 285-6383.

DEPARTMENT OF HEALTH & HUMAN SERVICES

Public Health Service

Phone: (304) 285-5751
Fax: (304) 285-5820

Centers for Disease Control
and Prevention (CDC)
National Institute for Occupational
Safety and Health (NIOSH)
1095 Willowdale Road
Morgantown, WV 26505-2888

May 17, 2006
HETA 2003-0257
Interim Letter X

Mr. James Doherty
Interim Director of Health, Safety and Environment
Alldyne Powder Technologies
7300 Highway 20
Huntsville, Alabama 35806

Dear Mr. Doherty:

The purpose of this letter is to report the progress of a National Institute for Occupational Safety and Health (NIOSH) industrial hygiene survey of airborne particulate exposures at the Alldyne Powder Technologies facilities located in Huntsville and Gurley, Alabama and the Firth Sterling facility located in Grant, Alabama. NIOSH surveyed these facilities in May 2004 and November 2004 in response to a confidential employee request concerning respiratory health effects and exposure to cobalt, nickel, chromium, and tungsten carbide.

Sincerely,

Nancy M. Sahakian, M.D., M.P.H.

Aleksandr Stefaniak, Ph.D., C.I.H.
Respiratory Disease Hazard Evaluation and
  Technical Assistance Program
Field Studies Branch
Division of Respiratory Disease Studies

cc:
Confidential Requesters

Survey goal:

Our goal was to better understand the characteristics (size, shape, chemistry) of bulk metal powders handled by employees and the characteristics of airborne particles generated in different work areas throughout the Alldyne Powder Technologies facilities located in Huntsville and Gurley, Alabama and the Firth Sterling facility located in Grant, Alabama. Exposure to airborne particles generated during the manufacture of cemented tungsten carbides can cause hard metal disease (HMD). Currently, it is thought that only particles with certain combinations of tungsten carbide and cobalt can cause HMD. Workers engaged in the manufacture of cemented tungsten carbides are also at risk of developing occupationally-induced asthma. It is thought that particles that contain only cobalt or particles that contain both cobalt and tungsten carbide may cause occupational asthma. Therefore, the characteristics of airborne particles generated during the manufacture of cemented tungsten carbides may be important exposure factors for HMD and occupational asthma.

Samples collected:

Bulk powders

As outlined in Interim Letter V (dated August 30, 2005), bulk samples of feed stock powders and process-generated materials were collected in May 2004. We determined the characteristics of five representative powders that span the cemented tungsten carbide manufacturing process: feed stock tungsten, tungsten carbide, and cobalt powders and process-generated spray drying powder and Chamfer grinder dust. The shapes of the particles were determined using a high-magnification microscope (scanning electron microscope). The identities of elements in the particles were determined using standard micro-analysis (energy dispersive x-ray spectrometry) and powder analysis (x-ray diffraction) techniques. Micro-analyses provided information on identities of elements (*e.g.*, cobalt, tungsten). Powder analyses provided information on the identities of elements, but only if they were present in crystalline form (*i.e.*, arranged in a regularly-repeating pattern). Knowledge of the particle shape and chemistry of feed stock and process powders provides insight into the observed airborne particles collected aerodynamically using micro-orifice uniform deposit impactor samplers.

Micro-orifice uniform deposit impactor (MOUDI)

Sixteen samples of airborne particles were collected in 13 different work areas using micro-orifice uniform deposit impactor (MOUDI) samplers (Model 110, MSP Corporation, Shoreview, MN). In each of 12 different work areas, one MOUDI sample was collected; in scrap reclamation, four MOUDI samples were collected. The MOUDI sampler collects airborne particles and separates them based on their size using different filter stages. The particle size cut points for the MOUDI sampler are in units of micrometers, μm, (1 μm = 1 millionth of 1 meter) and were >18 μm (inlet stage), 10 μm (stage 1), 5.6 μm (stage 2), 3.2 μm (stage 3), 1.8 μm (stage 4), 1.0 μm (stage 5), 0.56 μm (stage 6), 0.32 μm (stage 7), 0.18 μm (stage 8), 0.10 μm (stage 9), 0.056 μm (stage 10), and <0.056 μm (final filter). All samples were collected on mixed cellulose ester (MCE) filters. To minimize the potential for particle contamination with silicon, a known constituent of abrasive grinding wheels, only the stage 1 substrate of each sampler was sprayed with silicone to reduce particle bounce during sampling.

Characteristics of airborne particles that were collected on stage 1, stage 3, and stage 5 of each MOUDI sample were evaluated. These particle sizes were chosen because they have high probability of depositing in the deep lung. The shapes of particles were determined using the same type of high-magnification microscope and micro-analysis technique as for the bulk samples.

Results:

Bulk powder characteristics

The shape of each bulk powder is summarized in Figure 1. Bulk tungsten metal powder was loose agglomerates (particles weakly held together) of fairly round-shaped particles. Bulk tungsten carbide, cobalt feed stock powders, and the spray dryer powder were mostly aggregate clusters (particles held strongly together). The chamfer grinder dust was aggregate particles that were more compact than the feed stock or spray dryer powders.

The elements identified in the bulk powders are summarized in Table 1. Feed stock powders were high purity. For example, tungsten powder contained only tungsten metal. Powders from the spray dryer and the chamfer grinder contained tungsten, carbon, and cobalt.

Airborne particle physicochemical properties

The shape of airborne particles collected in five representative work areas that span the production process (reduction furnace, carburization furnace, charging, spray drying, and grinding) were similar to the associated bulk powder samples. In work areas that prepare and handle feed stock powders (reduction furnace, carburization furnace, powder mixing, spray drying, and screening), airborne particles appeared to be generally spherical individual particles, agglomerate particles, or aggregate particles. Airborne particles in the pressing and extrusion work areas were a mixture of agglomerates of mostly spherical particles, individual irregular shaped compact particles, and agglomerates of compact particles. In the sintering, grinding, and sand blasting work areas, airborne particles were irregular shaped compact particles.

The number of different elements identified in airborne particles collected from 13 work areas that span the manufacture of cemented tungsten carbides increased as manufacturing proceeded from production of feed stock powders through finishing of sintered product (see Table 2). Within each work area, the elements identified in particles were generally similar among the three evaluated particle sizes. (Carbon, a component of both the collection filters and several metal carbides used in the production process, and oxygen were identified in nearly all particles.)

Airborne particles in the autoreduction furnace, carburization furnace, and powder mixing work areas generally contained only a single chemical constituent. Nearly all particles characterized from the autoreduction work area were tungsten particles; only a few particles contained additive metals such as cobalt, chromium, nickel, and titanium or impurities such as iron, manganese, and silicon. Particles from the carburization furnace work area were predominantly tungsten particles and some particles contained the same metals and impurities identified in particles sampled from the reduction work area. In the powder mixing work area, particles were almost exclusively cobalt, with a few tungsten/cobalt particles and particles that contained metal additives such as nickel, tantalum, and titanium.

Particles generated in spray drying were a mixture of cobalt particles and tungsten/cobalt particles; some tungsten/cobalt particles contained the same metals and impurities identified in particles in the powder mixing work area. Airborne particles in screening, and all downstream, work areas were predominantly tungsten/cobalt particles, with some of these particles in each work area containing varying additive metals and impurities.

Airborne particles generated during reclamation of sintered scrap materials were a mixture of tungsten particles and tungsten/cobalt particles. Some tungsten/cobalt particles contained the same additive metals and impurities identified in the autoreduction furnace, carburization furnace, and powder mixing work areas.

Discussion:

We observed that airborne particles in spray drying and all downstream work areas were a mixture of cobalt particles and or tungsten/cobalt particles. This observation suggests that particles with combinations of tungsten carbide and cobalt that might cause HMD become airborne and are available for inhaling in both work areas that handle pre-sintered material and in work areas that handle post-sintered material. Additionally, our results suggest that tungsten and cobalt are in closer contact in post-sintered particles relative to pre-sintered particles. Pre-sintered tungsten/cobalt particles were often weakly held together, whereas in post-sintered material, tungsten and cobalt were probably physically bound on the same particle. Because of this greater physical closeness of tungsten and cobalt, the hazard potential of post-sintered particles for HMD could be greater than that of pre-sintered powder. Results from our medical surveys at the Grant, AL facility indicated that sintering and grinding were two higher risk work areas for HMD, despite low historical airborne cobalt exposure levels.

Cobalt was predominant in airborne particles generated in powder mixing and all downstream work areas, suggesting that particles that might cause occupational asthma become airborne and available for inhaling in work areas that handle pre-sintered material and in work areas that handle post-sintered material. As part of this Health Hazard Evaluation, both work areas that handle pre-sintered powders (milling/spray drying and maintenance at Gurley; pressing at Grant) and work areas that handle post-sintered materials (sintering, product testing) were higher risk work areas for occupational asthma.

Recommendations:

Building on our recommendations from previous interim letters, the following recommendations are made concerning inhalation exposure to cobalt at all three facilities:

- Routinely monitor inhalation exposure to metals
  - At least annually and whenever any major process change takes place
    - Inhalation exposure should be sampled in the personal breathing zone
- Exposure control
  - Continue ongoing efforts to reduce cobalt and tungsten exposures
    - Utilize the industrial hygiene hierarchy of controls (ranked in order of most preferred to least preferred control method): elimination> substitution> engineering>work practices> personal protective equipment

Table 1. Elemental and crystalline constituents of bulk powders samples

Powder	Constituents[a] Elements	Constituents[a] Crystalline (relative amount, %)
Tungsten metal	Tungsten	Tungsten (100%)
Tungsten carbide	Tungsten, Carbon	Tungsten monocarbide (98.3%), Tungsten carbide (1.7%)
Cobalt	Cobalt	Cobalt (87%), Cobalt oxide (13.1%)
Spray drying	Tungsten, Carbon, Cobalt	Tungsten monocarbide (82.6%), Cobalt (11.8%), Tungsten (4.6%), Tungsten carbide (1.0%)
Chamfer grinder	Tungsten, Carbon, Cobalt	Tungsten monocarbide (84.7%), Cobalt (11.2%), Carbon (4.1%)

Table 2. Elements identified in airborne particles from 13 different work areas (November 2004)

Work area	Elements identified in particles Major	Elements identified in particles Minor
Reduction furnace	Tungsten	Cobalt, Iron, Manganese, Nickel, Silicon
Carburization furnace	Tungsten	Cobalt, Iron, Manganese, Nickel, Silicon, Titanium
Scrap reclamation	Tungsten/Cobalt or Tungsten	Chromium, Iron, Nickel, Silicon, Vanadium
Powder mixing	Tungsten/Cobalt or Cobalt	Iron, Nickel, Tantalum, Titanium
Milling	Tungsten/Cobalt or Cobalt	Iron, Nickel, Silicon, Tantalum, Titanium
Spray drying	Tungsten/Cobalt or Cobalt	Iron, Nickel, Silicon, Titanium, Tantalum
Screening	Tungsten/Cobalt	Iron, Nickel, Tantalum, Titanium, Vanadium
Pressing (round cell)	Tungsten/Cobalt	Chromium, Iron, Manganese, Nickel, Silicon, Tantalum, Titanium
Pressing (CNC)	Tungsten/Cobalt	Iron, Nickel, Titanium
Extrusion	Tungsten/Cobalt	Chromium, Iron, Nickel, Tantalum, Titanium
Sintering	Tungsten/Cobalt	Iron, Nickel, Silicon
Grinding	Tungsten/Cobalt	Iron, Nickel, Silicon, Titanium
Sandblasting	Tungsten/Cobalt/Iron	Nickel, Silicon, Titanium

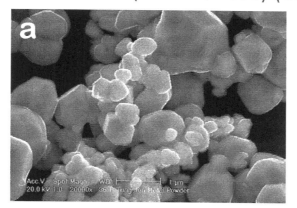

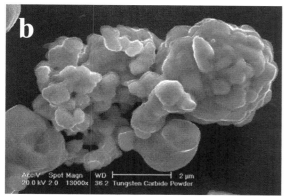

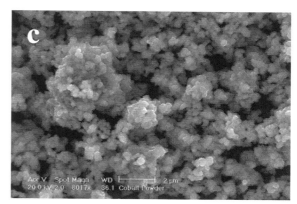

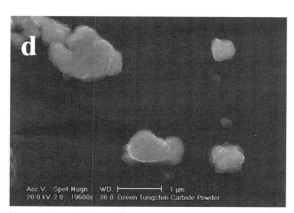

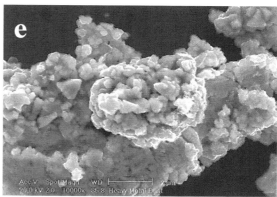

Figure 1. High magnification pictures illustrating the shape of bulk powder materials that span the cemented tungsten carbide manufacturing process: (a) bulk tungsten metal powder, (b) bulk tungsten carbide powder, (c) bulk cobalt powder, (d) bulk powder from spray dryer, and (e) bulk chamfer grinder powder. (No attempt was made to compare particle size among bulk powders, as such; the scale bars lengths differ among pictures, precluding direct comparison of particle sizes.)

DEPARTMENT OF HEALTH & HUMAN SERVICES

Phone: (304) 285-5751
Fax: (304) 285-5820

Public Health Service

Centers for Disease Control
and Prevention (CDC)
National Institute for Occupational
Safety and Health (NIOSH)
1095 Willowdale Road
Morgantown, WV 26505-2888

September 20, 2006
HETA 2003-0257
Interim Letter XI

Mr. Robert Whitaker
Director of Safety and Environment
Metalworking Products
1 Teledyne Place
La Vergne, Tennessee 37086

Dear Mr. Whitaker:

The purpose of this letter is to report the results of a National Institute for Occupational Safety and Health (NIOSH) industrial hygiene survey to characterize the levels and sizes of airborne metal particles at the Alldyne Powder Technologies plants located in Huntsville and Gurley, Alabama and the Firth Sterling plant located in Grant, Alabama. During this survey, conducted from October 25 to November 2, 2004, we also collected samples for airborne metal working fluids and total dust and metals and these results were previously reported to you in Interim Letter VII dated November 8, 2005. NIOSH surveyed these plants in response to a confidential employee request concerning respiratory health effects and exposure to cobalt, nickel, chromium, and tungsten carbide.

Sincerely,

Nancy M. Sahakian, M.D., M.P.H.

Aleksandr Stefaniak, Ph.D., C.I.H.
Respiratory Disease Hazard Evaluation and
  Technical Assistance Program
Field Studies Branch
Division of Respiratory Disease Studies

cc:
Confidential Requesters
Daryl Baker
Larry Hollingsworth
Junior Pugh
Alabama Department of Health
OSHA, Region 4
HETAB file
Close-out file (2003-0257)

Survey goal:

Estimate personal breathing zone full-shift exposure to cobalt, chromium, nickel, and tungsten using particle size-selective samplers in 21 pre-identified work areas throughout the Alldyne Powder Technologies plants located in Huntsville and Gurley, Alabama and the Firth Sterling plant located in Grant, Alabama.

Samples collected:

One hundred eight (108) samples of airborne particles were collected from employees in 21 different work areas using Marple series 290 8-stage cascade impactor samplers positioned in the personal breathing zones of employees during the course of their normal work activities. The Marple samplers collect and separate particles based on their size using different filter stages. Of the 108 samples, 27 (25%) were collected at Huntsville, 29 (27%) at Gurley, and 52 (48%) at Grant. The aerodynamic diameter cut points for the cascade impactor sampler at a flow rate of 2.0 liters per minute were >21.3 micrometers (μm) (stage 1), 14.8 μm (stage 2), 9.8 μm (stage 3), 6.0 μm (stage 4), 3.5 μm (stage 5), 1.55 μm (stage 6), 0.93 μm (stage 7), 0.52 μm (stage 8), and <0.52 (final filter). All impactor samples were collected on polyvinyl chloride (PVC) substrate that was sprayed with silicone to prevent particle bounce during sampling.

All impactor PVC filters and quality control samples (blank PVC filters) were submitted to a laboratory accredited for metals analysis by the American Industrial Hygiene Association Industrial Hygiene Laboratory Accreditation Program for quantification of cobalt, chromium, and nickel content in accordance with NIOSH Analytical Method 7300, and tungsten content in accordance with NIOSH Analytical Method 7074. The PVC substrates were analyzed in multiple batches. A new instrument calibration curve was established prior to analyzing each batch of samples. Because the analytical limit of detection (LOD) and limit of quantification (LOQ) are unique to a given calibration curve, ranges are provided for these reporting limits: cobalt, LOD = 0.06 to 0.4 μg/filter, LOQ = 0.2 to 1 μg/filter; chromium, LOD = 0.1 to 0.7 μg/filter, LOQ = 0.4 to 2 μg/filter; nickel, LOD = 0.06 to 1 μg/filter, LOQ = 0.2 to 4 μg/filter; and tungsten LOD = 0.4 to 0.8 μg/filter, LOQ = 1.0 to 3.0 μg/filter. The LOD is the minimum amount of a metal that may be detected by an analytical method. The LOQ is the minimum amount of a metal that can be detected with great confidence by an analytical method.

The concentration of each metal in air was determined by dividing the amount of metal collected on a filter by the amount of air sampled through the filter. To calculate concentration levels and estimates of particle size for samples with a mass level below the LOD, a value of one-half the appropriate LOD was assigned to the sample.

For the purpose of this Interim Letter, results of air samples were compared to the Occupational Safety and Health Administration (OSHA) permissible exposure limit (PEL) and the NIOSH recommended exposure limit (REL). The REL is a professionally recognized exposure limit and is among the lowest limits for cobalt. The PEL is higher than the REL and is a legally enforceable exposure limit in the United States. The OSHA PEL and NIOSH REL, expressed as 8-hour time-weighted averages, for cobalt, chromium, nickel, and tungsten are:

Limit	8-hour time-weighted average concentration (mg/m³)			
	Cobalt	Chromium	Nickel	Tungsten
PEL	0.1	1.0	1.0	--[A]
REL	0.05	0.5	0.5	5.0

[A] No PEL exists for this material

Note that other exposure recommendations exist for cobalt and for tungsten carbides that contain cobalt or nickel. For example, the World Health Organization (Concise International Chemical Assessment Document 69: Cobalt and inorganic cobalt compounds, World Health Organization, 2006. Available online at http://www.who.int/ipcs/publications/cicad/en/index.html) recommends 0.02 mg cobalt/m³, which is the commonly cited Threshold Limit Value proposed by the American Conference of Governmental Industrial Hygienists. NIOSH defines cemented tungsten carbide or "hard metal" as a mixture of tungsten carbide, cobalt, and sometimes metal oxides or carbides and other metals (including nickel). The NIOSH REL for cemented tungsten carbide containing >2% cobalt is 0.05 mg cobalt/m³ (expressed as a 10-hour time-weighted average). NIOSH considers cemented tungsten carbide containing nickel to be a potential occupational carcinogen and recommends a REL of 0.015 mg nickel/m³ (expressed as a 10-hour time-weighted average).

Results

Note that for purposes of this letter, the Gurley plant reprocessing and charging jobs were combined into a single category called "Powder Mixing", maintenance and janitor jobs were combined into a single category called "Maintenance", and the Building #2 Leadman job was grouped with Spray drying. The Grant plant round cell and shaping jobs were combined into a single category called "Shaping" and the receiving clerk and powder crib clerk jobs were combined into a single category called "Production Control."

Cobalt

Concentration Levels

Table I summarizes airborne cobalt concentration levels for the impactor samples by work area. At Huntsville, the concentration of airborne cobalt ranged from 0.0019 mg/m³ in the Powder Laboratory to 0.19 mg/m³ in Reclamation A. At the Gurley plant, cobalt concentrations ranged from 0.0061 mg/m³ in Inventory Control to 1.98 mg/m³ in Powder Mixing. At Grant, cobalt concentrations ranged from 0.00084 mg/m³ (Shipping) to 0.26 mg/m³ in Shaping.

The percentage of samples that exceeded the REL and PEL by work area are also summarized in Table 1. At Huntsville, the percentage of samples that exceeded the REL ranged from 0% (Powder Laboratory) to 30% (Reclamation B). The percentage of samples that exceeded the PEL by work area ranged from 0% (Powder Laboratory) to 15% (Reclamation B).

At Gurley, among the 29 samples, the percentage that exceeded the REL by work area ranged from 0% (Inventory Control, Shipping) to 34% (Powder Mixing); in comparison to the PEL, the percentage of all samples that exceeded this limit was 0% (Inventory Control, Milling, Spray Drying, Shipping, and Maintenance) to 34% (Powder Mixing).

Among the 52 samples collected at the Grant plant, the percentages that exceeded the REL or PEL was less than 2% in any work area sampled.

Relative to the REL, the least dusty areas (lowest average air concentration) tended to be areas where solid final product was handled and where engineering controls currently exist (e.g., Grinding, Sandblasting, Product Testing, and Shipping at Grant). Most dusty areas were areas where bulk powders were handled, e.g., Powder Mixing.

Particle Sizes

The mass median aerodynamic diameters (MMAD) and geometric standard deviations (GSD) of cobalt particles for the 105 samples with detectable levels of cobalt are summarized by work area in Table II. For the purposes of this letter, the MMAD can be thought of as the "average" particle diameter and the GSD is an estimate of the range of the particle sizes. At Huntsville and Gurley, the median MMAD was greater than 10 μm in all work areas, except Inventory Control at Gurley. At Grant, the median MMAD was below 10 μm in all work areas, except Pressing.

Chromium

Concentration Levels

Table III is chromium concentrations expressed as the sum of chromium mass on all impactor stages of each sample. At Huntsville, the concentration of airborne chromium ranged from 0.0007 mg/m^3 (Metal Separation) to 0.034 mg/m^3 (also in Metal Separation); chromium was not detected in samples collected in Reclamation A or the Powder Laboratory. At the Gurley plant, chromium concentrations ranged from 0.0010 mg/m^3 among Maintenance workers to 0.0043 mg/m^3 in Powder Mixing; chromium was not detected in any sample collected in Inventory Control, Milling, Spray Drying, or Shipping. At Grant, the chromium concentration was 0.031 mg/m^3 in Grinding; chromium was not detected in samples from Production Control, Pressing, Extrusion, Shaping, Breakdown, Sandblasting, Product Testing, Shipping, or Maintenance.

Among the 108 impactor samples collected at Huntsville, Gurley, and Grant none exceeded the REL or PEL for chromium.

Particle Sizes

The MMADs and GSDs of chromium particles for the 18 samples with detectable levels of chromium are summarized by work area in Table IV. The median chromium particle MMAD was greater than 10 μm in Metal Separation, Reclamation B, Powder Mixing, Screening, and Grinding. In Reclamation A and B (Huntsville) and Maintenance (Gurley), median MMADs were below 10 μm.

Nickel

Concentration Levels

Nickel concentration levels for the impactor samples are summarized by work area in Table V. At Huntsville, the concentration of airborne nickel ranged from 0.0022 mg/m^3 (Metal Separation) to 0.10 mg/m^3 (also in Metal Separation); nickel was not detected in samples collected in Reclamation A, Reclamation B, or the Powder Laboratory. At the Gurley plant, nickel concentrations ranged from 0.0035 mg/m^3 in Powder Mixing to 0.65 mg/m^3 (also in Powder Mixing); nickel was not detected in any sample collected in Inventory Control, Milling, Spray Drying, or Shipping. At Grant, nickel was only detected in one impactor sample collected from the Grinding work area.

None of the impactor samples collected at Huntsville or Grant exceeded the REL or PEL for nickel. At Gurley, among all 29 impactor samples, just 2 samples collected from the Powder Mixing work area (7%) exceeded the

REL for nickel; none of the samples exceeded the PEL.

Particle Sizes

The MMADs and GSDs of nickel particles for the 18 samples with detectable levels of nickel are summarized by work area in Table VI; nickel was only quantifiable in Metal Separation, Reclamation A and B, Powder Mixing, Screening, Production Control, and Grinding. Among these samples, the median MMADs were greater than 10 µm.

Tungsten

Concentration Levels

Table VII summarizes airborne tungsten concentration levels for the impactor samples by work area. At Huntsville, the concentration of airborne tungsten ranged from 0.016 mg/m³ in Powder Laboratory to 2.42 mg/m³ in Reclamation A and B. At the Gurley plant, tungsten concentrations ranged from 0.024 mg/m³ in Inventory Control to 1.98 mg/m³ in Powder Mixing. At Grant, tungsten concentrations ranged from 0.0078 mg/m³ (Sandblasting) to 2.73 mg/m³ in Shaping.

Among the 108 impactor samples collected at Huntsville, Gurley, and Grant none exceeded the REL for tungsten.

Particle Sizes

The MMADs and GSDs of tungsten particles for the 105 samples with detectable levels of tungsten are summarized by work area in Table VIII. At Huntsville and Gurley, median MMADs were greater than or equal to 10 µm in all work areas. At Grant, median MMADs were below 10 µm in all work areas, with the exception of Pressing.

Discussion

The concentrations of cobalt measured using impactor samplers were below the REL for airborne cobalt in the following 10 work areas: Powder Laboratory; Inventory Control, Shipping (Gurley); Production Control, Extrusion, Breakdown, Sandblasting, Product Testing, Shipping (Grant), and Maintenance (Grant). As presented in Table I, levels of airborne cobalt exceeded the REL (0.05 mg/m³) on at least one sample in the remaining 11 work areas sampled. Employee personal breathing zone cobalt exposures often exceeded the TLV in work areas where powder is handled or manipulated. Thus, efforts to minimize aerosolization of powders and implementation of controls to remove cobalt from air should help to reduce personal airborne cobalt exposure levels.

With the exception of two samples collected in Powder Mixing, which contained nickel at levels above the REL, airborne chromium, nickel, and tungsten were well below the REL and PEL (see Tables III, V, and VII).

Particles with aerodynamic diameters greater than 10 µm have a high probability of depositing in the upper airways where they can be cleared to the gastrointestinal tract then eliminated from the body. Particles with diameters less than 10 µm have high probability of depositing in the deep regions of the lung where it is difficult for the body to clear them. In nearly all work areas sampled at Huntsville and Gurley where powders were prepared or manipulated, the median cobalt and tungsten particle MMADs were greater than 10 µm; the one exception was that the cobalt particle MMAD in Inventory Control was less than 10 µm. At Grant, the median cobalt and tungsten particle MMAD in pressing, where powders are compacted, was above 10 μm. The median cobalt and tungsten particle MMAD was less than 10 μm in all work areas where solid compacts were handled, *i.e.*, downstream of pressing.

The observed particle size distributions may help to better understand the prevalence of asthma and hard metal disease at the Gurley and Grant facilities. For asthma, cobalt particles that deposit in any part of the lung may be important in developing sensitization (meaning the body responds to cobalt), thus all particle sizes that deposit in the lung may be important for exposure. In Interim Letter IX (reported to you on May 9, 2006) the higher risk work areas for asthma were Milling/Spray Drying, Maintenance at Gurley, Pressing, Sintering, and Product Testing. In these work areas, median cobalt particle MMADs ranged from 6.2 μm to 15.5 μm (no data were available from Sintering). It should be noted that differences in the amount of cobalt exposure and individual genetic susceptibility may also be risk factors for asthma and could help to explain why asthma is not observed in all work areas with cobalt exposure. For hard metal disease, tungsten carbide and cobalt particles that deposit in the deep region of the lung may be important in developing symptoms, thus particle sizes less than 10 μm may be important in exposure. Higher risk work areas for hard metal disease were Pressing, Sintering, and Grinding. In Grinding, the median cobalt particle MMAD was 6.9 μm and the median tungsten particle MMAD was 7.0 μm; however, in Pressing, median cobalt and tungsten particle MMADs were greater than 10 μm (no data were available from Sintering). The lack of a clear relationship between cobalt and tungsten median MMAD particle size and risk for hard metal disease suggests that in addition to the amount of exposure, other factors, such as a chemical interaction between cobalt and tungsten particles in the lung, may be important for exposure.

Recommendations

Building on our recommendations from previous interim letters sent to you, the following recommendations are made concerning inhalation exposure to cobalt at all three plants:

- Routinely monitor inhalation exposure to cobalt
  - o At least annually and whenever any major process change takes place
    - ▪ Inhalation exposure should be sampled in the personal breathing zone
- Engineering
  - o In work areas with elevated cobalt exposures, reduce cobalt exposure levels to below the current OSHA PEL (or to a lower professionally recognized level)
    - ▪ Utilize the industrial hygiene hierarchy of controls (ranked in order of most preferred to least preferred control method): elimination > substitution > engineering >work practices > personal protective equipment
- Work practices
  - o Provide a high-efficiency particulate air (HEPA) filtered vacuum in the pressing area for employees to clean their machines and work area. Use of a HEPA filtered vacuum will minimize transfer of cobalt from surfaces to air.
  - o Employees in grinding should stand at a reasonable distance away from grinding machines during operation. Distance between the operator and the machine will permit employees to oversee machine processes while minimizing the amount of cobalt in the breathing zone.
  - o Ensure and routinely check the integrity of the sandblasting glove box door seals, exhaust air hoses and gloves.
- Personal protective clothing and equipment
  - o Appropriate respiratory protection should be worn by properly trained personnel when job activities could result in cobalt aerosol exposure levels above the pertinent OSHA PEL (or a

lower feasible professionally recognized level) that could not be controlled to an acceptable level by engineering and work practice controls

o NIOSH, in the document "Pocket Guide to Chemical Hazards" recommends the following levels of respiratory protection for exposure to cemented tungsten carbides containing >2% cobalt by mass:

- Up to 0.25 mg Co/m^3: Any dust or mist respirator with an assigned protection factor (APF) of 5
- From 0.25 to 0.5 mg Co/m^3: Any dust and mist respirator (except single use and quarter-mask respirators) with an APF of 10; any dust, mist, and fume respirator with an APF of 10; or any supplied-air respirator with an APF of 10
- From 0.5 to 1.25 mg Co/m^3: Any supplied-air respirator operated in continuous-flow mode with an APF of 25; any powered, air-purifying respirator with a dust and mist filter with an APF of 25; or any powered, air-purifying respirator with a dust, mist, and fume filter with an APF of 25
- From 1.25 to 2.5 mg Co/m^3: Any air-purifying, full-facepiece respirator with a high-efficiency particulate air (HEPA) filter with APF of 50; any self-contained breathing apparatus with a full facepiece with APF of 50; or, any supplied-air respirator with a full facepiece with APF of 50
- Careful attention should be given to the use of respiratory and personal protection equipment to ensure that it is donned, used and maintained properly.

Table I. Cobalt concentration levels summarized by work area for samples collected in the personal breathing zone using Marple 8-stage impactor samplers (October 2004)

Plant	Work Area[1]	Samples Total[2]	Samples Cobalt[3]	Cobalt (mg/m³) Avg ± St Dev	Cobalt (mg/m³) Minimum	Cobalt (mg/m³) Maximum	%>REL[4]	%>PEL[4]
Huntsville	Metal Separation	8	8	0.035 ± 0.049	0.0030	0.13	7	7
Huntsville	Reclamation A	4	4	0.064 ± 0.085	0.0060	0.19	4	4
Huntsville	Reclamation B	8	8	0.11 ± 0.047	0.050	0.17	30	15
Huntsville	Reclamation A and B	3	3	0.13 ± 0.015	0.12	0.14	11	11
Huntsville	Powder Laboratory	4	4	0.026 ± 0.018	0.0019	0.041	0	0
Gurley	Inventory Control	1	1	0.0061			0	0
Gurley	Powder Mixing	14	14	0.44 ± 0.56	0.013	1.98	34	34
Gurley	Milling	2	2	0.052 ± 0.029	0.032	0.072	3	0
Gurley	Spray Drying	4	4	0.043 ± 0.014	0.025	0.058	3	0
Gurley	Screening	4	4	0.12 ± 0.078	0.040	0.20	10	7
Gurley	Shipping	1	1	0.017			0	0
Gurley	Maintenance	3	3	0.049 ± 0.042	0.025	0.097	3	0
Grant	Production Control	2	2	0.0042 ± 0.00023	0.0040	0.0043	0	0
Grant	Pressing	7	7	0.030 ± 0.015	0.011	0.060	2	0
Grant	Extrusion	2	2	0.0065 ± 0.0053	0.0028	0.010	0	0
Grant	Shaping	13	13	0.035 ± 0.071	0.0032	0.26	2	2
Grant	Breakdown	1	1	0.0081			0	0
Grant	Grinding	8	8	0.036 ± 0.056	0.0036	0.16	2	2
Grant	Sandblasting	4	4	0.0033 ± 0.0022	0.0015	0.0065	0	0
Grant	Product Testing	5	5	0.0057 ± 0.0037	0.0025	0.012	0	0
Grant	Shipping	5	5	0.013 ± 0.021	0.00084	0.045	0	0
Grant	Maintenance	5	5	0.0033 ± 0.0025	0.0015	0.0075	0	0

[1] Location that employee reported working on the day sample was collected
[2] Total number of samples collected in a given work area
[3] Number of samples with detectable amounts of cobalt in a given work area
[4] Samples in a work area that exceeded an occupational exposure limit, expressed as a percentage of the total number of samples collected in a given facility

Table II. Mass median aerodynamic diameters (MMAD) and geometric standard deviations (GSD) of cobalt particle summarized by work area for samples collected in the personal breathing zone using Marple 8-stage impactor samplers (October 2004)

Plant	Work Area[1]	Samples Total[2]	Samples Cobalt[3]	MMAD (μm) Median	MMAD (μm) Range	GSD Median	GSD Range
Huntsville	Metal Separation	8	8	15.2	7.4 - 23.2	3.0	2.7 - 3.5
Huntsville	Reclamation A	4	4	16.8	15.4 - 19.3	2.7	2.5 - 3.2
Huntsville	Reclamation B	8	8	18.5	15.7 - 22.7	2.7	2.5 - 2.8
Huntsville	Reclamation A and B	3	3	13.9	13.5 - 16.6	2.2	2.2 - 2.4
Huntsville	Powder Laboratory	4	4	15.9	11.8 - 26.9	3.0	2.7 - 3.5
Gurley	Inventory Control	1	1	8.7		2.5	
Gurley	Powder Mixing	14	14	11.9	9.4 - 15.3	2.4	2.2 - 3.0
Gurley	Milling	2	2	13.8	11.6 - 16.1	2.6	2.4 - 2.8
Gurley	Spray Drying	4	4	15.5	10.7 - 21.8	2.8	2.4 - 3.0
Gurley	Screening	4	4	11.4	9.6 - 15.4	2.3	2.1 - 2.5
Gurley	Shipping	1	1	10.3		2.5	
Gurley	Maintenance	3	3	10.9	9.1 - 16.4	2.9	2.4 - 3.1
Grant	Production Control	2	2	6.4	6.1 - 6.7	2.2	2.2 - 2.2
Grant	Pressing	7	7	14.6	6.0 - 16.4	2.6	2.2 - 3.3
Grant	Extrusion	2	2	6.3	6.0 - 6.7	2.4	2.2 - 2.6
Grant	Shaping	13	13	6.9	5.8 - 11.7	2.4	2.0 - 2.8
Grant	Breakdown	1	1	7.1		2.0	
Grant	Grinding	8	8	6.9	1.8 - 15.2	2.5	2.0 - 3.4
Grant	Sandblasting	4	4	6.0	5.0 - 6.5	2.2	2.0 - 2.3
Grant	Product Testing	5	5	6.2	5.6 - 9.6	2.3	2.0 - 3.0
Grant	Shipping	5	5	6.3	1.9 - 19.6	2.5	2.2 - 3.7
Grant	Maintenance	5	5	5.7	4.4 - 6.1	2.3	2.1 - 2.6

[1] Location that employee reported working on the day sample was collected
[2] Total number of samples collected in a given work area
[3] Number of samples with detectable amounts of cobalt in a given work area

Table III. Chromium concentration levels summarized by work area for samples collected in the personal breathing zone using Marple 8-stage impactor samplers (October 2004)

Plant	Work Area[1]	Samples Total[2]	Samples Chromium[3]	Chromium (mg/m^3) Avg ± St Dev	Chromium (mg/m^3) Minimum	Chromium (mg/m^3) Maximum	%>REL[4]	%>PEL[4]
Huntsville	Metal Separation	8	3	0.021 ± 0.018	0.00070	0.034	0	0
Huntsville	Reclamation B	8	1	0.0017			0	0
Huntsville	Reclamation A and B	3	3	0.0047 ± 0.0044	0.00084	0.0094	0	0
Gurley	Powder Mixing	14	3	0.0032 ± 0.0010	0.0026	0.0043	0	0
Gurley	Screening	4	1	0.0023			0	0
Gurley	Maintenance	3	1	0.0010			0	0
Grant	Grinding	8	1	0.031			0	0

[1] Location that employee reported working on the day sample was collected
[2] Total number of samples collected in a given work area
[3] Number of samples with detectable amounts of chromium in a given work area
[4] Samples in a work area that exceeded an occupational exposure limit, expressed as a percentage of the total number of samples collected in a given facility

Table IV. Mass median aerodynamic diameters (MMAD) and geometric standard deviations (GSD) of chromium particle summarized by work area for samples collected in the personal breathing zone using Marple 8-stage impactor samplers (October 2004)

Plant	Work Area[1]	Samples Total[2]	Samples Chromium[3]	MMAD (μm) Median	MMAD (μm) Range	GSD Median	GSD Range
Huntsville	Metal Separation	8	3	20.1	9.8 - 29.1	2.9	2.5 - 4.2
Huntsville	Reclamation B	8	1	12.0		4.5	
Huntsville	Reclamation A and B	3	3	7.5	4.7 - 10.8	3.0	2.2 - 5.5
Gurley	Powder Mixing	14	3	15.5	12.5 - 25.7	4.1	3.7 - 5.2
Gurley	Screening	4	1	12.0		3.9	
Gurley	Maintenance	3	1	7.3		4.8	
Grant	Grinding	8	1	20.1		2.5	

[1] Location that employee reported working on the day sample was collected
[2] Total number of samples collected in a given work area
[3] Number of samples with detectable amounts of chromium in a given work area

Table V. Nickel concentration levels summarized by work area for samples collected in the personal breathing zone using Marple 8-stage impactor samplers (October 2004)

Plant	Work Area[1]	Samples Total[2]	Samples Nickel[3]	Chromium (mg/m³) Avg ± St Dev	Chromium (mg/m³) Minimum	Chromium (mg/m³) Maximum	%>REL[4]	%>PEL[4]
Huntsville	Metal Separation	8	3	0.051 ± 0.050	0.0022	0.10	0	0
Huntsville	Reclamation A and B	3	1	0.0077			0	0
Gurley	Powder Mixing	14	10	0.18 ± 0.23	0.0035	0.65	7	0
Gurley	Screening	4	2	0.0096 ± 0.0082	0.0038	0.015	0	0
Gurley	Maintenance	3	1	0.0096			0	0
Grant	Grinding	8	1	0.068			0	0

[1] Location that employee reported working on the day sample was collected
[2] Total number of samples collected in a given work area
[3] Number of samples with detectable amounts of nickel in a given work area
[4] Samples in a work area that exceeded an occupational exposure limit, expressed as a percentage of the total number of samples collected in a given facility

Table VI. Mass median aerodynamic diameters (MMAD) and geometric standard deviations (GSD) of nickel particle summarized by work area for samples collected in the personal breathing zone using Marple 8-stage impactor samplers (October 2004)

Plant	Work Area[1]	Samples Total[2]	Samples Nickel[3]	MMAD (µm) Median	MMAD (µm) Range	GSD Median	GSD Range
Huntsville	Metal Separation	8	3	19.8	14.8 - 28.5	3.1	3.0 - 3.2
Huntsville	Reclamation A and B	3	1	11.4		2.7	
Gurley	Powder Mixing	14	10	17.1	13.3 - 28.1	2.3	2.2 - 3.2
Gurley	Screening	4	2	12.8	9.4 - 16.2	2.6	2.6 - 2.6
Grant	Production Control	3	1	18.2		2.6	
Grant	Grinding	8	1	10.8		4.7	

[1] Location that employee reported working on the day sample was collected
[2] Total number of samples collected in a given work area
[3] Number of samples with detectable amounts of nickel in a given work area

Table VII. Tungsten concentration levels summarized by work area for samples collected in the personal breathing zone using Marple 8-stage impactor samplers (October 2004)

Plant	Work Area[1]	Samples Total[2]	Samples Tungsten[3]	Tungsten (mg/m³) Avg ± St Dev	Tungsten (mg/m³) Minimum	Tungsten (mg/m³) Maximum	%>REL[4]	%>PEL[4]
Huntsville	Metal Separation	8	8	0.51 ± 0.41	0.051	1.22	0	0
Huntsville	Reclamation A	4	4	0.74 ± 0.77	0.070	1.63	0	0
Huntsville	Reclamation B	8	8	1.0 ± 0.36	0.58	1.51	0	0
Huntsville	Reclamation A and B	3	3	1.6 ± 0.75	0.94	2.42	0	0
Huntsville	Powder Laboratory	4	4	0.14 ± 0.090	0.016	0.23	0	0
Gurley	Inventory Control	1	1	0.024			0	0
Gurley	Powder Mixing	14	14	1.0 ± 0.74	0.050	1.98	0	0
Gurley	Milling	2	2	0.42 ± 0.25	0.25	0.60	0	0
Gurley	Spray Drying	4	4	0.34 ± 0.098	0.21	0.44	0	0
Gurley	Screening	4	4	1.17 ± 0.76	0.36	1.85	0	0
Gurley	Shipping	1	1	0.087			0	0
Gurley	Maintenance	3	3	0.33 ± 0.30	0.14	0.68	0	0
Grant	Production Control	2	2	0.025 ± 0.0062	0.021	0.030	0	0
Grant	Pressing	7	7	0.22 ± 0.12	0.10	0.44	0	0
Grant	Extrusion	2	2	0.039 ± 0.030	0.018	0.060	0	0
Grant	Shaping	13	13	0.30 ± 0.73	0.016	2.73	0	0
Grant	Breakdown	1	1	0.013			0	0
Grant	Grinding	8	7	0.31 ± 0.50	0.017	1.40	0	0
Grant	Sandblasting	4	4	0.017 ± 0.0083	0.0078	0.028	0	0
Grant	Product Testing	5	5	0.017 ± 0.0048	0.012	0.023	0	0
Grant	Shipping	5	3	0.12 ± 0.18	0.0089	0.36	0	0
Grant	Maintenance	5	5	0.022 ± 0.016	0.010	0.049	0	0

[1] Location that employee reported working on the day sample was collected
[2] Total number of samples collected in a given work area
[3] Number of samples with detectable amounts of tungsten in a given work area
[4] Samples in a work area that exceeded an occupational exposure limit, expressed as a percentage of the total number of samples collected in a given facility

Table VIII. Mass median aerodynamic diameters (MMAD) and geometric standard deviations (GSD) of tungsten particle summarized by work area for samples collected in the personal breathing zone using Marple 8-stage impactor samplers (October 2004)

Plant	Work Area[1]	Samples Total[2]	Samples Tungsten[3]	MMAD (µm) Median	MMAD (µm) Range	GSD Median	GSD Range
Huntsville	Metal Separation	8	8	17.1	7.6 - 24.7	2.8	2.5 - 3.9
Huntsville	Reclamation A	4	4	17.1	13.1 - 18.7	2.6	2.4 - 3.0
Huntsville	Reclamation B	8	8	16.6	14.1 - 18.6	2.5	2.4 - 2.7
Huntsville	Reclamation A and B	3	3	12.0	11.2 - 17.4	2.2	2.1 - 2.5
Huntsville	Powder Laboratory	4	4	17.4	8.6 - 27.4	3.1	2.8 - 3.3
Gurley	Inventory Control	1	1	10.0		2.8	
Gurley	Powder Mixing	14	14	13.9	7.7 - 21.6	2.5	2.2 - 2.8
Gurley	Milling	2	2	15.2	12.5 - 17.9	2.5	2.4 - 2.5
Gurley	Spray Drying	4	4	14.7	9.9 - 22.9	2.6	2.3 - 2.9
Gurley	Screening	4	4	11.7	10.3 - 15.1	2.2	2.1 - 2.3
Gurley	Shipping	1	1	11.2		2.5	
Gurley	Maintenance	3	3	11.2	10.1 - 17.8	2.8	2.4 - 3.1
Grant	Production Control	2	2	6.5	6.3 - 6.8	2.1	2.1 - 2.1
Grant	Pressing	7	7	14.5	6.3 - 18.2	2.5	2.2 - 3.0
Grant	Extrusion	2	2	6.5	6.1 - 6.8	2.2	2.2 - 2.2
Grant	Shaping	13	13	6.4	5.3 - 12.2	2.2	2.0 - 2.6
Grant	Breakdown	1	1	6.3	6.3 - 6.3	2.3	
Grant	Grinding	8	7	7.0	3.0 - 14.8	2.4	2.0 - 3.0
Grant	Sandblasting	4	4	5.9	5.2 - 6.8	2.2	2.0 - 2.4
Grant	Product Testing	5	5	5.8	5.4 - 6.2	2.3	2.0 - 2.4
Grant	Shipping	5	3	9.4	1.8 - 19.5	2.6	2.4 - 4.2
Grant	Maintenance	5	5	5.9	2.6 - 6.7	2.2	2.0 - 3.3

[1] Location that employee reported working on the day sample was collected
[2] Total number of samples collected in a given work area
[3] Number of samples with detectable amounts of tungsten in a given work area

Appendix A: Interim Letter XII (January 23, 2007)

DEPARTMENT OF HEALTH & HUMAN SERVICES

Phone: (304) 285-5751
Fax: (304) 285-5820

Public Health Service

Centers for Disease Control
and Prevention (CDC)
National Institute for Occupational
Safety and Health (NIOSH)
1095 Willowdale Road
Morgantown, WV 26505-2888

January 23, 2007
HETA 2003-0257
Interim Letter XII

Mr. Robert Whitaker
Director of Health, Safety, and Environment
Metalworking Products
1 Teledyne Place,
LaVergne, Tennessee 37086

Dear Mr. Whitaker:

The National Institute for Occupational Safety and Health (NIOSH) conducted industrial hygiene surveys at the Alldyne Powder Technologies plants located in Huntsville and Gurley, Alabama and the Firth Sterling plant located in Grant, Alabama in July 2003, May 2004, October 2004, and November 2004. These surveys were in response to a confidential employee request concerning respiratory health effects and exposure to cobalt, nickel, chromium, tungsten carbide, and metalworking fluids. The enclosed interim report includes the results for all airborne tungsten fiber samples which were collected from October 26 to November 4, 2004.

Sincerely,

Nancy Sahakian, M.D., M.P.H.
CDR, United States Public Health Service
Respiratory Disease Hazard Evaluation and
and Technical Assistance Program
Field Studies Branch
Division of Respiratory Disease Studies

Enclosure
CC:
Confidential requesters
Daryl Baker
Larry Hollingsworth
Junior Pugh
OSHA, Region 4
Alabama Department of Health
HETAB file
Close-out file (2003-0257)

Presence of Tungsten Oxide Fibers in Hard-Metal Processes

John McKernan, ScD, CIH
National Institute for Occupational Safety and Health
Division of Surveillance, Hazard Evaluations and Field Studies
Industry-wide Studies Branch
Phone: 513-841-4212
Email: JMcKernan@cdc.gov

January 23, 2007

Purpose

To date, the existence of tungsten oxide fibers in the tungsten-using industry has not been evaluated in the United States. The purpose of this research project was to collect air samples at various steps in the hard-metal production process and to analyze the samples for the presence of tungsten oxide fibers (*i.e.*, whiskers).

Background

Studies within the Swedish hard metal industry have shown that tungsten oxide fibers can be formed and become airborne as a byproduct of tungsten metal production. The tungsten oxide fibers created were small enough to be breathed deep into the lungs. It is unknown if there are any adverse health effects related to human exposure to airborne tungsten oxide fibers. However, one laboratory study conducted *in vitro* using human lung cells concluded that tungsten oxide fibers are capable of forming radicals that can damage or be toxic to lung cells (Leanderson and Sahle 1995). No new work on the toxicity of tungsten oxide fibers has been published since 1995.

Methods

Sampling Strategy

From the preliminary walk-through investigations of the facilities and available published data from the Swedish hard metal industry, 18 production processes among three plants with the potential to produce a broad range of fiber exposures were identified for air sampling (Sahle 1992; Sahle, Laszlo et al. 1994; Sahle, Krantz et al. 1996). Both personal breathing zone (PBZ) and general area samples for airborne tungsten oxide fibers were collected [see Table I]. Seven PBZ samples were collected to capture possible tungsten oxide fiber exposures during the course of normal employee work activities. Sixty-two area samples were collected at stationary locations in work areas to capture possible tungsten oxide fiber concentrations during specific process activities.

Sample Collection and Analysis

There is no specific validated method for the collection and analysis of airborne tungsten oxide fibers. As a result, all air samples were collected in accordance with National Institute for Occupational Safety and Health (NIOSH) Methods 7400 and 7402: Asbestos and Other Fibers by Phase Contrast and Transmission Electron Microscopy (NIOSH 2003), which are standard methods for sampling and analysis of airborne asbestos-containing fibers.

PBZ and area air samples were collected on 25 millimeter diameter electrically-conductive cassettes preloaded with mixed cellulose ester (MCE) 0.45 micrometer (μm) pore-size membrane filters (SKC Inc., Eighty Four, PA). The purpose of the electrically-conductive cassette was to ensure uniform deposition of fibers on the filter substrate. Air was drawn through the cassettes with battery operated pumps calibrated at 2 liters per minute (LPM) using a standard flow calibration device (BIOS International Corp., Butler, NJ).

In general, samples were collected over a full shift (e.g., 7 to 8 hours). The type (PBZ or area) and number of samples collected for each of the 18 production processes are provided in Table I.

Each MCE filter was removed from its sample cassette and prepared for analysis using the direct transfer method outlined in NIOSH Method 7402. After preparation, each sample was individually loaded into a transmission electron microscope [TEM] (Philips, Model CM 12, Eindhoven, Netherlands) for fiber analysis.

Fibers were defined as particles having an aspect ratio (length to diameter) of at least 5:1; that is, the fiber length was at least five times greater than the diameter. A modified version of the NIOSH Method 7400 counting rule "B" was used to count fibers on the samples (NIOSH 2003). The "B" rule prescribes counting all particles with ends that lie in the field of view with a length > 5 μm, a diameter < 3 μm, and an aspect ratio ≥ 5:1. The rule was modified to include counting fibers with lengths > 0.50 μm, > 5 μm, and > 15 μm. These size cuts were based on fiber size distribution data previously reported by Sahle and colleagues. The recommended quantitative working range of the method is 0.04 to 0.50 fibers per cubic centimeter of air (f/cm^3) per 1,000 liter air sample (NIOSH 2003). The recommended limit of detection (LOD) of NIOSH Method 7402 is 0.01 f/cm^3 for atmospheres free of interferences. The LOD/$\sqrt{2}$ was used for the below LOD samples when calculating average airborne concentrations (Hornung and Reed 1990).

The elemental composition of fibers was determined using an energy dispersive x-ray (EDX) spectrometer (Gresham Light Element Detector, Model 510 with IXRF software, Houston, TX) connected to the TEM. This EDX detector can identify elements having atomic numbers greater than 4 (beryllium).

Results

Tungsten oxide fibers with lengths > 0.50 μm, diameters < 3 μm, and aspect ratios ≥ 5:1 were detected in 32 of the 69 air samples that were analyzed (Table II). The concentration of airborne tungsten oxide fibers ranged from < 0.01 (ammonium paratungstate, ball mill, calcining [yellow], carburizing, charging, pressing/molding, reclamation [all], reduction, reprocessing [all], screening, sintering, and spray drying) to 0.26 (calcining [blue]) f/cm^3. The average airborne tungsten oxide fiber concentration for the 69 samples was 0.02 f/cm^3

Overall, the average airborne fiber lengths were approximately 4 μm, and diameters were approximately 0.40 μm. Figure 1 is a micrograph from an area sample collected near the reduction process at the Huntsville facility. The micrograph provides an example of an average tungsten oxide fiber, and is a good illustration of the way most fibers were found on the samples. In general, fibers were not in bundles, and were not agglomerated with other non-fibrous particles.

Using EDX analysis, it was determined that all fibers counted were composed of tungsten and oxygen. For the samples collected at processes where hard-metal binders were present (*i.e.*, charging, spray drying, and sintering), the number of cobalt-containing particles that were attached to tungsten oxide fibers was similar to the number of cobalt-containing particles that were not attached to tungsten oxide fibers. This result indicated that cobalt-containing particles were not attached preferentially to tungsten oxide fibers. Cobalt was not detected on filter samples collected in calcining, reduction, or carburizing processes. However, it is notable that airborne cobalt was present in the area where scrap products were being reprocessed (*i.e.*, reprocessing [screening]).

Summary

Results indicate that tungsten oxide fibers existed in the workplace air at concentrations up to 0.26 f/cm^3. Currently, the potential adverse health effects related to human exposure to tungsten oxide fibers are unknown. Among the samples analyzed, those collected from the calcining (blue) and reduction process areas resulted in the highest airborne concentrations of tungsten oxide fibers. The airborne tungsten oxide fibers observed were about 4 μm in length, and about 0.40 μm in diameter. Tungsten oxide fibers were not preferentially agglomerated to cobalt particles. Airborne tungsten oxide fiber concentrations were lowest for the processes we samples at the Gurley and Grant facilities.

Recommendations

Formation of tungsten oxide fibers may be the result of incomplete oxidation of ammonia paratungstate or aerosolization of these fibers during reduction of tungsten trioxide to tungsten metal. To be prudent, NIOSH recommends that engineering studies be undertaken to better understand the production process conditions (time, temperature, and oxygen content) under which tungsten oxide fibers are formed. Adjustment of any or all of these operating conditions may eliminate the formation of tungsten oxide fibers. In the interim, it is prudent to protect workers potentially exposed to tungsten oxide fibers since the health effects associated with exposure to these fibers are unknown. Protection can be provided to workers first through the recommended methods of ventilation control, or secondarily through implementation of a respiratory protection program that uses high-efficiency particulate air (HEPA) filters.

References

Hornung, R. W. and L. D. Reed (1990). "Estimation of Average Concentration in the Presence of Nondetectable Values." Appl. Occup. Environ. Hyg. **5**(1): 46-51.

Leanderson, P. and W. Sahle (1995). "Formation of Hydroxyl Radicals and Toxicity of Tungsten Oxide Fibers." Toxic. in Vitro **9**(2): 175-183.

NIOSH (2003). NIOSH Manual of Analytical Methods (NMAM). Cincinnati, OH, National Institute for Occupational Safety and Health.

Sahle, W. (1992). "Possible Role of Tungsten Oxide Whiskers in Hard-Metal Pneumoconiosis." Chest **102**: 1310.

Sahle, W., S. Krantz, et al. (1996). "Preliminary Data on Hard Metal Workers Exposure to Tungsten Oxide Fibers." Sci. Total Environ. **191**: 153-167.

Sahle, W., I. Laszlo, et al. (1994). "Airborne Tungsten Oxide Whiskers in a Hard-Metal Industry. Preliminary Findings." Ann. Occup. Hyg. **38**(1): 37-44.

Table I: Type and Number of Air Samples by Plant, Building, and Production Process

Plant	Building	Process	Sample Type *	Sample N
Huntsville	Metal Separation	Ammonium paratungstate	P	0
			A	1
Huntsville	Metal Separation	Calcining (blue)	P	0
			A	4
Huntsville	Metal Separation	Calcining (yellow)	P	0
			A	3
Huntsville	Carbide Plant	Carburizing	P	1
			A	5
Huntsville	Reclamation B	Reclamation (ball mill)	P	0
			A	2
Huntsville	Metal Separation	Reclamation (barrel dry)	P	0
			A	1
Huntsville	Reclamation B	Reclamation (crushing)	P	0
			A	1
Huntsville	Metal Separation / Reclamation A	Reclamation (screening)	P	0
			A	2
Huntsville	Reduction Plant	Reduction	P	1
			A	9
Huntsville	Autoreduction Plant	Reduction (automated)	P	0
			A	1
Gurley	Building B	Ball mill	P	1
			A	0
Gurley	Building A	Charging	P	1
			A	3
Gurley	Building A	Reprocessing (crushing)	P	0
			A	2
Gurley	Building A	Reprocessing (screening)	P	1
			A	2
Gurley	Building A	Screening	P	1
			A	6
Gurley	Building B	Spray Drying	P	1
			A	5
Grant	Manufacturing	Pressing/Molding	P	0
			A	7
Grant	Manufacturing	Sintering	P	0
			A	8
TOTAL				69

* A = Area air sample collected at stationary locations in work areas
P = Personal breathing zone air sample
N = Number of samples collected

APPENDIX A: INTERIM LETTER XII (JANUARY 23, 2007) (CONTINUED)

Table II: Airborne Tungsten Oxide Fiber Counts and Concentrations

Plant	Process	Type*	N	n	Fiber Count[A] Total	Fiber Count[A] >0.5μm	Fiber Count[A] >5μm	Fiber Count[A] >15μm	Concentration Average Airborne (f/cm³)[B]	Concentration Range	Concentration SD	Other Elements
Huntsville	Ammonium paratungstate	A	1	0	0	ND	ND	ND	<0.01	<0.01	-	-
	Calcining (blue)	A	4	4	199	166	32	1	0.10	0.01-0.26	0.12	-
	Calcining (yellow)	A	3	3	56	44	11	1	0.03	<0.01-0.05	0.02	-
	Carburizing	P	1	0	0	ND	ND	ND	<0.01	<0.01	-	-
		A	5	2	23	16	6	1	0.01	<0.01-0.01	<0.01	-
	Reclamation (ball mill)	A	2	1	2	2	ND	ND	<0.01	<0.01	<0.01	-
	Reclamation (barrel dry)	A	1	1	4	4	ND	ND	<0.01	<0.01	-	-
	Reclamation (crushing)	A	1	0	0	ND	ND	ND	<0.01	<0.01	-	-
	Reclamation (screening)	A	2	1	21	20	1	ND	0.02	<0.01-0.04	0.02	-
	Reduction	P	1	1	47	33	12	2	0.05	0.05	-	-
		A	9	8	155	103	41	11	0.03	<0.01-0.15	0.05	Cr, Ni
	Reduction (automated)	A	1	1	55	41	14	ND	0.09	0.09	-	-
Gurley	Ball mill	P	1	0	0	ND	ND	ND	<0.01	<0.01	-	-
	Charging	P	1	0	0	ND	ND	ND	<0.01	<0.01	-	-
	Reprocessing (crushing)	A	3	3	22	21	1	ND	<0.01	<0.01-0.01	0.01	Co
		A	2	1	1	1	ND	ND	<0.01	<0.01	-	Al, Co, Cr, Ti
	Reprocessing (screening)	P	1	1	2	1	1	ND	<0.01	<0.01	<0.01	Co
	Screening	A	2	2	7	7	ND	ND	<0.01	<0.01	<0.01	-
		P	1	0	0	ND	ND	ND	<0.01	<0.01	-	-
	Spray drying	A	6	0	0	ND	ND	ND	<0.01	<0.01	<0.01	-
		P	1	0	0	ND	ND	ND	<0.01	<0.01	-	-
Grant		A	5	1	5	4	1	ND	<0.01	<0.01	<0.01	Co
	Pressing/Molding	A	7	1	1	1	ND	ND	<0.01	<0.01	<0.01	-
	Sintering	A	8	1	5	4	1	ND	<0.01	<0.01	<0.01	Co
OVERALL			69	32	605	468	121	16	0.02	<0.01-0.26	0.04	Al, Co, Cr, Ni, Ti

* A = Area air sample collected at stationary locations in work areas
P = Personal breathing zone air sample
N = Number of samples collected
n = Number of samples with fibers detected
ND = Not detected
SD = Standard deviation
A = Fiber length > 0.50 μm, diameter < 3 μm and aspect ratio ≥ 5:1
B = The quantitative working range of this technique is 0.04 to 0.50 f/cm³ as calculated using the number of fibers with length > 0.50 μm; ND airborne concentration calculated using the limit of detection of the quantitative working range (0.01 f/cm³) divided by √2

Figure 1: Airborne Tungsten Oxide Fiber from Reduction Process

RDHETA 2003 - 0257
(Current Worker)

Interviewer: _____   Interview Date: __ __ / __ __ / __ __ __ __
                                                  (Month)   (Day)   (Year)

Section I: Identification and Demographic Information

Name: _____   _____   ____
                (Last name)   (First name)   (MI)

Address: _____
                (Number, Street, and/or Rural Route)

_____   _____   _____
        (City)   (State)   (Zip Code)

Home Telephone Number: (_____) _____ - _____

If you were to move, is there someone who would know how to contact you?

Name: _____   _____   ____
                (Last name)   (First name)   (MI)

Relationship to you: _____

Address: _____
                (Number, Street, and/or Rural Route)

_____   _____   _____
        (City)   (State)   (Zip Code)

Home Telephone Number: (_____) _____ - _____

1. Date of Birth: __ __ / __ __ / __ __ __ __
                                      (Month)   (Day)   (Year)

2. Sex: 1. ____ Male   2. ____ Female

3. Are you Spanish, Hispanic, or Latino?   1.____Yes   0.____No.

4. Select <u>one or more</u> of the following categories to describe your race:

                          1. ___ White
                          2. ___ African-American or Black
                          3. ___ Asian
                          4. ___ American Indian or Alaska Native
                          5. ___ Native Hawaiian or Other Pacific Islander

Section II: Health Information

I'm going to ask you some questions about your health. The answer to many of these questions will be "Yes" or "No." If you are in doubt about whether to answer "Yes" or "No," then please answer "No."

5.   Do you ever have trouble with your breathing? 1.___Yes   0.___No

IF YES:

a)	Which of the following statements best describes your breathing?
	  1. ___ I only rarely have trouble with my breathing
	  2. ___ I have regular trouble with my breathing but it always gets completely better
	  3. ___ My breathing is never quite right

6.   Do you usually have a cough? 1. ___ Yes   0. ___ No
(Count cough with first smoke or on first going out-of-doors. Exclude clearing of throat.)

IF YES:

a)	Do you usually cough on most days for 3 consecutive months or more during the year?	1. ___ Yes 0. ___ No
b)	In what month and year did this cough begin?	__ __ / __ __ __ __ (Month) (Year)
c)	When you are away from work on days off or on vacation, is this phlegm	1. ___ Better 2. ___ The same 3. ___ Worse 4. ___ N/A

7. Do you usually bring up phlegm from your chest?   1. ___ Yes   0. ___ No
   (Count phlegm with the first smoke or on first going out_of_doors. Exclude phlegm from the nose. Count swallowed phlegm.)

IF YES:

a) Do you usually bring up phlegm on most days for 3 consecutive months or more during the year?   1. ___ Yes   0. ___ No

b) In what month and year did this phlegm begin?   __ __ / __ __ __ __
   (Month)   (Year)

c) When you are away from work on days off or on vacation, is this phlegm
   1. ___ Better
   2. ___ The same
   3. ___ Worse
   4. ___ N/A

8. Have you ever had wheezing or whistling in your chest?   1. ___ Yes   0. ___ No

IF YES:

a) In what month and year did this wheezing or whistling begin?   __ __ / __ __ __ __
   (Month)   (Year)

b) Have you had wheezing or whistling in your chest at any time in the last 12 months?   1. ___ Yes   0. ___ No

c) Apart from when you have a cold, does your chest ever sound wheezy or whistling?   1. ___ Yes   0. ___ No

d) When you are away work on days off or on vacation, is this wheezing or whistling
   1. ___ Better
   2. ___ The same
   3. ___ Worse
   4. ___ N/A

9.   When you are in a dusty part of the house or with   1. ___ Yes   0. ___ No
     animals (such as dogs, cats, or horses), or near
     feathers (such as pillows, quilts, or down or feather
     comforters), do you ever get a feeling of tightness in your chest?

10. During the last 12 months have you ever been awakened   1. ___ Yes   0. ___ No
     from sleep by shortness of breath?

11. Are you troubled by shortness of breath when hurrying
     on level ground or walking up a slight hill?   1. ___ Yes   0. ___ No

IF YES:

a)	Do you get short of breath walking with people of your own age on level ground?	1. ___ Yes 0. ___ No
b)	Do you ever have to stop for breath when walking at your own pace on level ground?	1. ___ Yes 0. ___ No
c)	Do you ever have to stop for breath after walking about 100 yards (or after a few minutes) on level ground?	1. ___ Yes 0. ___ No
d)	In what month and year did this breathlessness start?	___ ___ / ___ ___ ___ ___ (Month)　　(Year)

I am now going to ask you some questions about your health during the last four weeks.

12. In the last four weeks if you run or climb stairs fast do you ever:
      a. Cough   1. ___ Yes   0. ___ No
      b. Wheeze   1. ___ Yes   0. ___ No
      c. Get chest tightness   1. ___ Yes   0. ___ No

13. In the last four weeks has your sleep ever been broken by:
      a. Wheeze?   1. ___ Yes   0. ___ No
      b. Difficulty with breathing?   1. ___ Yes   0. ___ No

14. In the last four weeks have you ever woken up in the
     morning (or from your sleep if a shift worker) with:
      a. Wheezing?   1. ___ Yes   0. ___ No
      b. Difficulty breathing?   1. ___ Yes   0. ___ No

15. In the last four weeks have you ever wheezed :
      a. If you were in a smoky room?   1. ___ Yes   0. ___ No
      b. If you were in a very dusty place?   1. ___ Yes   0. ___ No

16. Have you ever had to change your job, job duties, or work area at Allegheny Technologies because of breathing difficulties?

1. ___ Yes   0. ___ No

IF YES:

a) What month and year did you change your job, job duties, or work area?

___ ___ / ___ ___ ___ ___
(Month)   (Year)

b) What was your job, job duties, and/or work area before the change?

Describe: _____

c) How did your job, job duties, and/or work area differ after the change?

Describe: _____

d) Were your breathing problems after the change:

1. ___ Better
2. ___ The Same
3. ___ Worse

17. While working for Allegheny Technologies, have you had fever, chills or night-sweats?

1. ___ Yes   0. ___ No

IF YES:

a) How often have you had the fever, chills, or night-sweats?

1. ___ Rarely
2. ___ Monthly
3. ___ Weekly
4. ___ Daily

18. While working for Allegheny Technologies, have you had unusual tiredness or fatigue?

1. ___ Yes   0. ___ No

IF YES:

a) How often have you had the unusual tiredness or fatigue?

1. ___ Rarely
2. ___ Monthly
3. ___ Weekly
4. ___ Daily

IF YES:

a)	Was it confirmed by a doctor?	1. ___ Yes 0. ___ No
b)	While working for Allegheny Technologies, how many times have you had bronchitis?	_____ Times

20. Have you ever had chronic bronchitis?   1. ___ Yes 0. ___ No

IF YES:

a)	Was it confirmed by a doctor?	1. ___ Yes 0. ___ No
b)	How old were you when it began?	_____ Years old

21. Since you began working for Allegheny Technologies have you ever had pneumonia? (Include bronchopneumonia)   1. ___ Yes 0. ___ No

22. Have you ever had asthma?   1. ___ Yes 0. ___ No

IF YES:

a)	How old were you when it began?	_____ Years old
b)	Was it confirmed by a doctor?	1. ___ Yes 0. ___ No
c)	Do you still have it?	1. ___ Yes 0. ___ No

23. Have you ever had a pneumothorax, which is a collapsed lung?   1. ___ Yes 0. ___ No

24. Since working for Allegheny Technologies, have you had symptoms of nasal irritation such as a stuffy or blocked nose, an itchy nose, a stinging or burning nose, or a runny nose? (*apart from a cold*) 1. ___ Yes 0. ___ No

IF YES:

a) Is there an exposure at work that aggravates these nose symptoms? 1. ___ Yes 0. ___ No

b) Describe exposure(s):

_____

_____

25. Since working for Allegheny Technologies, have you had any symptoms of eye irritation such as: watering or tearing eyes, red or burning eyes, itching eyes, dry eyes? 1. ___ Yes 0. ___ No

IF YES:

a) Is there an exposure at work that aggravates these eye symptoms? 1. ___ Yes 0. ___ No

b) Describe exposure(s):

_____

_____

26. Since working for Allegheny Technologies, have you developed any new skin rash or skin problems? 1. ___ Yes 0. ___ No

27.   Have you ever had your blood tested for cobalt?   1. ___ Yes   0. ___ No

IF YES:

a)   How many times has your blood been tested for cobalt?   _____ times

b)   The first time you had your blood tested, what job were
     you assigned to?   _____

c)   The first time you had you blood tested, were you using a   1. ___ Yes   0. ___ No
     half-piece respirator with cartridges at work?

IF ANSWER TO a) >1:
   d)   Were you doing the same job all the times your   1. ___ Yes   0. ___ No
        blood was tested?

   IF NO to d):
   e)   What jobs were you assigned to at the time of this/these
        other test(s)?

        Job at test #2: _____
        Job at test #3: _____
        Job at test #4: _____
        Job at test #5: _____
        Job at test #6: _____

Section III. Work Information

28.   At which plant do you currently work?

1.___ Grant
2.___ Gurley
3.___ Huntsville

29.   What is your usual work shift?
        IF GRANT:

1.___ 7:00 am - 3:00 pm
2.___ 3:00 pm - 11:00 pm
3.___ 11:00 pm - 7:00 am
4.___ 7:00 am - 7:00 pm

        IF GURLEY:

1.___ 6:00 am - 6:00 pm
2.___ Other
(*specify*) _____

        IF HUNTSVILLE:

1.___ 6:30 am - 6:30 pm
2.___ 6:30 pm - 6:30 am

30.   Have you ever been exposed to a spill or unusual chemical release at work?

1.___ Yes   0.___ No

IF YES:

a)   Did you have any symptoms from it?   1.___ Yes   0.___ No

IF YES:
b)   What were your symptoms?

_____

31.   Do you use the company's service to have your work clothes cleaned?   1.___ Yes   0.___ No

IF YES:

a) When did you start using this service?   __ __ / __ __ __ __
                                                  (Month)   (Year)

32.   How many months out of the year are your arms covered at work?   _____Months

33.   How often do you shower within one hour of getting home from work?
        1.___ Never
        2.___ 1-2 days out of a 5-day work week (or 1 day out of a 3-day work week)
        3.___ 3-4 days out of a 5-day work week (or 2 days out of a 3-day work week)
        4.___ 5 days out of a 5-day work week (or 3 days out of a 3-day work week)

34. Do you take multivitamins or vitamin B12?   1. ___ Yes   0. ___ No
    (have you taken a multivitamin or vitamin B12 pill in the last week?)

35. Do you have an artificial joint?   1. ___ Yes   0. ___ No
    (for example an artificial knee or an artificial hip?)

36. Are you currently taking any medication for your breathing?   1. ___ Yes   0. ___ No

Section IV: Tobacco Use Information
I'm now going to ask you a few questions about tobacco use.

37. Have you ever smoked cigarettes?   1. ___ Yes   0. ___ No
    (NO if less than 20 packs of cigarettes in a lifetime or less than 1 cigarette a day for 1 year.)

IF YES:

a) How old were you when you first started smoking regularly?   _____ Years old

b) Over the entire time that you have smoked, what is the average number of cigarettes that you smoked per day?   _____ Cigarettes/day

c) Do you still smoke cigarettes?   1. ___ Yes   0. ___ No

     IF NO:

     d) How old were you when you stopped smoking regularly?   _____ Years old

     IF YES:

     e) Do you currently smoke cigarettes while at work (during breaks)?   1. ___ Yes   0. ___ No

         IF YES:
         f) On average, how many cigarettes per day do you smoke <u>while you are at work?</u>   _____ Cigarettes/day

         g) Where do you keep your cigarette pack <u>while you are at work?</u>
             1. ___ In your pocket
             1. ___ In your locker
             1. ___ Other (specify below)
             _____

---

38.   Currently at work, what percentage of the time do you:

IF NOT CURRENT SMOKER, SKIP TO c):

a)   Wash your hands before smoking?

1. _____ 0% to 25%
2. _____ 26% to 50%
3. _____ 51% to 75%
4. _____ 76% to 100%

b)   Wash your face before smoking?

1. _____ 0% to 25%
2. _____ 26% to 50%
3. _____ 51% to 75%
4. _____ 76% to 100%

c)   Wash your hands before eating?

1. _____ 0% to 25%
2. _____ 26% to 50%
3. _____ 51% to 75%
4. _____ 76% to 100%

d)   Wash your face before eating?

1. _____ 0% to 25%
2. _____ 26% to 50%
3. _____ 51% to 75%
4. _____ 76% to 100%

e)   Wash your hands before using
the restroom?

1. _____ 0% to 25%
2. _____ 26% to 50%
3. _____ 51% to 75%
4. _____ 76% to 100%

I am now going to ask you some questions about all the jobs that you have had at the Grant, Gurley and Huntsville plants. We will start with your current job and work back through time.

39. Work History:

Job #	Plant	Work Area	Job Title	Start Date (MM/YYYY)	End Date (MM/YYYY)	% of time (if more than 1 job title)
1						
2						
3						
4						
5						
6						
7						
8						
9						
10						
11						
12						
13						
14						
15						

For each job ask: Job Number:_____

40.   Have you worn a half-face respirator with cartridges   1.___ Yes   0.___ No
      while working as a {JobTitle} in {WorkArea}
      between {StartDate} and {EndDate}?

IF YES:

a)   Were you fit tested prior to using the respirator?   1.___ Yes   0.___ No

b)   On average, what percentage of your total work   _____%
      time did you use a respirator?

c)   Did you wear the respirator for only certain tasks?   1.___ Yes   0.___ No

d)   What were those tasks?

      _____

      _____

41.   Have you worn vinyl, latex, or nitrile gloves while working 1.___ Yes   0.___ No
      as a {JobTitle} in {WorkArea} between {StartDate}
      and {EndDate}?

IF YES:

a)   On average, what percentage of your total work   _____%
      time did you wear gloves?

Thank you for participating in this survey!

ID: _____   Interviewer Initials: _____   Interview Date: ____ / ____ / _____

Form Approved
OMB No.: 0920-0260
Expiration Date: 11/30/2007

National Institute for Occupational Safety and Health (NIOSH)
Centers for Disease Control and Prevention (CDC)
U.S. Department of Health and Human Services

UPDATED WORK HISTORY AND MEDICAL QUESTIONNAIRE
Metalworking Products: Grant, Gurley, and Huntsville, Alabama
HETA 2003-0257 (January, 2005)

Name: _____   ____   _____
          (First name)   (MI)   (Last name)

Address: _____

_____   _____   _____
    (City)   (State)   (Zip Code)

Home Telephone Number: (____) _____ - _____

----

1. Have you ever had asthma?   1. ___ Yes   0. ___ No

        —————————— IF *Yes* TO QUESTION 1: ——————————
        | 1 a) How old were you when it began?   _____ Years old |
        | 1 b) Was it confirmed by a doctor?   1. ___ Yes   0. ___ No |
        | 1 c) Do you still have it?   1. ___ Yes   0. ___ No |

2. Are you currently taking any medication for your breathing?   1. ___ Yes   0. ___ No

3. **In the last four weeks,**
    3a. if you run or climb stairs fast do you ever cough?   1. ___ Yes   0. ___ No
    3b. if you run or climb stairs fast do you ever wheeze?   1. ___ Yes   0. ___ No
    3c. if you run or climb stairs fast do you ever get chest tightness?   1. ___ Yes   0. ___ No

4. **In the last four weeks,**
    4a. has your sleep ever been broken by wheeze?   1. ___ Yes   0. ___ No
    4b. has your sleep ever been broken by difficulty with breathing?   1. ___ Yes   0. ___ No

ID: _____

5. **In the last four weeks,**
   5a. have you ever woken up in the morning (or from your sleep if a shift worker) with wheezing?　　1. ___ Yes　0. ___ No
   5b. have you ever woken up in the morning (or from your sleep if a shift worker) with difficulty breathing?　　1. ___ Yes　0. ___ No

6. **In the last four weeks,**
   6a. have you ever wheezed if you are in a smoky room?　　1. ___ Yes　0. ___ No
   6b. have you ever wheezed if you are in a very dusty place?　　1. ___ Yes　0. ___ No

7. Since you began working for Allegheny Technologies have you ever had pneumonia? *(include bronchopneumonia)*　　1. ___ Yes　0. ___ No

8. Have you ever smoked cigarettes?
   (Choose NO if less than 20 packs of cigarettes in a lifetime or less than 1 cigarette a day for 1 year.)　　1. ___ Yes　0. ___ No

---
IF *Yes* TO QUESTION 8:

8 a) How old were you when you first started smoking regularly?　　_____ Years old

8 b) Over the entire time that you have smoked, what is the average number of cigarettes that you smoked per day?　　_____ Cigarettes/day

8 c) Do you still smoke cigarettes?　　1. ___ Yes　0. ___ No

IF *No* TO QUESTION 8 c:

8 d) How old were you when you stopped smoking regularly?　　_____ Years old

---

9. Do you take multivitamins or vitamin B12? *(have you taken a multivitamin or vitamin B12 pill in the last week?)*　　1. ___ Yes　0. ___ No

10. Do you have an artificial joint? *(for example an artificial knee or artificial hip?)*　　1. ___ Yes　0. ___ No

ID: _____

WORK HISTORY

Please list all the jobs you have ever worked at the Grant, Gurley, and Huntsville plants since the NIOSH September 2003 survey and half-face respirator and glove usage. Please BEGIN with the job you were working September 2003 and work forward in time up to today (January 2005).

JOB #	PLANT	WORK AREA	JOB TITLE	START DATE (Month/Year)	END DATE (Month/Year)	Did you wear a half-face respirator?	Did you wear vinyl, latex, or nitrile gloves?
Example	GRANT	PRESSING	PRESSING OPERATOR	9/2003	1/ 2005 (TODAY)	1. ___ Yes 0. _X_ No	1. ___ Yes 0. _X_ No
JOB #	PLANT	WORK AREA	JOB TITLE	START DATE (Month/Year)	END DATE (Month/Year)	Did you wear a half-face respirator?	Did you wear vinyl, latex, or nitrile gloves?
1				9/2003		1. ___ Yes 0. ___ No	1. ___ Yes 0. ___ No
2						1. ___ Yes 0. ___ No	1. ___ Yes 0. ___ No
3						1. ___ Yes 0. ___ No	1. ___ Yes 0. ___ No
4						1. ___ Yes 0. ___ No	1. ___ Yes 0. ___ No
5						1. ___ Yes 0. ___ No	1. ___ Yes 0. ___ No
6						1. ___ Yes 0. ___ No	1. ___ Yes 0. ___ No

METHODS

Metal Antibodies

Metal-bound proteins were analyzed using matrix-assisted laser desorption/ionization time-of-flight mass spectrometry (MALDI-TOF MS) to identify the number of metals bound to each protein. Mass spectra of metal-bound SOD showed 0–3 cobalt ions, 0–3 zinc ions, and 0–1 nickel ions bound per SOD molecule. Poor resolution of mass spectra for metal-bound HSA prevented characterization of these haptens by MALDI-TOF MS. Differences in the color of metal-bound and metal-free HSA was used as evidence of binding to the HSA protein.

Exposure-Response Analyses

Urine and wrist cobalt and cobalt, nickel, and tungsten in exhaled breath condensate

We tested whether workers who participated in the 2005 medical survey (n=150) were more likely to report three or more asthma-like symptoms [Venables et al. 1993] if they had higher amounts of cobalt on the skin of their wrists, higher concentrations of cobalt in their urine, or higher concentrations of cobalt, nickel, or tungsten in their exhaled breath condensate. These analyses were initially controlled for age, gender, tenure, smoking (pack-years), and race and were reanalyzed with both current asthma included and race removed from the statistical models. For marginally significant results we reanalyzed the data again using categorical exposure metrics based on cutpoints defined by the Classification and Regression Tree (CART) algorithm (JMP, version 5.1, SAS Institute Inc., Cary, NC).

Air measurements of cobalt, tungsten, nickel, chromium, and dust

Among workers who participated in either the 2003 or 2005 medical surveys (n=232), we tested whether specific respiratory health outcomes were related to estimates of work area exposures for the work areas they worked in at the time they completed their spirometry tests or questionnaires (whichever was applicable). For workers who participated in both surveys, we used results from their most recent spirometry test or questionnaire in this analysis.

APPENDIX C: METHODS (CONTINUED)

Health outcomes tested included: 1) FEV_1; 2) FVC; 3) FEV_1/FVC ratio; 4) percent predicted FEV_1; 5) percent predicted FVC; 6) three or more asthma-like symptoms; 7) usual cough that improved away from work; and 8) shortness of breath when hurrying on level ground or walking up a slight hill. Work area exposures were based on air sample measurements obtained historically by the company (from 1985 to 2003) and by NIOSH for total cobalt particles or on air samples obtained by NIOSH for all other concentrations of metals in air. Work area exposure indices included in statistical models were: 1) mean, median, and highest measured cobalt and tungsten air concentrations for all particles (total), inhalable-sized particles, thoracic-sized particles, and respirable-sized particles; 2) mean, median, and highest measured concentrations of nickel, chromium, and dust particles; and 3) the ratio of respirable cobalt to respirable tungsten (excluding workers with multiple current jobs at the time of spirometry test or questionnaire). For percent predicted FEV_1 and percent predicted FVC outcomes, statistical models controlled for differences in smoking (pack-years) and tenure; for FEV_1, FVC, and FEV_1/FVC outcomes, they controlled for differences in age, gender, height, race, smoking (pack-years), and tenure; and for respiratory symptoms outcomes, they controlled for differences in age, gender, race, smoking (pack-years), and tenure.

We performed similar analyses for estimated cumulative exposures; controlled variables were similar to those above, but did not include tenure. We assessed whether workers who participated in either the 2003 or 2005 medical survey (n=232) were more likely to have specific respiratory health outcomes if they had a greater estimated cumulative exposure to cobalt based on mean cobalt measurements, or a greater estimated cumulative exposure to tungsten based on mean tungsten measurements. We also looked for associations between respiratory health outcomes and the highest recorded levels of cobalt or tungsten from air samples collected in all areas where a worker had ever worked. For these analyses, we included workers for whom less than 10% of their work history was missing an exposure estimate and we used results from the workers' most recent spirometry test or questionnaire. For each worker, estimated cumulative exposures to cobalt and tungsten in a specific work area were calculated by multiplying the number of years in that work area by the average exposure in that work area. Each worker's estimated cumulative exposure was calculated by adding up all the of that workers' area-specific cumulative exposures up to the time that the spirometry test or questionnaire was completed or the onset time the worker reported for specific respiratory symptoms. Estimated cumulative exposures were calculated and tested for each of the metal and dust air exposures described in the preceding paragraph. Health outcomes assessed included: 1) airways obstruction; 2) restriction (on spirometry); 3) FEV_1; 4) FVC; 5) FEV_1/FVC ratio; 6) percent predicted FEV_1; 7) percent predicted FVC; 8) three or more asthma-like symptoms; 9) usual cough that improved away from work; and 10) shortness of breath when hurrying on level ground or walking up a slight hill. For models with a respiratory symptom outcome, we controlled for gender, age, race, and smoking (pack-years). For models with FEV_1, FVC, or FEV_1/FVC ratio as the outcome, we controlled for gender, race, age, height, and smoking (pack-years). For models with percent predicted FEV_1 or percent predicted FVC as the outcome, we controlled for smoking (pack-years).

NIOSH Human Subjects Review Board Approval and Centers for Disease Control 308(d) Protection of Confidentiality

Due to the experimental nature of the exhaled breath condensate assays, the analyses for metal antibodies in blood, and the genetic analyses, the study protocol was reviewed and approved by the NIOSH Human Subjects Review Board. We obtained a 308(d) assurance of confidentiality from the Centers for Disease Control and Prevention to protect the results of genetic analyses from release to anyone other than the individual tested.

Occupational Exposures Limits and Health Effects

Chromium

The toxic effects of chromium are primarily related to hexavalent chromium (chromium VI) compounds which more easily penetrate the skin and mucous membranes than the trivalent (chromium III) form. The hexavalent form (but not the trivalent form or chromium metal) has been associated cancer of the lung and nose [IARC 1990].

Skin exposure to chromium mist, dust, or solutions can cause skin irritation and skin ulceration. Chromium compounds can cause a skin allergy (allergic contact dermatitis). Inhalation of chromium mist, dust, or solution can cause irritation and temporary constriction of the airways (acute bronchospasm) and infrequently occupational asthma.

The OSHA PEL for chromium metal and insoluble chromium salts is 1,000 $\mu g/m^3$ (8-hour TWA) and the NIOSH REL is 500 $\mu g/m^3$ (10-hour TWA).

Cobalt

Cobalt can be absorbed by the lungs, gastrointestinal tract, and skin. Absorption of cobalt by the lungs is greatly increased in the presence of tungsten carbide [Lasfargues et al. 1992]. Absorption of cobalt by the skin will occur with prolonged skin contact with cobalt dust or cobalt-contaminated metalworking fluid. Absorption is probably much higher with exposure to cobalt-contaminated metalworking fluid than with exposure to cobalt dust alone. In a human experiment, a subject who held his hand in a mixture of cobalt and tungsten carbide powder for 90 minutes, demonstrated a 10-fold increase in urinary cobalt levels [Scansetti et al. 1994]. Absorbed cobalt is rapidly excreted in the urine for the first few days; cobalt still remaining in the bloodstream after several weeks is then slowly excreted over a number of years [Elinder et al. 1986]. Urine cobalt levels obtained prior to the work shift at the beginning of the work week reflect long-term exposure, whereas urinary levels obtained at the end of the shift on the last day of the work week additionally reflect cumulative exposures from the week.

Cobalt exposure has been associated with upper airway irritation, cough, poor lung function, occupational asthma, interstitial lung disease (hard metal disease), heart muscle damage (cardiomyopathy), skin allergy (allergic contact dermatitis), and lung cancer (when also exposed to tungsten).

Hard metal disease occurs in cemented tungsten carbide workers exposed to both cobalt and tungsten carbide and in diamond polishers exposed to cobalt. Common early symptoms include a dry cough and shortness of breath on exertion. The disease may develop after as little as 2 years from the time of first exposure, but usually 10 to 12 years is required [Barceloux 1999]. As the disease progresses, lung function tests demonstrate a restrictive pattern and decreased DL_{CO}. The disease is usually not reversible, even when there is no further exposure. If a lung biopsy is performed on a worker with hard metal disease, large cells with many nuclei (giant cells) may be seen in the alveoli (air sacs); this finding has also been referred to as giant cell pneumonitis [Cugell et al. 1990]. Giant cell pneumonitis has been identified in cemented tungsten carbide workers exposed in grinding, powder mixing, and shaping work areas [Ohori et al. 1989].

An immune-mediated etiology has been proposed for both cobalt asthma and hard metal disease based on the following findings: 1) the presence of cobalt antibodies in some workers with cobalt asthma [Shirakawa et al. 1989]; and 2) the recurrence of giant cell pneumonitis in one affected worker following lung transplantation [Frost et al. 1993].

Several cases of cardiomyopathy have been diagnosed in workers with elevated cobalt levels in heart tissue or blood [Jarvis et al. 1992; Barborik et al. 1972; Kennedy et al. 1981]. Two studies in cemented tungsten carbide workers demonstrated an association between cobalt exposure and poor heart function (decreased left ventricular ejection fraction) [Horowitz et al. 1988; D'Adda et al. 1994]. Animal studies have confirmed this association [Mohiuddin et al. 1970; Speijers et al. 1982; Morvai et al. 1993]. An allergic skin rash may result from skin exposure to cobalt. Cobalt exposure may also result in an increased number of red blood cells and thyroid enlargement.

The International Agency for Research on Cancer (IARC) has determined that cobalt metal with tungsten carbide probably can cause cancer and that cobalt metal without tungsten carbide possibly causes cancer [IARC 2006]. Epidemiological studies have identified an increased risk of lung cancer among cemented tungsten carbide workers.

The OSHA PEL for cobalt metal, dust, and fume is 100 µg/m³ (8-hour TWA) and the NIOSH REL for cobalt metal, dust, or fume is 50 µg/m³ (10-hour TWA). The NIOSH REL is based on skin effects and pulmonary fibrosis [NIOSH 1992]. The 1981 NIOSH document *Criteria for Controlling Occupational Exposure to Cobalt* cites two studies among cemented tungsten carbide workers [NIOSH 1981]. A Swedish study of 155 workers identified pulmonary function declines during the work week that improved over the weekend in workers who dry polished sintered material (average cobalt exposure = 10 µg/m³) and in workers who wet polished sintered material (average cobalt exposure = 8 µg/m³) [Alexandersson 1979a,b,c]. A Czechoslovakian study found that 6 of 61 workers who worked near grinding machines had pulmonary fibrosis (average cobalt exposure = 43 µg/m³; range = 6 to 90 µg/m³)[Jirkova 1971].

In October 1988, NIOSH submitted testimony to the Department of Labor for a proposed change to the OSHA PEL. This document mentioned two recent studies. Findings from one, a mortality study among electrochemical plant workers who produced cobalt, suggested an increased lung cancer risk [Mur et al. 1987]. Findings from the other, a cross-sectional study among cemented tungsten carbide workers, documented two cases of occupational cobalt asthma with mean cobalt exposures of 18 and 24 µg/m³ [Kusaka et al. 1986]. The document indicated that an occupational limit of 50 µg/m³ would not be protective against the development of cobalt-induced asthma for all workers.

Biological exposure measurements reported to correspond to the OSHA and NIOSH occupational limits are listed below.

Occupational Exposure Limit	Cobalt air concentration	Equivalent urine cobalt concentration	Equivalent blood cobalt concentration
NIOSH REL	50 µg/m³	30 µg/L	2.5 µg/L
OSHA PEL	100 µg/m³	60 µg/L	5 µg/L

Modified from Lauwerys and Hoet [2001].

Metalworking Fluids

Exposure to metalworking fluids is associated with respiratory symptoms, decreased lung function [Robins et al. 1997; Eisen et al. 2001], asthma [Chan-Yeung et al. 1995; Savonius et al. 1994; Rosenman et al. 1997; Kriebel et al. 1997], and hypersensitivity pneumonitis [Kreiss et al. 1997; Hodgson et al. 2001].

Hypersensitivity pneumonitis symptoms include cough and shortness of breath on exertion, fever, chills, fatigue, decreased appetite, and weight loss. Lung scarring may result if workers continue to be exposed. When this occurs, lung function tests typically show a pattern of restriction and decreased DL_{CO}. Important exposures related to the use of metalworking fluids include biocides, metals, and microbial contamination (*Mycobacteria*, Gram-positive bacteria, and fungi).

Metalworking fluid-related asthma can present as new-onset asthma or as aggravation of pre-existing asthma. Important exposures related to the use of metalworking fluid that are associated with asthma include metalworking fluid components (ethanolamine, colophony, pine oil, tall oil), additives (formaldehyde, chlorine), and contaminants (chromium, nickel, cobalt, tungsten carbide, bacteria, fungi, and endotoxin). The usual latency period for MWF asthma is 12 years with a range from under 1 year to up to 41 years [Robertson et al. 1988].

The OSHA PEL for metalworking fluid (mineral oil mists) is 500 $\mu g/m^3$ (8-hour TWA). The NIOSH REL for metalworking fluids is 400 $\mu g/m^3$ (i.e., 0.4 mg/m^3) for thoracic particulate mass (10-hour TWA), which corresponds to approximately 500 $\mu g/m^3$ for total particulate mass [NIOSH 1998].

No occupational exposure limits exist for the amounts of endotoxin, bacteria, or cobalt in metalworking fluid. Researchers suggest that well-maintained metalworking fluids have bacterial contamination of less than 10^6 colony forming units (CFU)/mL fluid. Typical bacterial counts are 10^5 to 10^7 CFU/mL fluid. Cobalt in metalworking fluid may have a greater toxicity than cobalt in the form of a dry powder. Cobalt levels in metalworking fluid can increase to 200 $\mu g/g$ (approximately 200 mg/L) in some MWFs within the first few weeks of use [Sjögren et al. 1980].

Nickel

Nickel compounds and nickel metal can cause allergic contact dermatitis. Exposure to nickel compounds can cause occupational asthma. Based on studies among nickel refinery workers, exposure to nickel oxides and nickel sulfides may cause cancer of the lung and nose. IARC considers that exposure to metallic nickel and alloys to possibly cause cancer in humans [IARC 1990]. NIOSH considers cemented tungsten carbide that contains nickel to be a potential occupational carcinogen [NIOSH 2008].

The OSHA PEL for nickel metal and insoluble nickel compounds is 1000 µg/m³ (8-hour TWA), and the NIOSH REL for nickel metal and nickel compounds is 15 µg/m³ (10-hour TWA).

Cemented Tungsten Carbide

Cemented tungsten carbide refers to a mixture of tungsten carbide, cobalt, and sometimes metal oxides or carbides and other metals (including nickel). When the cobalt content of cemented tungsten carbide exceeds 2%, its contribution to the potential hazard is judged to exceed that of tungsten carbide, and the NIOSH REL for cobalt [50 µg Co/m³ (10-hour TWA)] would apply. The applicable OSHA PEL is 100 µg Co/m³ (8-hour TWA).

Tungsten

Workers exposed to only tungsten (and not to cobalt) are not thought to develop hard metal disease. There is no OSHA PEL for tungsten. The NIOSH REL for tungsten metal is 5,000 µg/m³ (10-hour TWA) and the NIOSH 15-minute short-term exposure limit (STEL) is 10,000 µg/m³.

Heptane (Used in Milling) and Plasticizers (Used in Extrusion)

The health effects associated with heptane include neurological symptoms of dizziness, vertigo, incoordination, and inappropriate behavior. The chemical structure of heptane is similar to that of hexane, which is known to cause a sensory and motor loss of function in the limbs. Because of this, NIOSH has recommended the same occupational exposure limits for all 5 to 8 carbon alkanes (pentane, hexane, heptane, and octane).

The OSHA PEL for heptane (n-heptane) is 2,000,000 µg/m³ (8-hour TWA). The NIOSH REL is 350,000 µg/m³ (8-hour TWA) and the NIOSH STEL is 1,800,000 µg/m³. There are no OSHA or NIOSH occupational exposure limits for the plasticizers used in extrusion.

Silicon Carbide

Silicon carbide is an abrasive that has hardness close to that of diamonds. In the granular (non-fibrous) form, silicon carbide is considered relatively inert dust. The OSHA PELs (8-hour TWAs) for silicon carbide are 15,000 µg/m³ for total dust and 5,000 µg/m³ for respirable dust. The NIOSH RELs (10-hour TWAs) for silicon carbide are 10,000 µg/m³ for total dust and 5,000 µg/m³ for respirable dust.

Alexandersson R [1979a]. [Studies on the effects of exposure to cobalt. II. Reactions of the respiratory organs of various exposure levels in the hard metal industry.] Arbete och Halsa 2:1–34. (Swe)

Alexandersson R [1979b]. [Studies on the effects of exposure to cobalt. II. Exposure, uptake, and pulmonary effects of cobalt in the hard metal industry.] Arbete och Halsa 10:1–24. (Swe)

Alexandersson R [1979c]. [Studies on the effects of exposure to cobalt. II. Ventilation capacity, distribution of inhaled gas, and closing of repiratory passages during ongoing work and after periods of nonexposure.] Arbete och Halsa 7:1–25. (Swe)

Barborik M, Dusek J [1972]. Cardiomyopathy accompanying industrial cobalt exposure. Br Heart J 34:113–116.

Barceloux D [1999]. Cobalt. Clin Toxicol 37:201–216.

Chan-Yeung M, Malo J-L [1995]. Compendium I: table of the major inducers of occupational asthma. In: Bernstein IL, Chan-Yeung M, Malo J-L, Bernstein DI, eds. Asthma in the workplace. New York, NY: Marcel-Dekker, Inc., pp. 595–623.

Cugell DW, Morgan KC, Perkins DG, Rubin A [1990]. The respiratory effects of cobalt. Arch Intern Med 150:177–183.

D'Adda F, Borleri D, Migliori M, Mosconi G, Medolago G, Virotta G, Colombo F, Seghizzi P [1994]. Cardiac function study in hard metal workers. Sci Total Environ 150:179–186.

Eisen E, Smith T, Kriebel D, Woskie SR, Meyers DJ, Kennedy SM, Shalat S, Monson RR [2001]. Respiratory health of automobile workers and exposures to metal-working fluid aerosols: lung spirometry. Am J Ind Med 39:443–453.

Elinder CG, Friberg L [1986]. Cobalt. In: Friberg L, Norbers G, Vouk V, eds. Handbook on the toxicology of metals. 2nd ed. Vol II. Amsterdam, Belgium: Elsevier Science Publishers, pp. 211–232.

Frost AE, Keller CA, Brown RW, Noon GP, Short HD, Abraham JL, Pacinda S, Cagle PT [1993]. Giant cell interstitial pneumonitis. Am Rev Respir Dis 148:1401–1404.

Hodgson M, Bracker A, Yang C, Storey E, Jarvis BJ, Milton D, Lummus Z, Bernstein D, Cole S [2001]. Hypersensitivity pneumonitis in a metal-working environment. Am J Ind Med 39:616–628.

Horowitz SF, Fischbein A, Matza D, Rizzo JN, Stern A, Machac J, Solomon SJ [1988]. Evaluation of right left ventricular function in hard metal workers. Br J Ind Med 45:742–746.

International Agency for Research on Cancer (IARC) [1990]. Chromium, nickel and welding. Monographs on the evaluation of carcinogenic risks to humans, vol. 49. Lyon, France: IARC.

International Agency for Research on Cancer (IARC) [2006]. Cobalt in hard metals and cobalt sulfate, gallium arsenide, indium phosphide and vanadium pentoxide. Monographs on the evaluation of carcinogenic risks to humans, vol. 86. Lyon, France: IARC.

Jarvis JQ, Hammond E, Meier R, Robinson C [1992]. Cobalt cardiomyopathy: a report of two cases from mineral assay laboratories and a review of the literature. J Occup Env Med 34:620–626.

Jirkova H [1971]. [Dust hazards when grinding tools made of sintered carbides.] Prac Lek 23:114–116. (Cze)

Kennedy A, King R, Dornan JD [1981]. Fatal cardiac disease associated with industrial exposure to cobalt. Lancet 1(8217):412–414.

Kriebel D, Sama S, Woskie S, Christiani DC, Eisen EA, Hammond SK, Milton D, Smith M, Virgi MA [1997]. A field investigation of the acute respiratory effects of metalworking fluids. I: Effects of aerosol exposures. Am J Ind Med 31:756–766.

Kreiss K, Cox-Ganser J [1997]. Metalworking fluid-associated hypersensitivity pneumonitis: a workshop summary. Am J Ind Med 32:423–432.

Kusaka Y, Yokoyama K, Sera Y, Yamamoto S, Sone S, Kyoto H, Shirakawa T, Goto S [1986]. Respiratory diseases in hard metal workers: an occupational hygiene study in a factory. Br J Ind Med 43:474–485.

Lasfargues G, Lison D, Maldague P, Lauwerys R [1992]. Comparative study of the acute lung toxicity of pure cobalt powder and cobalt-tungsten carbide mixture in rat. Toxicol Appl Pharmacol 112:41–50.

Lauwerys RR, Hoet P [2001]. Industrial chemical exposure: guidelines for biological monitoring. 3rd ed., Boca Raton, FL: Lewis Publishers. p. 93.

Mohiuddin SM, Taskar PK, Rheault M, Roy PE, Chenard J, Morin Y [1970]. Experimental cobalt cardiomyopathy. Am Heart J 80:532–543.

Morvai V, Szakmary E, Tatrai E, Unjvary G, Folly G [1993]. The effects of simultaneous alcohol and cobalt chloride administration on the cardiovascular system of rats. Acta Physiol Hung 81:253–261.

Mur JM, Moulin JJ, Charruyer-Seinerra MP, Lafitte J [1987]. A cohort mortality study among cobalt and sodium workers in an electrochemical plant. Am J Ind Med 11:75–81.

NIOSH [1981]. Occupational hazard assessment: criteria for controlling occupational exposure to cobalt. Washington, DC: U.S. Department of Health and Human Services, Public Health Service, Centers for Disease Control, National Institute for Occupational Safety and Health [http://www.cdc.gov/niosh/82-107.html].

NIOSH [1992]. Recommendations for occupational safety and health: Compendium of policy documents and statements. Cincinnati, OH: U.S. Department of Health and Human Services, Public Health Service, Centers for Disease Control, National Institute for Occupational Safety and Health, DHHS (NIOSH) Publication No. 92-100. p. 62. [http://www.cdc.gov/niosh/pdfs/92-100-c.pdf].

NIOSH [1998]. Criteria for a recommended standard: Occupational exposure to metalworking fluids. Cincinnati, OH: U.S. Department of Health and Human Services, Public Health Service, Centers for Disease Control and Prevention, National Institute for Occupational Safety and Health [http://www.cdc.gov/niosh/pdfs/98-102-b.pdf].

NIOSH [2008] Pocket guide to chemical hazards, Appendix C: Supplementary exposure limits. U.S. Department of Health and Human Services, Public Health Service, Centers for Disease Control and Prevention, National Institute for Occupational Safety and Health. Accessed March 6, 2008. [http://www.cdc.gov/niosh/npg/nengapdx.html#c].

Ohori NP, Sciurba FC, Owens GR, Hodgson MJ, Yousem SA [1989]. Giant-cell interstitial pneumonia and hard-metal pneumoconiosis. Am J Surg Pathol 13:581–587.

Robertson AS, Weir DC, Burge PS [1988]. Occupational asthma due to oil mists. Thorax 43:200–205.

Robins T, Seixas N, Franzblau A, Abrams L, Inc. S, Burge S, Schork MA. [1997]. Acute respiratory effects on workers exposed to metalworking fluid aerosols in an automotive transmission plant. Am J Ind Med 31:510–524.

Rosenman K, Reilly M, Kalinowski D [1997]. Work-related asthma and respiratory symptoms among workers exposed to metal-working fluids. Am J Ind Med 32:325–331.

Savonius B, Keskinen H, Tuppurainen M, Kanerva L [1994]. Occupational asthma caused by ethanolamines. Allergy 49:877–881.

Scansetti G, Botta GC, Spinelli P, Reviglione L, Ponzetti C [1994]. Absorption and excretion of cobalt in the hard metal industry. Sci Total Environ 150:141–144.

Shirakawa T, Kusaka Y, Fujimura N, Goto S, Kato M, Heki S, Morimoto K [1989]. Occupational asthma from cobalt sensitivity in workers exposed to hard metal dust. Chest 95:29–36.

Sjögren I, Hillerdal G, Andersson A, Zetterström O [1980]. Hard metal lung disease: importance of cobalt in coolants. Thorax 35:653–659.

Speijers GJA, Krajnc EI, Berkvens JM, van Logten MJ [1982]. Acute oral toxicity of inorganic cobalt compounds in rats. Food Chem Toxicol 20:311–314.

Acknowledgements and Availability of Report

The Respiratory Disease Hazard Evaluations and Technical Assistance Program (RDHETAP) of the National Institute for Occupational Safety and Health (NIOSH) conducts field investigations of possible health hazards in the workplace. These investigations are conducted under the authority of Section 20(a)(6) of the Occupational Safety and Health (OSH) Act of 1970, 29 U.S.C. 669(a)(6) which authorizes the Secretary of Health and Human Services, following a written request from any employers or authorized representative of employees, to determine whether any substance normally found in the place of employment has potentially toxic effects in such concentrations as used or found. RDHETAP also provides, upon request, technical and consultative assistance to federal, state, and local agencies; labor; industry; and other groups or individuals to control occupational health hazards and to prevent related trauma and disease.

The findings and conclusions in this report are those of the authors and do not necessarily represent the views of NIOSH. Mention of any company or product does not constitute endorsement by NIOSH. In addition, citations to websites external to NIOSH do not constitute NIOSH endorsement of the sponsoring organizations or their programs or products. Furthermore, NIOSH is not responsible for the content of these websites. All Web addresses referenced in this document were accessible as of the publication date.

This report was prepared by Nancy Sahakian, MD MPH, Aleksandr Stefaniak, PhD CIH, and Gregory Day, PhD, of the RDHETAP, Division of Respiratory Disease Studies (DRDS), and Richard Kanwal, MD MPH (contractor). Laboratory collaboration was provided by Paul Siegel, PhD, Toni Bledsoe, MS, James Ensey, BS, Bonnie Frye, MS, John McKernan, PhD, and Masssimo Corradi, PhD. Field assistance was provided by Diana Freeland, Jim Taylor, David Spainhour, Marty Pflock, Rachel Sparks, Sandra White, Terry Rooney, Dan Yereb, BS, Chris Piacitelli, BS, Randy Boylstein, BS, Jennifer Mosby, BS, Thomas Jefferson, and Kathleen Kreiss MD. Analytical support was provided by Nicole Edwards, Brian Tift, Jean Cox-Ganser, PhD, and Anthony Billings, PhD. Desktop publishing was performed by Tia McClelland.

Copies of this report have been sent to management representatives at Metalworking Products, HHE requestors,

ACKNOWLEDGEMENTS AND AVAILABILITY OF REPORT (CONTINUED)

Alabama Department of Public Health, and the OSHA Regional Office. This report is not copyrighted and may be freely reproduced. The report may be viewed and printed from the following internet address: http://www.cdc.gov/niosh/hhe. Copies may be purchased from the National Technical Information Service (NTIS) at 5825 Port Royal Road, Springfield, Virginia 22161.